AF251537

Myocardial Perfusion Imaging - Beyond the Left Ventricle

M. Elizabeth Oates • Vincent L. Sorrell

Myocardial Perfusion Imaging - Beyond the Left Ventricle

Pathology, Artifacts and Pitfalls in the Chest and Abdomen

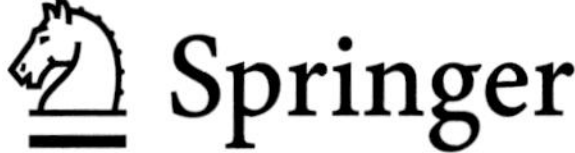

M. Elizabeth Oates
Division of Nuclear Medicine and
Molecular Imaging
Department of Radiology
University of Kentucky
Lexington, Kentucky
USA

Vincent L. Sorrell
Division of Cardiovascular Medicine
Department of Internal Medicine
Gill Heart Institute
University of Kentucky
Lexington, Kentucky
USA

Videos to this book can be accessed at http://link.springer.com/book/10.1007/978-3-319-25436-4

ISBN 978-3-319-25434-0   ISBN 978-3-319-25436-4   (eBook)
DOI 10.1007/978-3-319-25436-4

Library of Congress Control Number: 2016941597

© Springer International Publishing Switzerland 2017
This work is subject to copyright. All rights are reserved by the Publisher, whether the whole or part of the material is concerned, specifically the rights of translation, reprinting, reuse of illustrations, recitation, broadcasting, reproduction on microfilms or in any other physical way, and transmission or information storage and retrieval, electronic adaptation, computer software, or by similar or dissimilar methodology now known or hereafter developed.
The use of general descriptive names, registered names, trademarks, service marks, etc. in this publication does not imply, even in the absence of a specific statement, that such names are exempt from the relevant protective laws and regulations and therefore free for general use.
The publisher, the authors and the editors are safe to assume that the advice and information in this book are believed to be true and accurate at the date of publication. Neither the publisher nor the authors or the editors give a warranty, express or implied, with respect to the material contained herein or for any errors or omissions that may have been made.

Printed on acid-free paper

This Springer imprint is published by Springer Nature
The registered company is Springer International Publishing AG Switzerland

Dr. Oates acknowledges the invaluable help of her staff (notably, Lisa Cunningham, Joyce McCown, Sharon Rayburn, and Jeff Richards) during the preparation of this book. I thank the many nuclear technologists at the University of Kentucky and other academic medical centers with whom I have worked throughout my career, for they are the ones who create the images for us to make critical diagnoses for our patients. This book is a tribute to the patience and support of my husband and children who sustain me. To the Winfreys: Don, Victoria, Olivia, and Cecilia, thank you!

Dr. Sorrell recognizes the consistent efforts by the residents and fellows in training to learn the techniques necessary to become competent and then expert in nuclear cardiology. It is these efforts that fuel the energy necessary to spend hours teaching, mentoring, and writing books such as this one. Most importantly, it is our families who support these choices and sacrifice so many evenings and weekends. To Mandy, Zoe, and Jack, thanks again. P.S., I will be late for dinner.

Drs. Oates and Sorrell extend their deepest gratitude to Paul Anaya, M.D., Ph.D., Associate Professor of Medicine, Division of Cardiovascular Medicine, Department of Internal Medicine, Director of Nuclear Cardiology, Gill Heart Institute, University of Kentucky, for his careful and insightful critique of the manuscript and its figures.

Foreword

Myocardial Perfusion Imaging – Beyond the Left Ventricle. Pathology, Artifacts and Pitfalls in the Chest and Abdomen by Oates and Sorrell is a new addition to the many books that have been published on the subject of nuclear cardiology. This however is one contribution that simply must be among whichever others a nuclear cardiology lab chooses to use for reference. Certainly, no teaching facility should be without it. It distinguishes itself in several important respects. First, it is an e-book, so that the reader sees both static and dynamic data as it would look on the interpretive computer screen. Second, it focuses on "all the other things" that are commonly seen in a contemporary myocardial perfusion imaging study, even when performed with CT for attenuation correction. No other resource that I am aware of covers this increasingly important aspect of study interpretation. Third, it is both comprehensive and detailed, devoting separate chapters to each of numerous organs within the field of view of a myocardial perfusion study. Most nuclear cardiologists will not need to know how to differentiate appearances of various types of organ abnormality, but this book is excellent in showing what is normal and what is not, as well as documenting the various possibilities that need to be considered. Fourth, the references are an important resource for those who want to go to some primary descriptive data and investigations. Fifth, the combined expertise of a nuclear cardiologist and a nuclear radiologist provides a unique perspective on what to look for, how to describe the findings, and the diagnostic significance. Finally, an especially important aspect of this book is that the authors offer helpful reporting recommendations in each chapter to assist with how to communicate these non-cardiac findings in a way that the referring physician can know how or whether further investigation should be undertaken.

There are nearly 30 well-illustrated and well-referenced chapters, including hundreds of high quality, state-of-the-art figures and cine images. This book is organized to provide an interactive format, including many annotated videos, that allows the reader to learn as if "at the workstation" alongside an expert teacher. A particular strength of this novel e-book is the set of 36 "real-life" challenging cases in the last three chapters that one can work through to self-assess recognition and interpretation of the many common and uncommon findings within the imaging field of view.

The final three chapters increase in difficulty from 12 relatively simple, straightforward case examples to 12 moderately difficult and then 12 expert level illustrations.

This book should be kept nearby for easy access during routine cardiac SPECT MPI interpretation sessions. Mine is one teaching lab that will require this e-book to be read by all rotating cardiology fellows and radiology residents. My bet is that this will be the most popular among the other "required reading" books.

Timothy M. Bateman, MD
University of Missouri – Kansas City School of Medicine
Missouri, USA

Preface

This book presents a dedicated, comprehensive review of incidental pathology, imaging artifacts, and interpretative pitfalls apart from the left ventricle on conventional nuclear stress single-photon emission computed tomography (SPECT) myocardial perfusion imaging, the most commonly performed diagnostic test for the most common cause of morbidity and mortality in the world today (i.e., coronary artery disease).

With its systematic approach, it serves as an image-rich resource (including many cinematic images) and self-assessment guide for practicing physicians and trainees (including cardiologists, nuclear medicine physicians, and diagnostic radiologists) as well as nuclear technologists and students.

Readers will learn to identify a wide variety of "hot" and "cold" physiologic or pathologic findings in the chest ("above the diaphragm") and in the abdomen ("below the diaphragm") that might be encountered in daily practice. While some may be clinically relevant and related to the reason for the imaging examination, others are incidental, with or without clinical ramifications. Readers will be able to recognize typical confounding artifacts that may appear "hot" or "cold" on the raw (unprocessed) and processed SPECT images and, in so doing, can avoid potential interpretative pitfalls.

The two authors—a nuclear radiologist and a nuclear cardiologist—have many years of clinical experience with all cardiac radiopharmaceuticals, different gamma camera systems, and a vast array of clinical cases.

Contents

Part III   The Abdomen ("Below the Diaphragm")

Part IV   Case Challenges: A Self-Assessment Tool

Abbreviations by Convention

AC	Attenuation correction
AP	Anterior-posterior
CAD	Coronary artery disease
CT	Computed tomography
ECG	Electrocardiogram
EDV	End-diastolic volume
HLA	Horizontal long-axis
IV	Intravenous
LAD	Left anterior descending [coronary artery]
LAO	Left anterior oblique
LPO	Left posterior oblique
LV	Left ventricle
LVEF	Left ventricular ejection fraction
METS	Metabolic equivalents
MPI	Myocardial perfusion imaging
PA	Posterior-anterior
RAO	Right anterior oblique
RCA	Right coronary artery
ROI	Region-of-interest
RV	Right ventricle
SA	Short-axis
SPECT	Single-photon emission computed tomography
VLA	Vertical long-axis

Introduction 1

Cardiac stress testing with radionuclide myocardial perfusion imaging (MPI) is an essential diagnostic tool in patients with suspected coronary artery disease (CAD) and confers prognosis in patients with known CAD for risk stratification and management optimization. MPI is performed using one of several available radiopharmaceuticals (^{99m}Tc sestamibi, ^{99m}Tc tetrofosmin, ^{201}Tl chloride). Today, MPI uses single-photon emission computed tomography (SPECT) with or without a radionuclide or x-ray attenuation correction source. Myocardial perfusion is assessed at rest and at peak stress; left ventricular function (ejection fraction, wall motion, wall thickening) is assessed with ECG-gated SPECT as an integral component of the examination.

While the goal of SPECT MPI is assessment of perfusion and function of the left ventricular myocardium and the left ventricle, the imaging field-of-view includes some or all of the chest and the abdomen. Thus, a wide variety of localized and systemic noncardiac conditions that present "above the diaphragm" and "below the diaphragm" may be demonstrated—or even discovered—on SPECT MPI apart from the target left heart. The raw (unprocessed) projection data are particularly rich in findings and should be comprehensively reviewed during image interpretation.

This book describes and illustrates a wide variety of common and uncommon pathologies as well as typical imaging artifacts and potential interpretative pitfalls which might be encountered in daily clinical practice. Throughout the chapters, many images are shown in cinematic mode for optimal visualization and anatomic localization. Pathologies include focal lesions (such as benign and malignant neoplasms) and organ/systemic diseases (such as emphysema, cirrhosis and its sequelae, cholecystitis, and end-stage renal disease), all of which may be identified with SPECT MPI. Some findings will be clinically relevant and related to the reason for the cardiac stress test while others will be incidental. All may present as "hot" [relatively increased radioactivity] or "cold" [relatively decreased radioactivity] compared to normal patterns on SPECT MPI. Such findings often merit direct communication with the patient's care provider.

© Springer International Publishing Switzerland 2017
M.E. Oates, V.L. Sorrell, *Myocardial Perfusion Imaging - Beyond the Left Ventricle: Pathology, Artifacts and Pitfalls in the Chest and Abdomen*, DOI 10.1007/978-3-319-25436-4_1

Section I provides an overview of the technical principles behind image acquisition and general guidelines regarding image interpretation for SPECT MPI. Sections II and III describe and illustrate incidental findings representing potential pathologies, imaging artifacts, and interpretative pitfalls in the chest and in the abdomen, respectively. Key points are summarized at the end of each chapter. Part IV challenges readers to apply their knowledge and skills gained from reading the chapters and studying the case examples to solve a set of collected "unknown cases" that range in difficulty from basic to advanced.

Part I

The Fundamentals

Technical Principles

2

Understanding the normal biodistribution and kinetics of the three most common cardiac radiopharmaceuticals ([99mTc] sestamibi, [99mTc] tetrofosmin, [201Tl] chloride) is fundamental to the practice of gamma camera-based MPI. The [99mTc] radiopharmaceuticals localize into the myocardium more slowly with a 60 % first-pass extraction fraction compared to 85 % for [201Tl]. They enter the myocardial cells by passive diffusion; uptake is proportional to blood flow at the time of the injection and cellular mitochondrial content. They are cleared by the liver, thus gallbladder and intestinal visualization is expected; the urinary tract is the secondary route of physiologic elimination. The hepatic clearance of [99mTc] tetrofosmin is more rapid compared to [99mTc] sestamibi. Conversely, as a potassium analog, [201Tl] chloride is actively transported into the myocardial cells via the Na-K ATPase pump; it is cleared primarily by the urinary system and the gastrointestinal route is the alternate route. Another important difference is that [201Tl] chloride redistributes relatively quickly (within minutes), while the [99mTc] radiopharmaceuticals redistribute relatively slowly (4 h or longer) (Chamarthy and Travin 2010; Henzlova et al. 2009; Holly et al. 2010; Wackers et al. 1989).

The gamma camera instrumentation may be dedicated to imaging the heart with two small perpendicularly oriented detectors, or it may be a system with general purpose large field-of-view detectors that can be configured for SPECT MPI. The axis of rotation of the detectors is typically 180° from the right anterior oblique position to the left posterior oblique position in order to image the left-sided heart. Typically, for a 180° axis, 32 raw planar images are acquired by each of the two detectors (for a total of 64 images) with computer reconstruction of the projection data to create the SPECT MPI images. Some gamma camera systems are capable of attenuation correction, using either a radionuclide or an x-ray source, to correct for anterior soft-tissue attenuation (e.g., breast tissue) or inferior soft-tissue attenuation (e.g., diaphragm).

During image acquisition, the perfusion data may be gated to the R-R interval of the ECG monitor to create gated SPECT images. Gated SPECT images permit

© Springer International Publishing Switzerland 2017
M.E. Oates, V.L. Sorrell, *Myocardial Perfusion Imaging - Beyond the Left Ventricle: Pathology, Artifacts and Pitfalls in the Chest and Abdomen*, DOI 10.1007/978-3-319-25436-4_2

evaluation of global and regional left ventricular function and regional wall thickening. The end-systolic and end-diastolic left ventricular volumes and left ventricular ejection fraction (LVEF) can be calculated using automated contour software available from multiple vendors. The validity of these reported values are dependent upon the accuracy of the contours.

There are many accepted SPECT MPI stress test protocols (ACR–SNM–SPR 2009; Henzlova et al. 2009; Hesse et al. 2005; Holly et al. 2010; Strauss et al. 2008). Traditionally, patients undergo two scans, one during rest and the other after stress. Most protocols use the same intravenous radiopharmaceutical for both scans; however, some combine ^{201}Tl chloride at rest with a ^{99m}Tc radiopharmaceutical for the stress test. Patients are stressed either by treadmill exercise or with one of several available pharmacologic agents (adenosine, regadenoson, dipyridamole, or dobutamine). Administered activities of the ^{99m}Tc MPI radiopharmaceuticals typically range from 7 to 12 mCi (259 to 444 MBq) at rest, with an approximate threefold increase from 22 to 30 mCi (814 to 1110 MBq) during stress for a one-day protocol. Morbidly obese patients undergoing two-day protocols are typically administered up to 40 mCi (1480 MBq) each day. For a ^{201}Tl chloride stress/rest (redistribution) protocol, a single intravenous injection of 3–4 mCi (111–148 MBq) is required. Scan patterns, incidental findings, and imaging artifacts may vary considerably depending on the protocol followed. For example, the degree of gallbladder visualization is influenced by the fasting state which is usually different on a two-day stress/rest protocol compared to a one-day rest/stress protocol.

Regarding image acquisition, intravenous injection-to-imaging time intervals are quite variable. Traditionally, imaging commences immediately after stress for ^{201}Tl chloride because of its rapid redistribution; delayed redistribution images are acquired 3–4 h later. After intravenous administration of a ^{99m}Tc radiopharmaceutical, the interval ranges anywhere from 15 to 90 minutes, with longer intervals after pharmacologic stress compared to exercise to allow for greater liver clearance (because increased splanchnic blood flow occurs during pharmacologic stress compared to exercise, thereby delivering more radiopharmaceutical to the liver). Persistent liver activity often results in cardiac reconstruction processing artifacts; thus, it is important to maximize liver clearance before cardiac imaging (Germano et al. 1994). Various strategies have been proposed to optimize liver clearance (Cherng et al. 2006).

Gastric activity is usually related to duodenogastric bile reflux and can be quite problematic because of the reconstruction processing artifacts related to the "hot" gastric fundus adjacent to the inferior myocardial wall. To remedy this confounding effect, different strategies to reduce or eliminate gastric activity have been tried with variable success (Boz et al. 2003; Hassan et al. 1991; Hofman et al. 2006; Hurwitz et al. 1993; Malhotra et al. 2010; Middleton and Williams 1994, 1996; Rehm et al. 1996; van Dongen and van Rijk 2000; Weinmann and Moretti 1999). No intervention is able to eliminate completely the possibility, and therefore, the reader must be able to recognize this finding and understand the potential ramifications.

Processing of the raw projection data is generally performed with iterative reconstruction. Limits are set around the heart and the long-axis from base to apex is defined. Currently, dedicated computer software packages for SPECT MPI and gated SPECT analysis are standard and readily available from the vendors. In selected situations, reconstruction of the entire field-of-view data set—without limiting the reconstruction to the heart ("whole-field reconstruction" as is routine in noncardiac SPECT)—can be helpful to clarify and localize an extracardiac finding (Gedik et al. 2007; Seo et al. 2005). Figure 10.2 is one representative example highlighting the value of this additive technique.

There are many sources of imaging artifacts, including patient motion, soft-tissue attenuation, filtering and windowing, and subdiaphragmatic activity (Burrell and MacDonald 2006; Sorrell et al. 1996). Systems with attenuation correction mitigate the soft-tissue effects to a great extent, but are imperfect. Many representative clinical examples of such artifacts are shown throughout this book.

Image Interpretation **3**

The first step in image interpretation is careful review of the rest raw and stress raw planar projection data sets in a cinematic format, ideally side-by-side (Gholamrezanezhad and Mirpour 2007; Hendel et al. 1999; Holly et al. 2010; Strauss et al. 2008). As outlined in Table 3.1, one should routinely and systematically assess the quality of each acquisition for patient motion, positioning in the detectors' field-of-view, sources of soft-tissue attenuation, and technical performance of the gamma camera system. Despite close attention given to consistent positioning, breast tissue can shift between image acquisitions and can create artifactual findings on the reconstructed SPECT images (Holly et al. 2010). Such variable soft-tissue attenuation (breasts, obesity) may result in variable stress and rest defects that can lead to misinterpretation of reversibility (i.e., ischemia).

The next steps in image interpretation are identification and description of the cardiac and noncardiac findings, followed by interpretation of their etiology and significance. The raw data allow for an initial evaluation of the heart: the left ventricular axis and orientation, size and uptake pattern, the right ventricular size and degree of uptake, and recognition of the frequently prominent right auricular appendage (refer to Chap. 13).

A representative normal 1-day rest/stress gated SPECT MPI is shown in Fig. 3.1. The heart is positioned in the middle of the field-of-view on the rest raw (a) and stress raw (b) projection images, and there is only quiet respiratory motion during the approximately 15-minute acquisition. Note the normal right auricular appendage (c), the commonly seen minimal gastric activity (e), and normally visualized liver (a, b), gallbladder (d), small intestine (a, b), and left kidney (f). The processed

Electronic supplementary material The online version of this chapter (doi:10.1007/978-3-319-25436-4_3) contains supplementary material, which is available to authorized users.

© Springer International Publishing Switzerland 2017
M.E. Oates, V.L. Sorrell, *Myocardial Perfusion Imaging - Beyond the Left Ventricle: Pathology, Artifacts and Pitfalls in the Chest and Abdomen,* DOI 10.1007/978-3-319-25436-4_3

SPECT images (g, h) show a uniform myocardial uptake pattern without reversible or fixed perfusion defects. On the gated SPECT images (i, j), there is normal global left ventricular systolic function with a normal left ventricular ejection fraction, normal regional wall motion evidenced by appropriate excursion during the cardiac cycle, and normal wall thickening evidenced by brightening of the color within the

Table 3.1 Structured approach to evaluation of SPECT MPI raw projection data

Step-by-step approach to interpretation			
Step	Domain	General checklist	Specific observations
1	Quality of acquisition	Patient motion	Horizontal vs. vertical or both
		Positioning within field-of-view	Centered vs. off-center
		Soft-tissue attenuation	Regional body fat or muscle, breasts, diaphragm
		Technical performance	Excess vs. loss of counts, mechanical failure
2	Heart	Left ventricle	Axis and orientation
			Chamber size and shape
			Myocardial uptake pattern (uniformity, defects)
		Right ventricle	Chamber size and shape
			Myocardial uptake pattern (intensity, thickness)
3	Chest	Biodistribution pattern	Normal structures/tissues
			Abnormal findings ("hot" or "cold")
4	Abdomen	Biodistribution pattern	Normal structures/tissues
			Abnormal findings ("hot" or "cold")

Fig. 3.1 Typical normal 1-day rest/stress gated SPECT MPI. This patient exercised well on a treadmill. Left ventricular ejection fraction was 73 %. The rest raw (**a**) and stress raw (**b**) images were acquired on a standard field-of-view gamma camera. Anatomic landmarks are identified (**c–f**). The processed SPECT (**g, h**) and gated SPECT (**i, j**) images are normal.

(**a**) Rest raw projection image (Video 3.1a, frame 1), ^{99m}Tc sestamibi. (**b**) Stress raw projection image (Video 3.1b, frame 1), ^{99m}Tc sestamibi. (**c**) Stress raw projection image (Video 3.1c, frame 13), ^{99m}Tc sestamibi, right auricular appendage (*yellow box*). (**d**) Stress raw projection image (Video 3.1c, frame 29), ^{99m}Tc sestamibi, gallbladder (*blue lines*). (**e**) Stress raw projection image (Video 3.1c, frame 43), ^{99m}Tc sestamibi, stomach (*blue oval*). (**f**) Stress raw projection image (Video 3.1c, frame 57), ^{99m}Tc sestamibi, left kidney (*blue lines*). (**g**) Stress (top row A)/rest (bottom row B) processed SPECT images (from left to right: *SA* short-axis from apex to base, *VLA* vertical long-axis from septum to lateral wall, *HLA* horizontal long-axis from inferior wall to anterior wall), myocardial walls labeled in schematics along right margin of image (Note: The conventional orientation and display are used throughout this book.) (**h**) Stress (top row A)/rest (bottom row B) processed SPECT images (*SA* short-axis, *VLA* vertical long-axis, *HLA* horizontal long-axis), stomach (*blue ovals*), right ventricle (*yellow box*). (**i**) Stress gated SPECT image (Video 3.1d, frame 1) (SA, VLA, HLA). (**j**) Stress gated SPECT image (Video 3.1e, frame 1) (SA, VLA, HLA), stomach (*blue ovals*), membranous septum (*yellow box*)

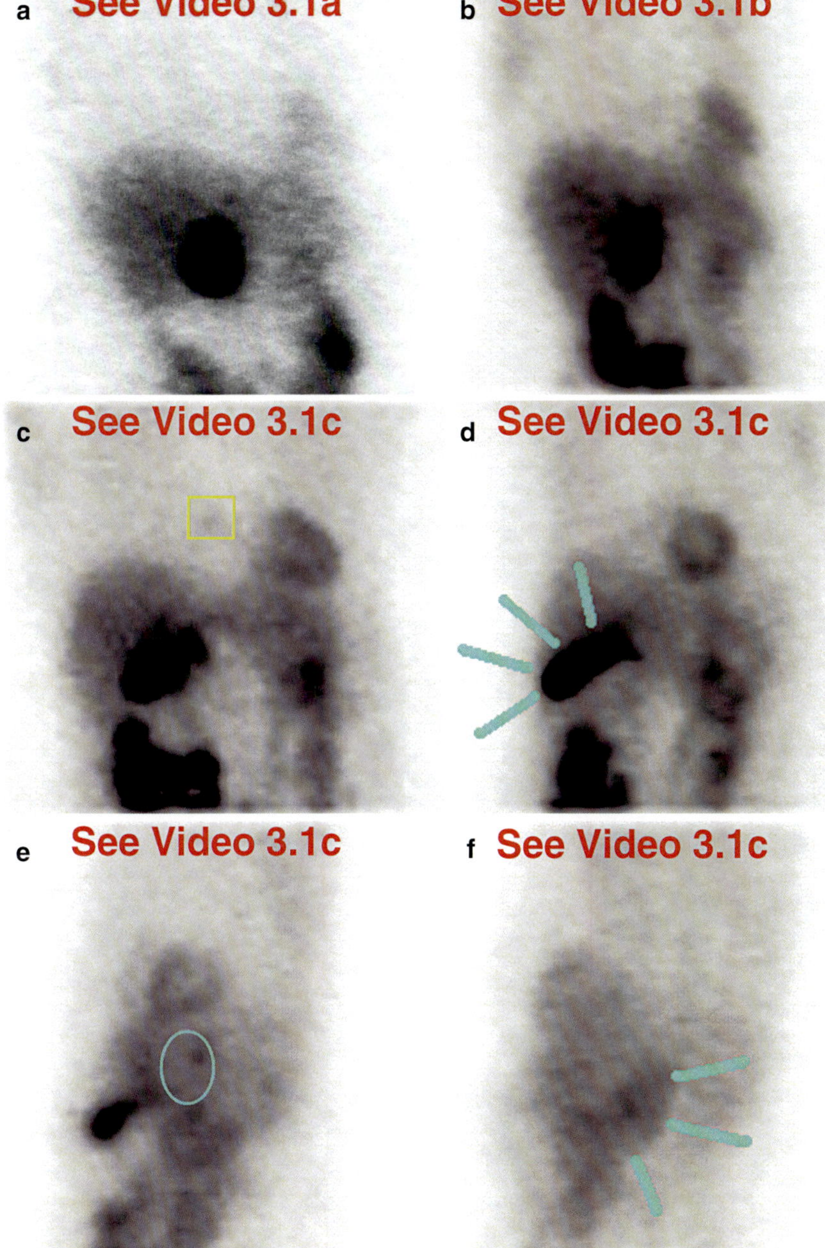
See Video 3.1a
See Video 3.1b
See Video 3.1c
See Video 3.1c
See Video 3.1c
See Video 3.1c
a
b
c
d
e
f

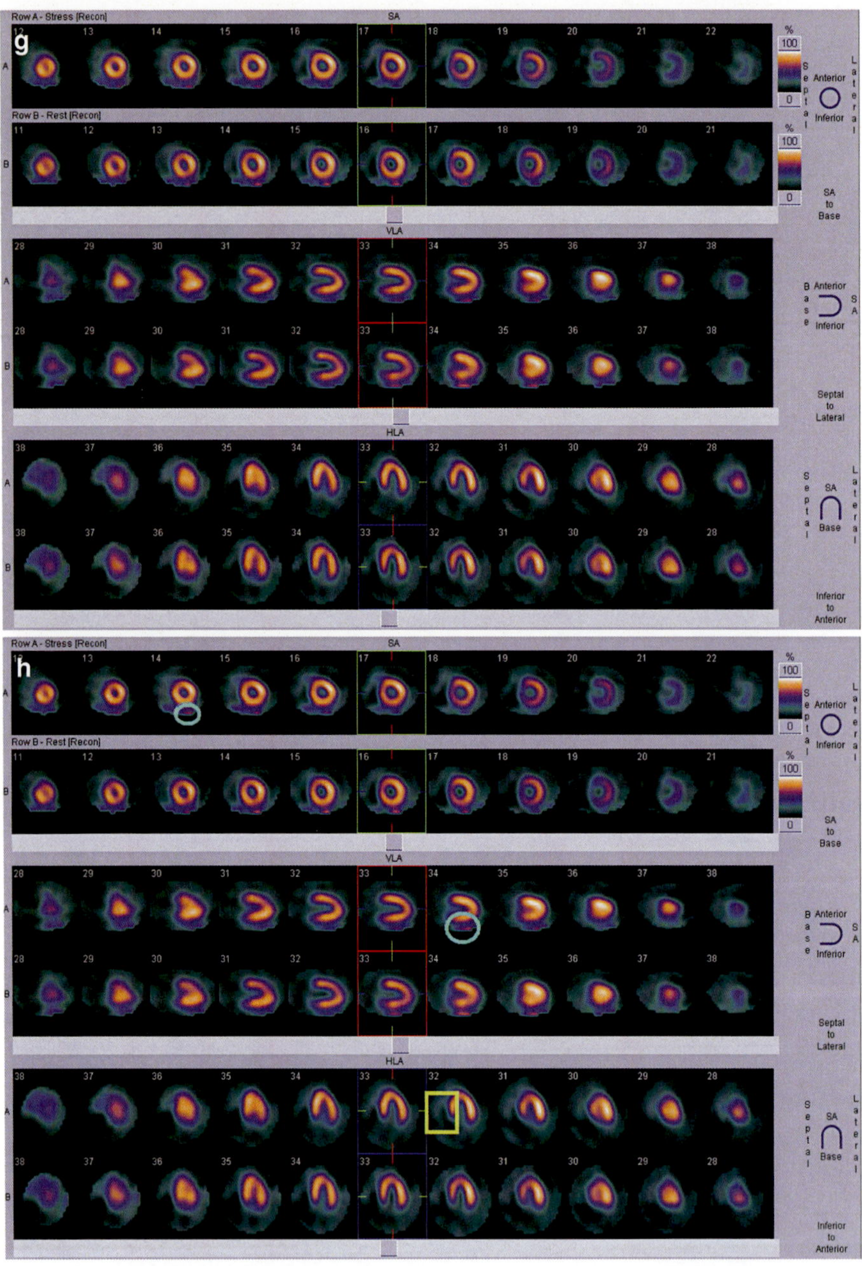

Fig. 3.1 (continued)

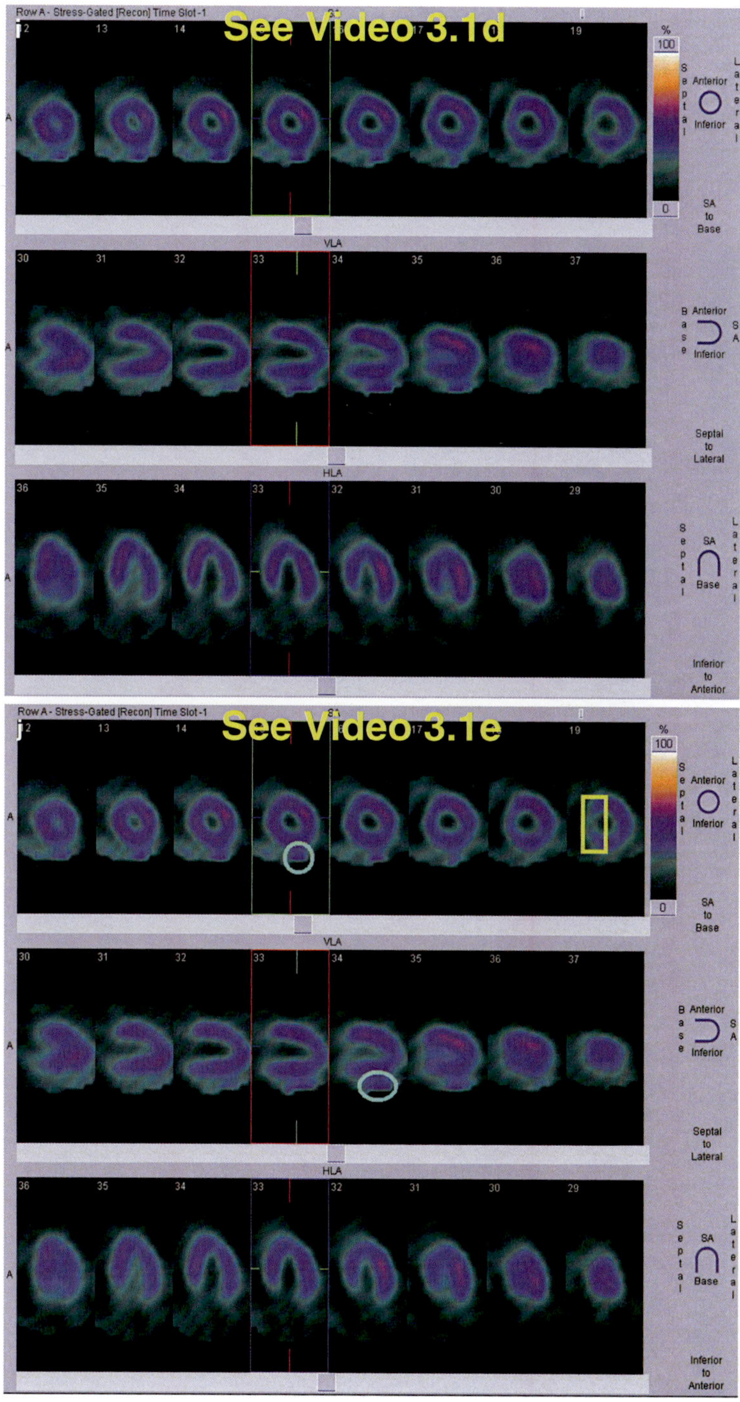

Fig. 3.1 (continued)

myocardial walls during systole. With experience, the subsequent SPECT MPI reconstructions can, and should, be predicted with a high degree of confidence and consistency.

One should also be able to recognize normal tissues and variants, including the thyroid gland, skeleton (faint), skeletal muscle, and brown adipose tissue (Chamarthy and Travin 2010; Henzlova et al. 2009; Holly et al. 2010; Mohr et al. 1996; Wackers et al. 1989). Figure 3.2 shows normal skeletal muscle about the

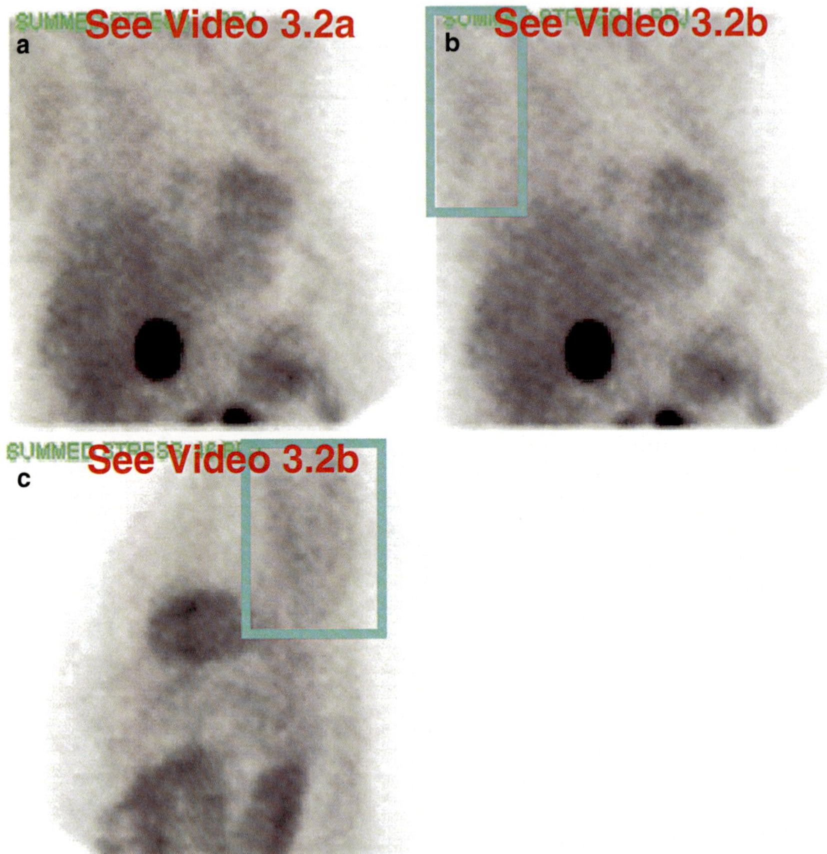

Fig. 3.2 Normal skeletal muscle in chest wall, shoulders, and back. This patient exercised on a treadmill for 6 minutes to 87 % of the maximal predicted heart rate and achieved 11.5 METS (metabolic equivalents). This stress SPECT MPI (**a–c**) acquired with his arms raised alongside his head shows normal shoulder musculature.

(**a**) Stress raw projection images (Video 3.2a, frame 1), ^{99m}Tc sestamibi. (**b**) Stress raw projection image (Video 3.2b, frame 1), ^{99m}Tc sestamibi, right shoulder musculature (*blue box*). (**c**) Stress raw projection image (Video 3.2b, frame 46), ^{99m}Tc sestamibi, left shoulder musculature (*blue box*)

left shoulder and upper chest wall. Patients are routinely imaged with both arms raised alongside their head to permit positioning of the gamma camera detectors as close as possible to their chest. The shoulder musculature can be more prominent, especially after a high exercise workload (because the patient's arms grip the handrails while walking on the treadmill) and could be misleading to the inexperienced.

Regardless of the radiopharmaceutical, one should consistently inspect the SPECT MPI raw projection data for incidental extracardiac findings that can signal underlying pathology (including unsuspected neoplasms), be physiologic, or be artifactual in nature. Incidental findings have been reported in up to 6 % of patients undergoing MPI (Chamarthy and Travin 2010; Gedik et al. 2007; Gentili et al. 1994; Gholamrezanezhad et al. 2006; Hendel et al. 1999; Howarth et al. 1996; Raza et al. 2005a, b; Shih et al. 2002, 2005; Williams et al. 2003). Such incidental findings can be expected (i.e., related to known clinical conditions) or unexpected and can be significant enough to warrant communication to the referring physician. Sources of "hot" artifacts (such as radiopharmaceutical or radioactive urine contamination, liver activity, and/or stomach activity) and "cold" artifacts (such as metallic objects, breast tissue, fluid collections, left hemidiaphragm) may have significant bearing on the accurate interpretation of cardiac findings (Burrell and MacDonald 2006; Chamarthy and Travin 2010; Holly et al. 2010). Correlation with medical and surgical history and other imaging may be required for optimal interpretation and is beneficial for quality assurance in clinical practice (and especially valuable for teaching students, residents, and fellows in training).

There are many potential pathologies and imaging artifacts related to the organ systems that lie within the SPECT MPI field-of-view. Tables 3.2 and 3.3 classify these imaging findings as "hot" or "cold" and organize them by location: "above the diaphragm" in the chest and "below the diaphragm" in the abdomen. Italicized text items may warrant personal communication to the primary or referring physician. The written report should contain language along the lines of the following example:

> On both rest and stress raw projection images, there is an intense focus of abnormal radioactivity in the left lung posterior to the heart; the differential diagnosis for this finding includes malignancy, and correlation with other imaging is recommended.

Table 3.2 Differential diagnosis of "hot" and "cold" imaging findings in the chest

"Above the Diaphragm"			
Organ system	"Hot" finding	"Cold" finding	References

Thyroid gland	Multinodular goiter
	Diffuse toxic goiter
	Substernal goiter
	*Nodule/neoplasm,
	  benign*
	*Nodule/neoplasm,
	  malignant*
	Lymphoma
	Free ^{99m}Tc pertechnetate
		Cyst
		Neoplasm, primary
		Neoplasm, metastasis
			Chamarthy and Travin
			  (2010)
			Gedik et al. (2007)
			Seabold et al. (1999)
			Seo et al. (2005)
			Smith and Oates
			  (2004a)
			Sundram and Mack (1995)
			Williams et al. (2003)

Parathyroid
  glands
	Adenoma
	Hyperplasia
	Carcinoma
		Cystic adenoma	Chamarthy and Travin
			  (2010)
			Coakley et al. (1989)
			Gedik et al. (2007)
			Lazar et al. (2005)
			O'Doherty et al. (1992)
			Smith and Oates
			  (2004b)

Breasts	Cystic disease
	Fibroadenoma
	Microcalcifications
	Hematoma
	Scar
	Lactation
	Gynecomastia
	  (periareolar pattern)
	Carcinoma
		Cyst
		Implants
		Prosthesis
		Soft tissue/shifting
		  breasts (positional)
		Mastectomy
			Arbab et al. (1995)
			Burrell and MacDonald
			  (2006)
			Chamarthy and Travin
			  (2010)
			García-Talavera et al.
			  (2013)
			Gedik et al. (2007)
			Hendel et al. (1999)
			Hesse et al. (2005)
			Holly et al. (2010)
			Howarth et al. (1996)
			Mlikotic and Mishkin
			  (2000)
			Ramakrishna and
			  Miller (2004)
			Raza et al. (2005a, b)
			Shih et al. (2002)
			Taillefer et al. (1995,
			  1998)
			Waxman (1997)
			Williams et al. (2003)

Table 3.2 (continued)

"Above the Diaphragm"			
Organ system	"Hot" finding	"Cold" finding	References
Chest wall	Brown adipose tissue Shoulder/upper chest skeletal musculature (due to arterial injection) Contamination (radiopharmaceutical, urine) Cross talk from nearby radioactive source (another patient on treadmill)	Soft-tissue mass Internal metal objects (pacemaker, defibrillator, vascular port) External metal objects (jewelry, chain, coin, keys, belt buckle) Arms by sides (positioning) Cracked crystal Malfunctioning photomultiplier tube	Afzelius and Henriksen (2008) Burrell and MacDonald (2006) Chamarthy and Travin (2010) Gedik et al. (2007) Gentili et al. (1994) Goetze et al. (2008) Hendel et al. (1999) Howarth et al. (1996) Vijayakumar et al. (2005) Williams et al. (2003)
Skeleton	Anemia/thalassemia Fracture/sternotomy Osteomyelitis Gaucher disease Paget disease Myelofibrosis/ myelodysplastic process *Multiple myeloma* *Osteosarcoma/sarcoma* *Neoplasm, metastasis*	*Neoplasm, metastasis*	Caner et al. (1992) Chamarthy and Travin (2010) Fisher et al. (2000) Gowda et al. (2006) Mariani et al. (2003) Maurea et al. (1995) Mohr et al. (1996) Onsel et al. (1996) Shih et al. (2005) Soderlund et al. (1997) Williams et al. (2003)
Pleura	*Neoplasm, malignant/ mesothelioma* *Pleural effusion, malignant*	Pleural effusion, benign *Pleural effusion, malignant*	Chamarthy and Travin (2010) Chin et al. (1995) Eftekhari and Gholamrezanezhad (2006) Gedik et al. (2007) Joy et al. (2007) Shih et al. (2002) Williams et al. (2003)

(continued)

Table 3.2 (continued)

"Above the Diaphragm"

Organ system	"Hot" finding	"Cold" finding	References
Lungs	*Congestive heart failure (diffuse pattern)* Interstitial lung disease Smoking Atelectasis Hematoma Pneumonia Fibrosing alveolitis Actinomycosis Granulomatous disease (sarcoidosis/ tuberculosis) *Neoplasm, primary malignant (lung carcinoma, carcinoid)* *Neoplasm, metastasis* Lymphangitic carcinomatosis	Hyperinflation/ emphysema Pneumonectomy/ elevated right hemidiaphragm Elevated left hemidiaphragm	Aras et al. (2003) Bom et al. (1998) Chamarthy and Travin (2010) Chin et al. (1995) Eftekhari and Gholamrezanezhad (2006) Gedik et al. (2007) Hendel et al. (1999) Mohr et al. (1996) Nishiyama et al. (1997) Onsel et al. (1996) Reyhan et al. 2004) Seo et al. (2005) Shih et al. (2002) Takekawa et al. (1999)
Mediastinum	Gastroesophageal reflux Hiatal hernia (refluxed duodenogastric bile) *Neoplasm, primary malignant (esophageal cancer, thymoma)* Extramedullary hematopoiesis (paravertebral masses)	Cyst Dilated esophagus Fluid- or food-filled hiatal hernia	Bhambhvani et al. (2010a) Burrell and MacDonald (2006) Chadika et al. (2005) Chamarthy and Travin (2010) García-Talavera et al. (2013) Gedik et al. (2007) Hawkins et al. (2007) Niederkohr et al. (2009) Raza et al. (2005c) Seo et al. (2005) Slavin et al. (1998) Vijayakumar et al. (2005) Watanabe et al. (1997)
Myocardium and pericardium	*Myocardial mass* *Pericardial mass*	*Pericardial effusion*	Chamarthy and Travin (2010) Kasi et al. (2002) Williams et al. (2003)

Table 3.2 (continued)

"Above the Diaphragm"			
Organ system	"Hot" finding	"Cold" finding	References
Right atrium and right ventricle	Prominent right ventricular wall (coronary artery disease, valvular disease, pulmonary hypertension) Brown adipose tissue Prominent right auricular appendage *Neoplasm*, *primary or metastatic*	Enlarged atria	Chamarthy and Travin (2010) Goetze et al. (2008) Mlikotic and Mishkin (2000) Mohr et al. (1996) Williams and Schneider (1999) Wosnitzer et al. (2012)
Vascular system	Contamination during injection Extravasation at injection site Retention in central veins Retention in central venous catheters/ports Pulmonary arterial wall	Dilated pulmonary arteries	Aras et al. (2003) Burrell and MacDonald (2006) Chamarthy and Travin (2010) Gedik et al. (2007) Gentili et al. (1994) Howarth et al. (1996) Shih et al. (2002) Strauss et al. (2008) Tallaj and Iskandrian (2000)
Lymphatic system	Sarcoidosis *Neoplasm*, *metastasis* (*e.g.*, *breast carcinoma*) Lymphoma Venous extravasation resulting in visualization of axillary lymph node(s)	Necrotic lymph node(s) *Neoplasm*, *metastasis*	Aktolun et al. (1994) Aktolun and Bayhan (1994) Chamarthy and Travin (2010) Gedik et al. (2007) Gentili et al. (1994) Mlikotic and Mishkin (2000) Shih et al. (1999, 2002) Taillefer et al. (1995, 1998) Waxman (1997) Williams et al. (2003)
Diaphragm	Elevated liver (due to right-sided eventration) Elevated bile-containing stomach (due to left-sided eventration) Herniated small or large intestine	Muscular diaphragm (causes inferior wall attenuation artifact)	Chamarthy and Travin (2010) Friedman et al. (1989) Gedik et al. (2007) Hendel et al. (1999) Howarth et al. (1996) Pitman et al. (2005)

Table 3.3 Differential diagnosis of "hot" and "cold" imaging findings in the abdomen

"Below the diaphragm"

Organ system	"Hot" finding	"Cold" finding	References
Abdominal wall	Contamination (radiopharmaceutical, urine)	Internal metal objects (implanted devices) External metal objects (jewelry, coin, key, belt buckle) Arms by sides and superimposed on abdominal wall (positioning) Cracked crystal Malfunctioning photomultiplier tube	Burrell and MacDonald (2006) Chamarthy and Travin (2010) Hendel et al. (1999)
Peritoneum	Not reported	Ascites (decompensated cirrhosis, malignancy) Peritoneal dialysate	Chamarthy and Travin (2010) Joy et al. (2007) Raza et al. (2005a, b) Shih et al. (2002, 2005) Tallaj et al. (2000) Williams et al. (2003)
Liver	Slow physiologic clearance Hepatomegaly Misshapen dome (elevated right hemidiaphragm) Intrahepatic gallbladder Pericholecystic rim sign (acute cholecystitis) *Neoplasm, primary (hepatocellular carcinoma)* *Neoplasm, metastasis (e.g., colon carcinoma)*	Rapid physiologic clearance Cyst/hydatid cyst Post-thermal ablation cyst Polycystic disease *Neoplasm, primary* *Neoplasm, metastasis* Postoperative change	Bhambhvani et al. (2010b) Burrell and MacDonald (2006) Chamarthy and Travin (2010) Chatziioannou et al. (1999) Fukushima et al. (1997) Gedik et al. (2007) Ghanbarinia et al. (2008) Hardebeck et al. (2013) Howarth et al. (1996) Joy et al. (2007) Lamont et al. (1996) Raza et al. (2005a, b) Shih et al. (2002, 2005) Tallaj et al. (2000)
Biliary system and gallbladder	Biliary ectasia with stasis Common bile duct obstruction	Inadequate or prolonged fasting *Cholecystitis (acute, chronic)* Biliary stricture/stone at ampulla of Vater	Chamarthy and Travin (2010) Gedik et al. (2007) Hesse et al. (2005) Howarth et al. (1996) Meesala et al. (2006) Panjrath et al. (2004) Shih et al. (2002, 2005) Toran et al. (1997)

Table 3.3 (continued)

"Below the diaphragm"

Organ system	"Hot" finding	"Cold" finding	References
Spleen	Splenomegaly	Cyst Infarct	Chamarthy and Travin (2010) Joy et al. (2007) Shih et al. (2002, 2005) Tallaj et al. (2000)
Stomach	Duodenogastric reflux Gastroparesis Gastropathy (dyspepsia/ gastritis, cirrhosis) Free ^{99m}Tc pertechnetate	Ingestion of fluids Distension, acute or chronic	Burrell and MacDonald (2006) Cote and Dumont (2004) Gedik et al. (2007) Gholamrezanezhad et al. (2006) Gupta et al. (2015) Khary et al. (1995) Middleton and Williams (1994, 1996)
Small intestine and large intestine	Herniation Stasis/slow peristalsis Neoplasm, primary (e.g., duodenal leiomyosarcoma) Previous radiopharmaceutical	Barium	Chamarthy and Travin (2010) Gedik et al. (2007) Hendel et al. (1999) Shuke et al. (1995)
Adrenal glands	Not reported	Cyst *Neoplasm, primary* *Neoplasm, metastasis*	Not applicable
Kidneys and female reproductive system	Retention of excreted radioactivity in dilated collecting system Stone disease Urinary catheters Physiologic in hepatic failure	Congenital absence/ nephrectomy Ptotic or small kidney Atrophy/end-stage renal disease Scar/pyelonephritis Cyst/polycystic disease *Neoplasm, primary* (*kidney*, uterine leiomyoma) *Neoplasm, metastasis*	Chamarthy and Travin (2010) Garg et al. (2013) Gedik et al. (2007) Ghanbarinia et al. (2008) Howarth et al. (1996) Raza et al. (2005d) Shih et al. (2002, 2005)
Vascular system	Contamination from injection/ extravasation at injection site	Not reported	Chamarthy and Travin (2010) Gentili et al. (1994) Strauss et al. (2008)

Part II

The Chest ("Above the Diaphragm")

Thyroid Gland

4

MPI radiopharmaceuticals normally localize in the thyroid gland. Benign and malignant thyroid conditions may accumulate these radiopharmaceuticals. Accordingly, apart from MPI, they have been used diagnostically for the evaluation of non-iodine-avid thyroid cancer and for the evaluation of thyroid nodules (Seabold et al. 1999; Sundram and Mack 1995). "Hot" lesions tend to be more easily recognized, but, at times, the degree of localization may actually be less than the surrounding or adjacent normal thyroid tissue, and the lesion may appear relatively "cold."

Situated in the lower neck, the thyroid gland is often included at the top of the imaging field-of-view during routine SPECT MPI (Fig. 4.1), particularly when using large detectors. The degree of uptake is usually relatively faint, but images can be manipulated to enhance its visualization (Fig. 4.1b, d). Review of the raw projection images can lead to identification of a variety of underlying thyroid conditions (Williams et al. 2003). Table 4.1 lists potential "hot" and "cold" imaging findings related to the thyroid gland.

On occasion, primary malignancies of the thyroid gland as well as other head and neck cancers may be discovered (Chamarthy and Travin 2010; Gedik et al. 2007). Benign conditions include enlargement of the thyroid gland associated with diffuse toxic goiter and toxic or nontoxic multinodular goiter. Also, goitrous tissue can migrate from the neck deep into the substernal chest. Such ectopic thyroid tissue can interfere with cardiac interpretation (Gedik et al. 2007; Seo et al. 2005). Figure 4.2 illustrates a large ^{9m}Tc sestamibi-avid multinodular thyroid gland predominantly located in the mediastinum just superior to the heart (Smith and Oates 2004a).

Electronic supplementary material The online version of this chapter (doi:10.1007/978-3-319-25436-4_4) contains supplementary material, which is available to authorized users.

© Springer International Publishing Switzerland 2017
M.E. Oates, V.L. Sorrell, *Myocardial Perfusion Imaging - Beyond the Left Ventricle: Pathology, Artifacts and Pitfalls in the Chest and Abdomen*, DOI 10.1007/978-3-319-25436-4_4

Fig. 4.1 Normal thyroid gland at top of field-of-view. Normal thyroid activity can be identified on rest (**a, b**) and stress (**c–e**) images.

(**a**) Rest raw projection images (Video 4.1a, frame 1) at usual contrast setting for the heart, ^{99m}Tc sestamibi. (**b**) Rest raw projection images (Video 4.1b, frame 1) with enhanced contrast for the thyroid gland, ^{99m}Tc sestamibi. (**c**) Stress raw projection images (Video 4.1c, frame 1) at usual contrast setting for the heart, ^{99m}Tc sestamibi. (**d**) Stress raw projection images (Video 4.1d, frame 1) with enhanced contrast for the thyroid gland, ^{99m}Tc sestamibi. (**e**) Stress raw projection image (Video 4.1e, frame 16) with enhanced contrast for the thyroid gland, ^{99m}Tc sestamibi, bilobed thyroid gland (*yellow box*), heart for anatomic reference only (*blue lines*)

Table 4.1 Differential diagnosis of "hot" and "cold" imaging findings related to the thyroid gland

Organ system	"Hot" finding	"Cold" finding	References
Thyroid gland	Multinodular goiter Diffuse toxic goiter Substernal goiter *Nodule/neoplasm, benign* *Nodule/neoplasm, malignant* *Lymphoma* Free ^{99m}Tc pertechnetate	Cyst *Neoplasm, primary* *Neoplasm, metastasis*	Chamarthy and Travin (2010) Gedik et al. (2007) Seabold et al. (1999) Seo et al. (2005) Smith and Oates (2004a) Sundram and Mack (1995) Williams et al. (2003)

In the event of an enlarged or heterogeneous thyroid gland with a prominent focal or multifocal "hot" or "cold" pattern, one should correlate the findings with medical history and other relevant imaging to narrow the differential diagnosis. Depending on the outcome of that investigation, one should consider reporting such findings personally to the referring physician. As one example, the written report could include wording along the lines of:

> Incidentally noted is an enlarged, heterogeneous thyroid gland which extends into the superior mediastinum; this finding correlates with a benign-appearing substernal goiter on recent CT scan.

Free ^{99m}Tc refers to ^{99m}Tc pertechnetate which may be present in the radiopharmaceutical preparation if there was a problem with the radiolabeling of ^{99m}Tc sestamibi or ^{99m}Tc tetrofosmin (Gedik et al. 2007). [99m]Tc pertechnetate normally localizes to the thyroid gland, the salivary glands, and the stomach wall. A particularly well-visualized thyroid gland and stomach should prompt one to investigate the purity of the administered radiopharmaceutical. For example, if more than one patient exhibits this finding on the same day, one should contact the radiopharmaceutical supplier to query the quality control testing of that lot. As a corollary, this same principle holds for radiolabeled red blood cells used for cardiac gated blood pool imaging in that a well-labeled preparation will not show the thyroid gland, salivary glands, and stomach; directed imaging of those regions can confirm the presence of excess free ^{99m}Tc pertechnetate in the administered radiopharmaceutical preparation. However, the key difference is that the ^{99m}Tc MPI radiopharmaceuticals *normally* localize in those tissues; thus, one has to appreciate often subtle relatively greater activity than usual; this skill develops with experience.

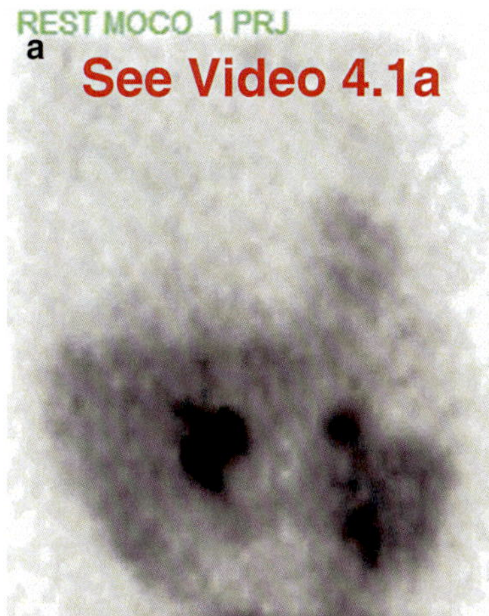
REST MOCO 1 PRJ
a
See Video 4.1a

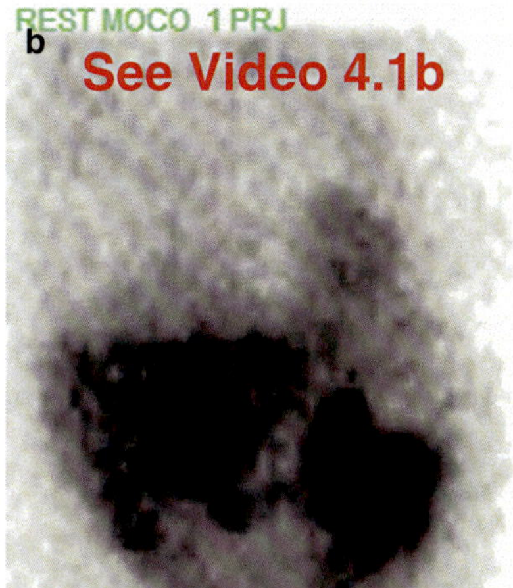
REST MOCO 1 PRJ
b
See Video 4.1b

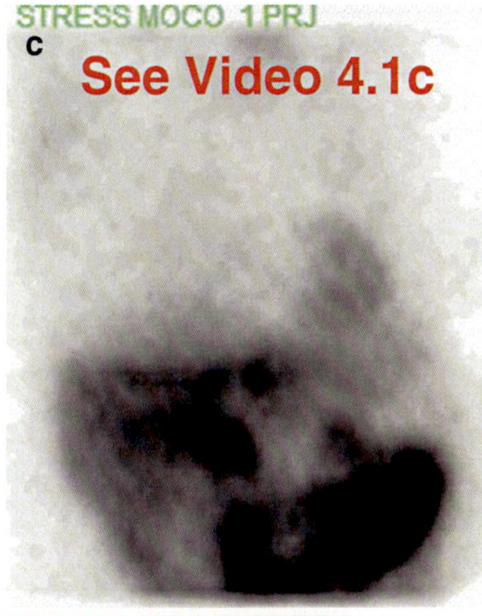
STRESS MOCO 1 PRJ
c
See Video 4.1c

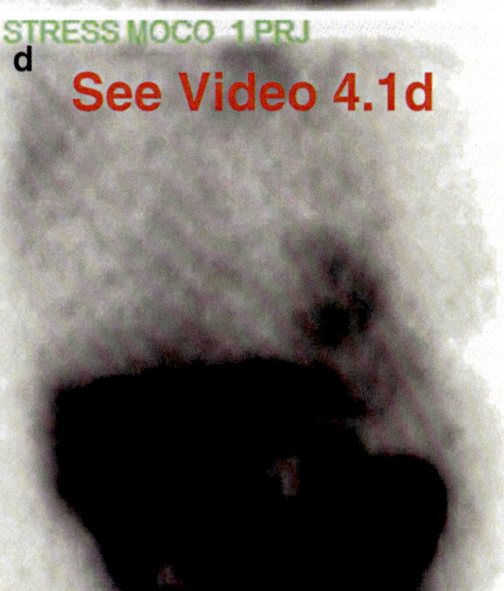
STRESS MOCO 1 PRJ
d
See Video 4.1d

STRESS MOCO 1 PRJ
e
See Video 4.1e

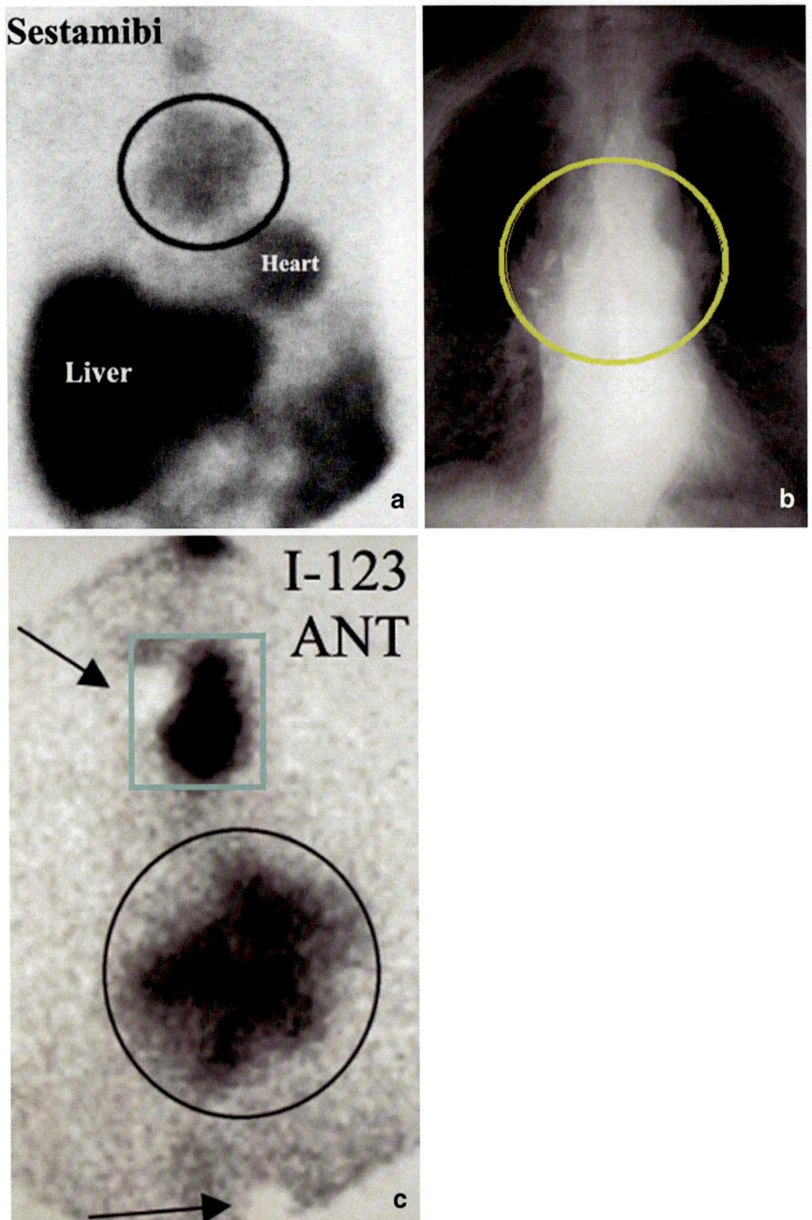

Fig. 4.2 Substernal multinodular goiter. The degree of radiopharmaceutical localization in the substernal goiter is of similar intensity to the myocardium (**a**). The chest radiograph (**b**) confirms a mediastinal mass. The tissue is radioiodine-avid (**c**), clinching the diagnosis of ectopic thyroidal tissue.

(**a**) Anterior planar chest image, ^{99m}Tc sestamibi, heart and liver labeled, substernal thyroid (*black circle*). (**b**) PA chest radiograph, substernal thyroid (*yellow circle*). (**c**) Anterior planar chest image, ^{123}I sodium iodide, thyroid in neck/superior mediastinum at sternal notch (*blue box*), substernal thyroid (*black circle*), "cold" marker at sternal notch (*superior arrow*), and "cold" marker at xiphoid process (*inferior arrow*) placed by technologist as anatomic landmarks (Reprinted with permission Smith and Oates (2004a). Wolters Kluwer Health, Inc.)

Key Points
- The thyroid gland can be faintly visible during routine SPECT MPI, typically seen at the top of the imaging field-of-view.
- Ectopically located thyroid tissue can present a pitfall during image interpretation.
- Free ^{99m}Tc pertechnetate normally localizes to the thyroid gland, salivary glands, and stomach wall; enhanced visualization of these tissues should prompt investigation of the purity of the administered radiopharmaceutical.

Parathyroid Glands

5

Normal parathyroid glands are too small to be visualized by routine radionuclide imaging using MPI radiopharmaceuticals. However, benign or malignant enlarged parathyroid glands typically accumulate and retain sufficient activity for imaging detection. Historically, ^{201}Tl chloride was used diagnostically for preoperative identification and localization of culprit glands causing primary and secondary hyperparathyroidism; ^{99m}Tc sestamibi is the most widely used radiopharmaceutical today (Coakley et al. 1989; O'Doherty et al. 1992; Smith and Oates 2004b). The hallmark pattern is early uptake with relatively delayed ("differential") washout from the enlarged parathyroid gland(s) compared to the thyroid gland. However, some lesions may washout more rapidly; since MPI typically commences anywhere from 15 to 90 minutes after injection, be aware that these lesions may appear "warm" rather than the more characteristic "hot" uptake pattern due to the washout kinetics.

Table 5.1 provides a short list of potential "hot" and "cold" imaging findings related to the parathyroid glands. Particularly if ectopic in location, the enlarged parathyroid gland(s) harboring adenoma, hyperplasia, or carcinoma might be included in the field-of-view during routine MPI (Chamarthy and Travin 2010; Gedik et al. 2007). Figure 5.1 illustrates a "hot" ectopic parathyroid adenoma in the anterior mediastinum just superior to the heart. Mediastinal parathyroid adenomas can be occult during cardiac surgery and may require imaging localization for subsequent directed surgery (Lazar et al. 2005). If large enough, parathyroid lesions can appear "cold" if there is central cystic change or necrosis (Fig. 5.2).

Electronic supplementary material The online version of this chapter (doi:10.1007/978-3-319-25436-4_5) contains supplementary material, which is available to authorized users.

© Springer International Publishing Switzerland 2017

M.E. Oates, V.L. Sorrell, *Myocardial Perfusion Imaging - Beyond the Left Ventricle: Pathology, Artifacts and Pitfalls in the Chest and Abdomen*, DOI 10.1007/978-3-319-25436-4_5

Table 5.1 Differential diagnosis of "hot" and "cold" imaging findings related to the parathyroid glands

Organ system	"Hot" finding	"Cold" finding	References
Parathyroid glands	*Adenoma* *Hyperplasia* *Carcinoma*	Cystic adenoma	Chamarthy and Travin (2010) Coakley et al. (1989) Gedik et al. (2007) Lazar et al. (2005) O'Doherty et al. (1992) Smith and Oates (2004b)

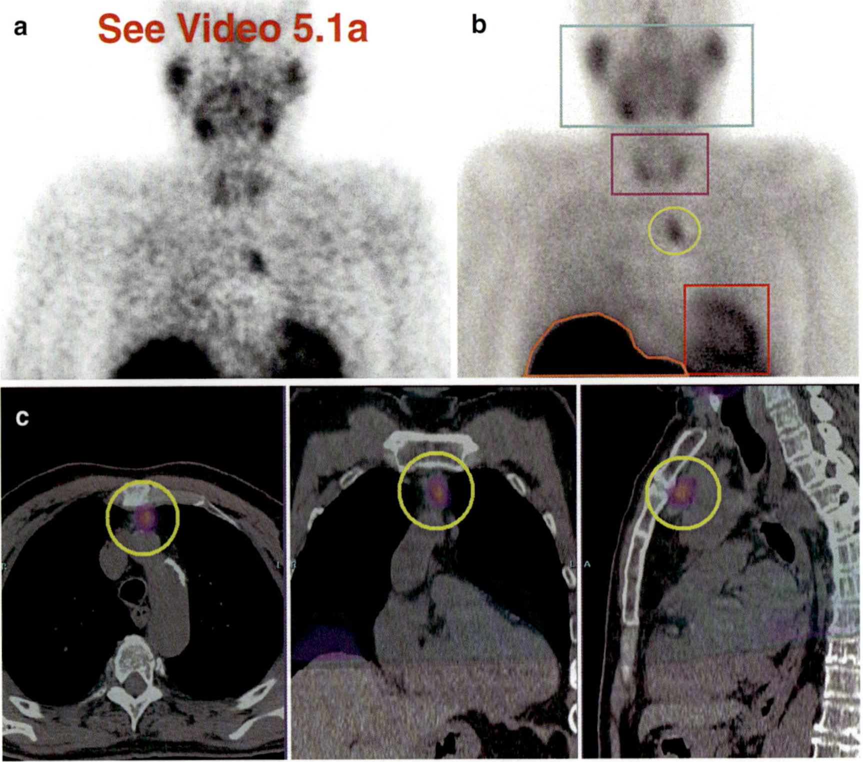

Fig. 5.1 Ectopic sestamibi-avid anterior mediastinal parathyroid adenoma. The enlarged ectopic parathyroid gland (**a**, **b**) is localized by SPECT/CT fusion images (**c**) in the anterior mediastinum. It weighed 5 g on surgical resection. Note normal salivary glands, thyroid gland, liver, and left ventricular myocardium (**b**).

(**a**) Raw projection images (360°, Video 5.1a, frame 1), ^{99m}Tc sestamibi. (**b**) Anterior early planar chest image, ^{99m}Tc sestamibi, salivary glands (*blue box*), thyroid gland (*pink box*), ectopic parathyroid adenoma (*yellow circle*), liver (*orange outline*), left ventricle (*red box*). (**c**) Axial, coronal, and sagittal SPECT/CT fusion images, ectopic parathyroid adenoma (*yellow circles*)

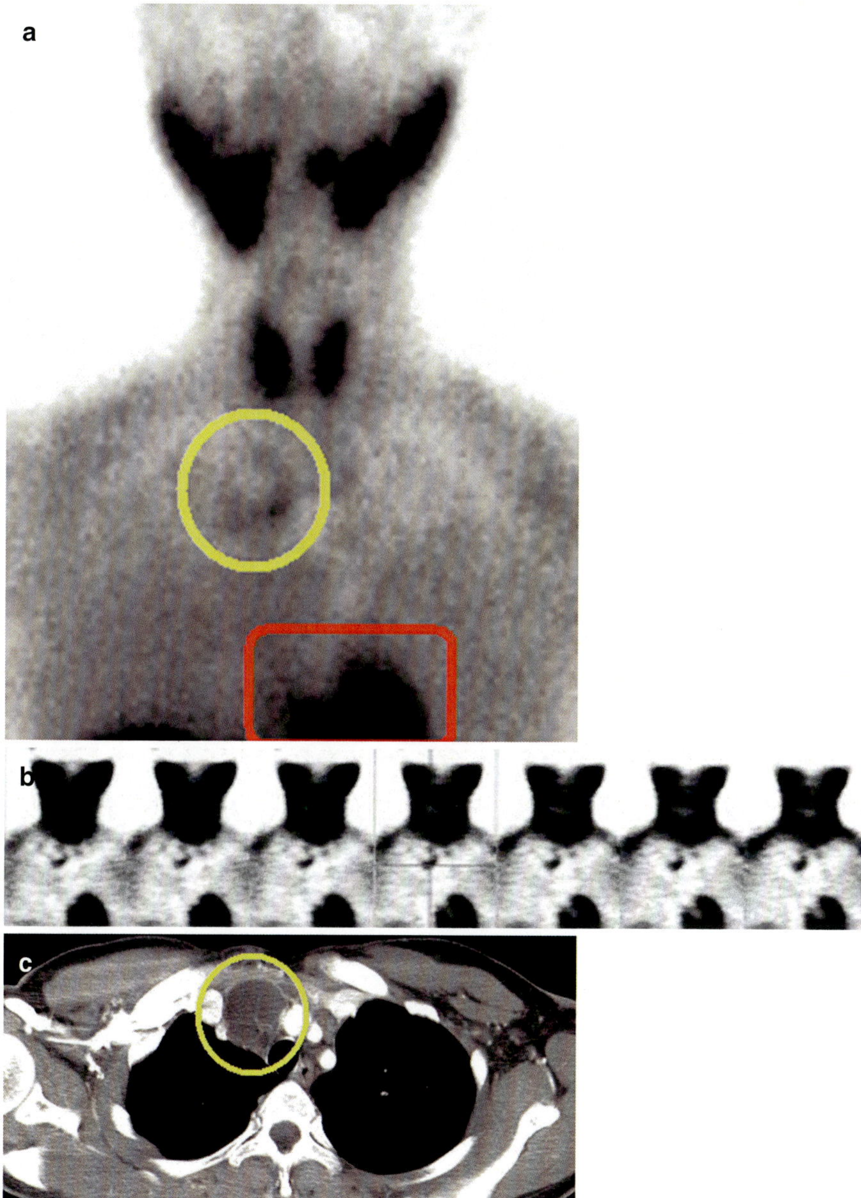

Fig. 5.2 "Cold" rim-like sestamibi-avid anterior superior mediastinal parathyroid adenoma. The enlarged cystic mediastinal mass has a distinctive "cold" center and rim-like uptake (**a**, **b**). The salivary glands and thyroid gland appear intensely "hot" because the image contrast has been adjusted to enhance visualization of the lesion (**a**). Note the correlative CT finding of a low-attenuation cystic center with internal septations (**c**).

(**a**) Anterior early planar chest image, contrast-adjusted for the lesion, ^{99m}Tc sestamibi, lesion (*yellow circle*), myocardium (*red box*). (**b**) Subsequent coronal SPECT images, anterior to posterior, contrast-adjusted for the lesion, ^{99m}Tc sestamibi, lesion (cross-hairs in middle image), myocardium (left lower chest in each image). (**c**) Axial CT image at level of lesion (*yellow circle*) (Reprinted with permission Smith and Oates (2004b), Radiological Society of North America)

One should correlate such an abnormal focal finding with the patient's medical history and laboratory values (e.g., calcium, parathormone levels) and consider reporting it personally to the referring physician. The written report should mention the incidental finding and suggest further evaluation of suspected underlying parathyroid gland pathology. For example:

On review of the raw projection data, there is an incidental focal abnormality in the superior mediastinum just to the left of midline; in light of an elevated calcium level on today's blood laboratory report, this finding suggests a hyperfunctional parathyroid gland that may warrant follow-up.

Key Points
- Normally, the parathyroid glands are not visible by routine radionuclide imaging using MPI radiopharmaceuticals.
- A pathologic (usually benign) parathyroid gland typically demonstrates the hallmark pattern of early uptake and delayed washout relative to the thyroid gland.
- Ectopically located parathyroid tissue can present a pitfall during image interpretation.

Review of the raw projection data from routine MPI may reveal incidental breast pathology (Table 6.1) (Gedik et al. 2007; Raza et al. 2005a, b). The left and most of the right breast are included in the field-of-view during routine SPECT MPI. A variety of benign conditions tend to show a diffuse and symmetric pattern (Fig. 6.1) (Chamarthy and Travin 2010). Lactating breasts (Fig. 6.2) will show varying degrees of bilaterally symmetric increased uptake depending on the postpartum state and breastfeeding status (Ramakrishna and Miller 2004). Breastfeeding does not need to be stopped for the examination; ^{99m}Tc radiopharmaceuticals are preferred in this setting (Hesse et al. 2005). In males, gynecomastia may be evident (Fig. 6.3) and is often associated with underlying liver disease or associated with hormonal therapy or medical therapy for congestive heart failure (e.g., spironolactone).

^{99m}Tc sestamibi has been long used clinically to evaluate the breast for malignancy (Taillefer et al. 1995, 1998; Waxman 1997). Breast-specific gamma imaging (BSGI) remains under active investigation as a molecular approach adjunctive to mammography, ultrasonography, and magnetic resonance imaging, particularly in mammographically dense breasts (Holbrook and Newel 2015). Thus, the differential diagnosis for focal increased uptake in the breasts includes primary, metastatic, or recurrent breast malignancy, particularly if it is unilateral and intensely avid for ^{201}Tl chloride and ^{99m}Tc sestamibi (Fig. 6.4) (Arbab et al. 1995; Chamarthy and Travin 2010; García-Talavera et al. 2013; Hendel et al. 1999; Mlikotic and Mishkin 2000; Shih et al. 2002; Williams et al. 2003). The rest raw acquisition might be more revealing and should be reviewed, ideally with a whole-field-of-view reconstruction for three-dimensional characterization of a suspected lesion (Seo et al. 2005). The written report should include wording along the lines of:

Electronic supplementary material The online version of this chapter (doi:10.1007/978-3-319-25436-4_6) contains supplementary material, which is available to authorized users.

© Springer International Publishing Switzerland 2017
M.E. Oates, V.L. Sorrell, *Myocardial Perfusion Imaging - Beyond the Left Ventricle: Pathology, Artifacts and Pitfalls in the Chest and Abdomen,*
DOI 10.1007/978-3-319-25436-4_6

Table 6.1 Differential diagnosis of "hot" and "cold" imaging findings related to the breasts

Organ system	"Hot" finding	"Cold" finding	References

Breasts	Cystic disease
	Fibroadenoma
	Microcalcifications
	Hematoma
	Scar
	Lactation
	Gynecomastia
	  (periareolar
	  pattern)
	Carcinoma
		Cyst
		Implants
		Prosthesis
		Soft-tissue/shifting
		  breasts
		  (positional)
		Mastectomy
			Arbab et al. (1995)
			Burrell and MacDonald (2006)
			Chamarthy and Travin (2010)
			García-Talavera et al. (2013)
			Gedik et al. (2007)
			Hendel et al. (1999)
			Hesse et al. (2005)
			Holly et al. (2010)
			Howarth et al. (1996)
			Mlikotic and Mishkin (2000)
			Ramakrishna and Miller (2004)
			Raza et al. (2005a, b)
			Shih et al. (2002)
			Taillefer et al. (1995, 1998)
			Waxman (1997)
			Williams et al. (2003)

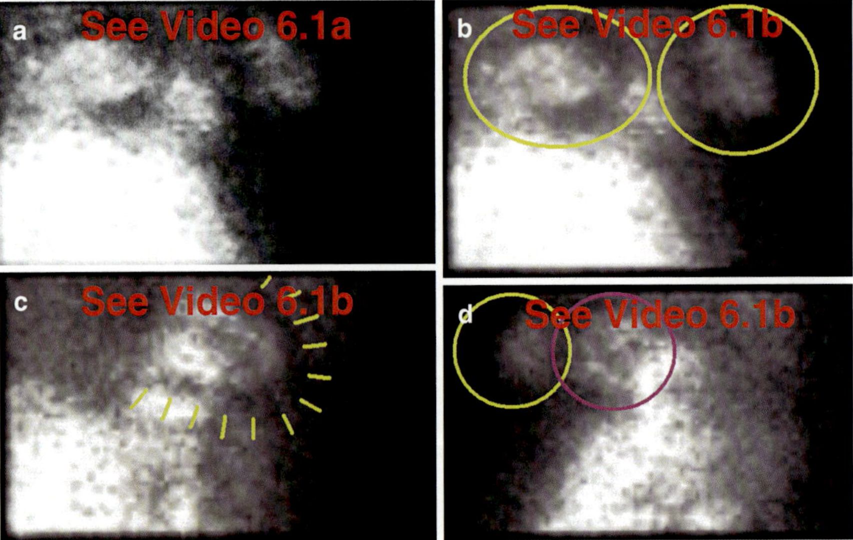

Fig. 6.1 Symmetric, diffusely "hot" breasts. The breast uptake is relatively intense and extensive but localizes to the central subareolar tissues (**a–d**). A 47-year-old female has benign-appearing "dense" breasts by ultrasound; she opted out of conventional mammography.

(**a**) Stress raw projection images (Video 6.1a, frame 1), ^{99m}Tc sestamibi. (**b**) Stress raw projection image (Video 6.1b, frame 1, RAO), ^{99m}Tc sestamibi, both breasts (yellow ovals). (**c**) Stress raw projection image (Video 6.1b, frame 25, Anterior), ^{99m}Tc sestamibi, left breast contour (*yellow lines*) extends well beyond internal breast uptake. (**d**) Stress raw projection image (Video 6.1b, frame 44, LAO), ^{99m}Tc sestamibi, both breasts (right, *yellow oval*; left, *pink oval*)

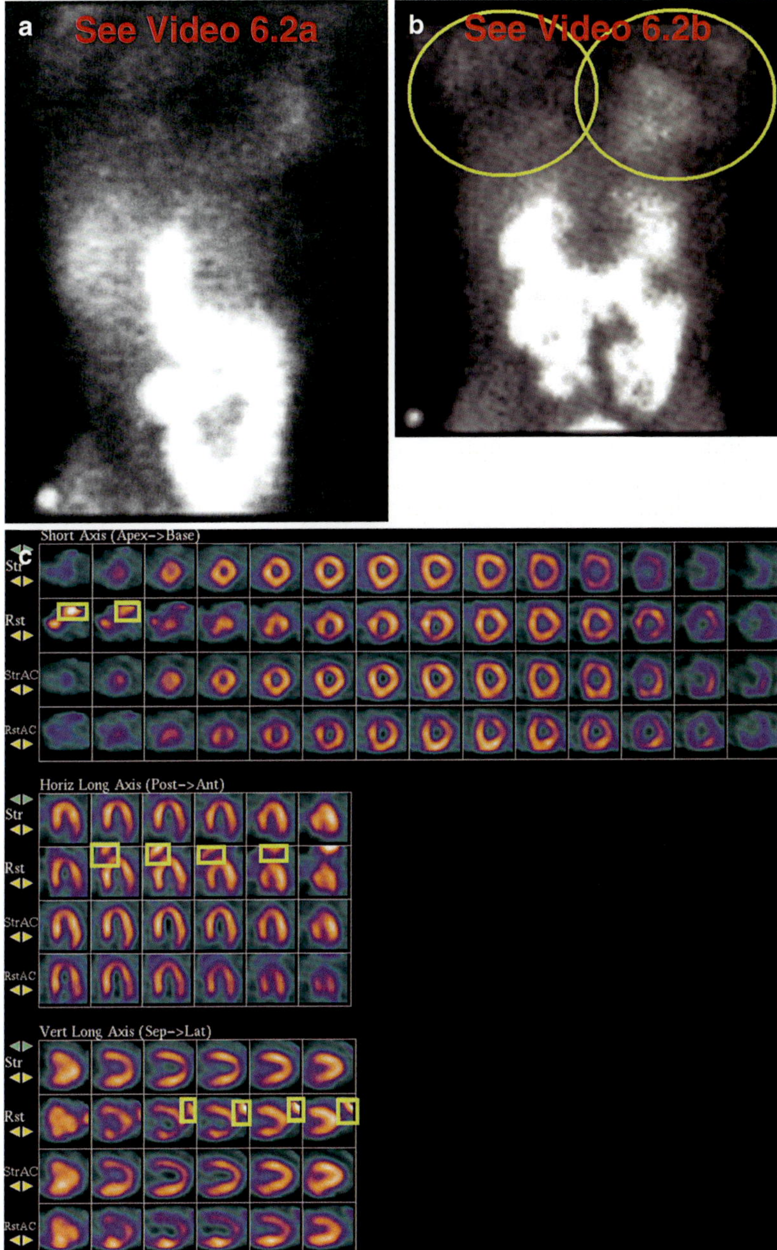

Fig. 6.2 Lactation. Diffusely "hot" breasts (**a, b**) in a lactating 38-year-old female. The anterolateral extracardiac activity has much greater relative intensity on rest processed images (**c**); this pattern is likely related to relative differences in cardiac-to-breast activity after treadmill exercise.

(**a**) Rest raw projection images (Video 6.2a, frame 1), ^{99m}Tc tetrofosmin; breasts appear spread out due to arms raised and supine position for imaging. (**b**) Rest raw projection image (Video 6.2b, frame 18, Anterior), ^{99m}Tc tetrofosmin, breasts (*yellow ovals*); note left breast overlies left ventricle. (**c**) Stress/rest processed SPECT images (SA, HLA, VLA) (without and with AC), left breast uptake (*yellow boxes* on representative images)

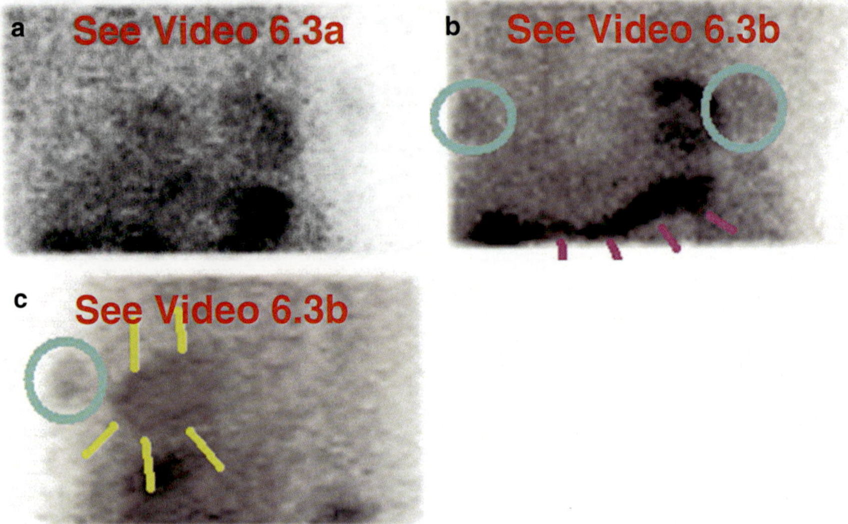

Fig. 6.3 Gynecomastia. There is well-defined localized periareolar activity creating "hot" breasts (**a–c**) in a cirrhotic male. Note the "hot" stomach which is related to the associated gastropathy (**b**). The left breast activity is anteriorly situated relative to the heart (**c**).

(**a**) Stress raw projection images (Video 6.3a, frame 1), ^{99m}Tc sestamibi. (**b**) Stress raw projection image (Video 6.3b, frame 18, Anterior), ^{99m}Tc sestamibi, areolar regions of both breasts (*blue ovals*), stomach (*pink lines*). (**c**) Stress raw projection image (Video 6.3b, frame 62, Lateral), ^{99m}Tc sestamibi, areolar region of left breast (*blue circle*), left ventricular myocardium (*yellow lines*)

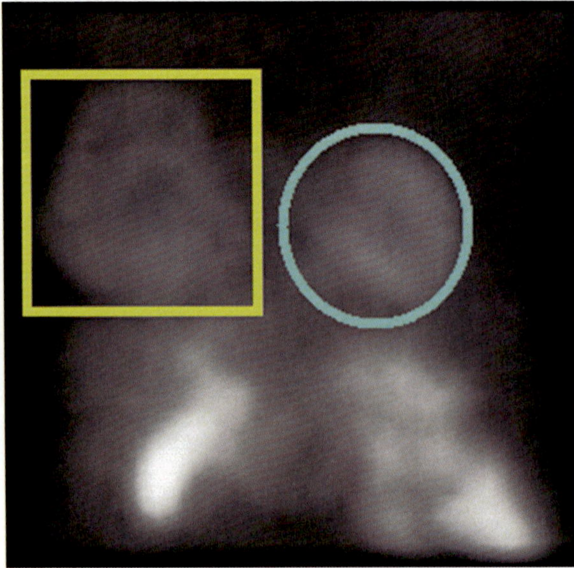

Fig. 6.4 Right breast cancer. A 64-year-old female has a diffusely "hot" right breast. (**a**) Stress raw projection image, ^{99m}Tc sestamibi, right breast (*yellow box*), heart (*blue circle*)

There is an intense, well-defined focus of abnormal radioactivity in the left breast that may warrant further diagnostic investigation; primary malignancy is included in the differential diagnosis.

Personal communication with the referring physician is appropriate in those circumstances.

Frankly decreased ("cold") uptake in the breasts may be related to prostheses or implants (Fig. 6.5), and the nuclear technologist should ask the patient to remove

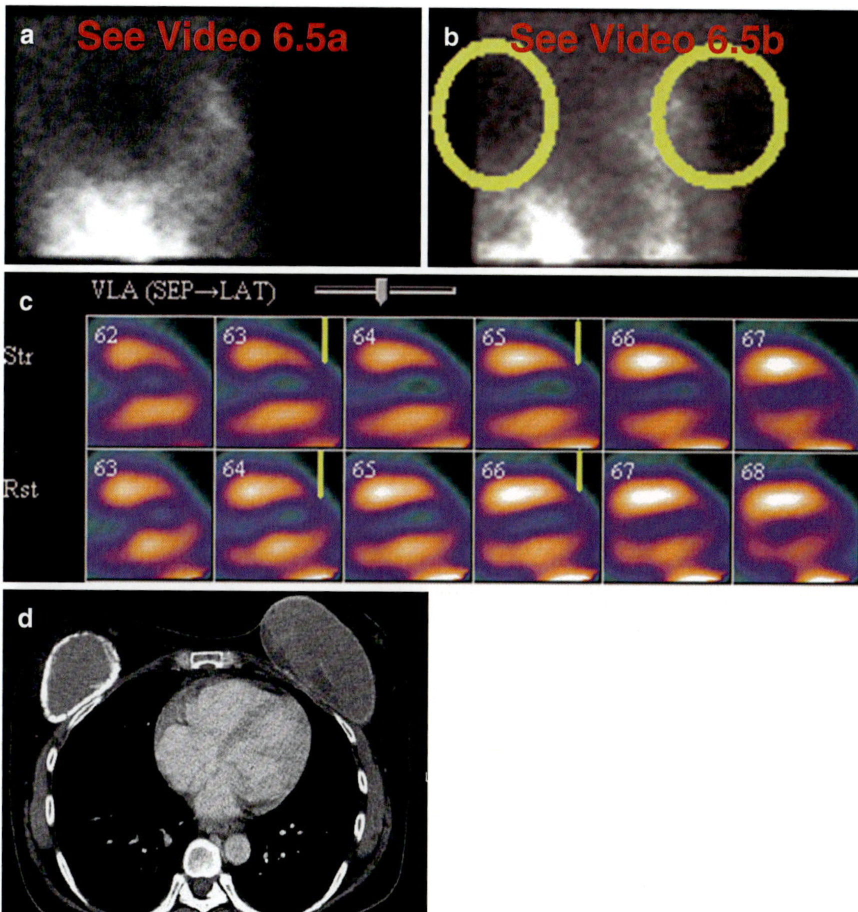

Fig. 6.5 Breast implants. Note the sharply demarcated "cold" defects in both breasts (**a, b**). There is an associated fixed defect in the anteroapical wall (**c**). The relationship of the implants to the heart is demonstrated on the CT scan (**d**).

(**a**) Stress raw projection images (Video 6.5a, frame 1), ^{99m}Tc sestamibi. (**b**) Stress raw projection image (Video 6.5b, frame 16, RAO/Anterior), ^{99m}Tc sestamibi, "cold" implants (*yellow ovals*). (**c**) Stress/rest processed SPECT images (VLA), anteroapical fixed defect (*yellow lines*, selected images). (**d**) Axial CT image through lower chest at level of breasts

the prosthesis if it is removable (Burrell and MacDonald 2006; Hendel et al. 1999; Howarth et al. 1996). However, normal breast tissue creates a commonly problematic and often unpredictable soft-tissue attenuation artifact overlying the heart (Burrell and MacDonald 2006; Chamarthy and Travin 2010; Hendel et al. 1999). This typically results in a characteristic, sometimes severe, fixed perfusion defect that may or may not completely normalize with an attenuation correction technique. Normal wall motion and preserved wall thickening on gated SPECT imaging assists in differentiating such a fixed perfusion defect from myocardial scar/infarction. Breast attenuation artifact generally includes the most basal aspect of the anterior wall, may spare the apex, and has a sharp crescentic edge effect conforming to the shape of the breast (Figs. 6.6 and 6.7). This is contrary to the most common pattern of LAD coronary artery disease which has less distinct borders, spares the most basal anterior segment, and usually includes the apex.

At times, however, the soft-tissue attenuation defect produced can appear reversible, simulating anterior, septal, apical, or even lateral wall ischemia and may be misinterpreted as LAD coronary artery disease. Normal wall motion and preserved wall thickening on gated SPECT imaging would be expected and are not incrementally clarifying when evaluating reversible defects. This pattern occurs when the position of the breasts, particularly the left breast, is substantially different between the rest and stress image acquisitions. Attention should be paid to reproduce the patient position exactly (Fig. 6.8) (Burrell and MacDonald 2006; Hendel et al. 1999; Holly et al. 2010). A repeat acquisition may be appropriate when the cause for the variability is obvious (e.g., bra left on during stress imaging but not on rest imaging).

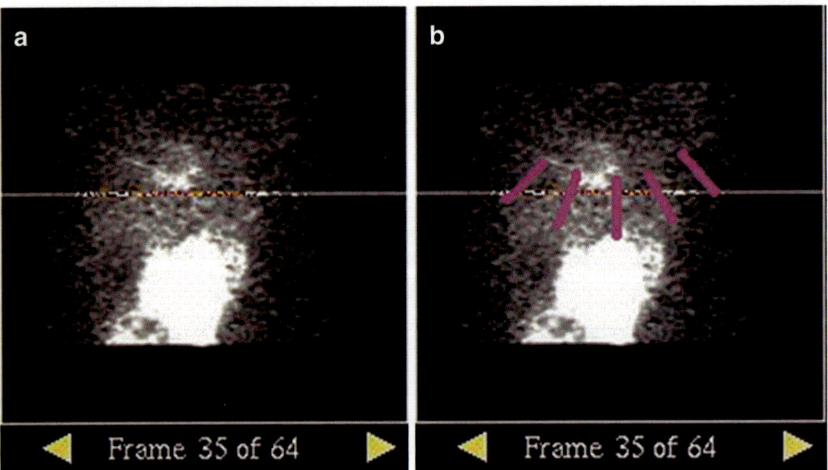

Fig. 6.6 "Cold" breast attenuation artifact. There is a typical "cold" soft-tissue pattern for the breasts on the raw data (**a–d**). The SPECT images demonstrate a characteristic fixed anterior wall defect that clearly normalizes on attenuation-corrected stress and rest images (**e**) in a 34-year-old female.

(**a**) Rest raw projection image, ⁹⁹ᵐTc tetrofosmin, lower limit of heart (*white line*). (**b**) Rest raw projection image, ⁹⁹ᵐTc tetrofosmin, left breast contour (*pink lines*). (**c**) Stress raw projection image, ⁹⁹ᵐTc tetrofosmin, lower limit of heart (*white line*). (**d**) Stress raw projection image, ⁹⁹ᵐTc tetrofosmin, left breast contour (*pink lines*). (**e**) Stress/rest processed SPECT images (VLA) (without and with AC), anterior wall defect, selected non-AC vs. AC images (*yellow ovals*)

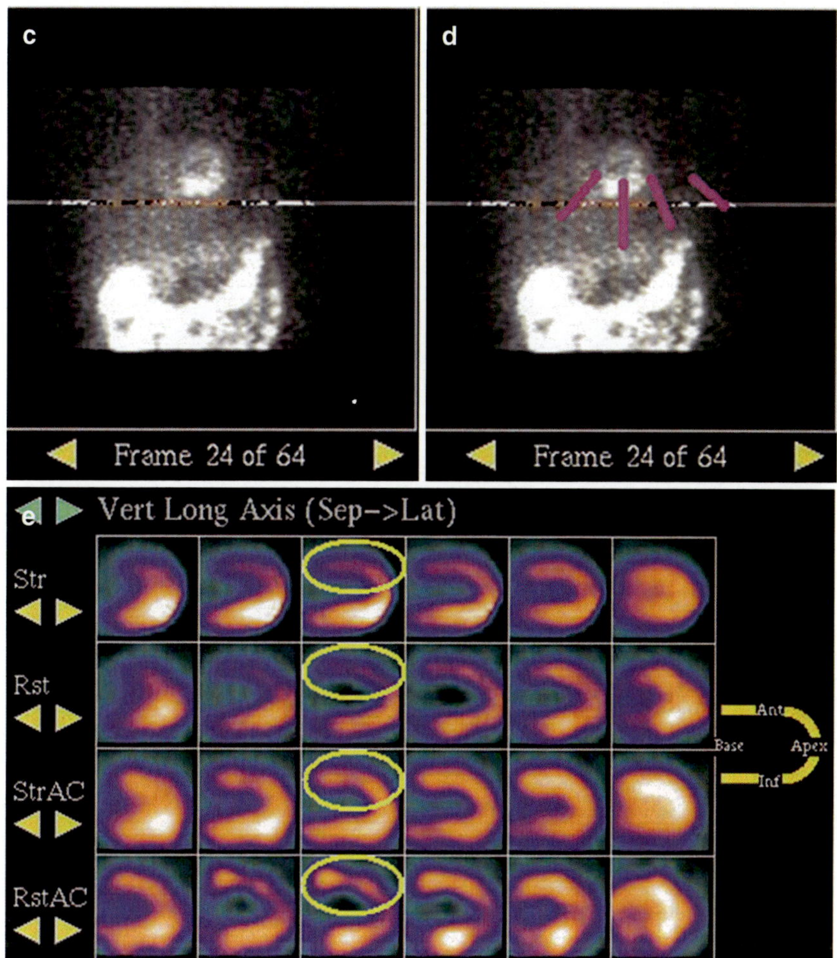

Fig. 6.6 (continued)

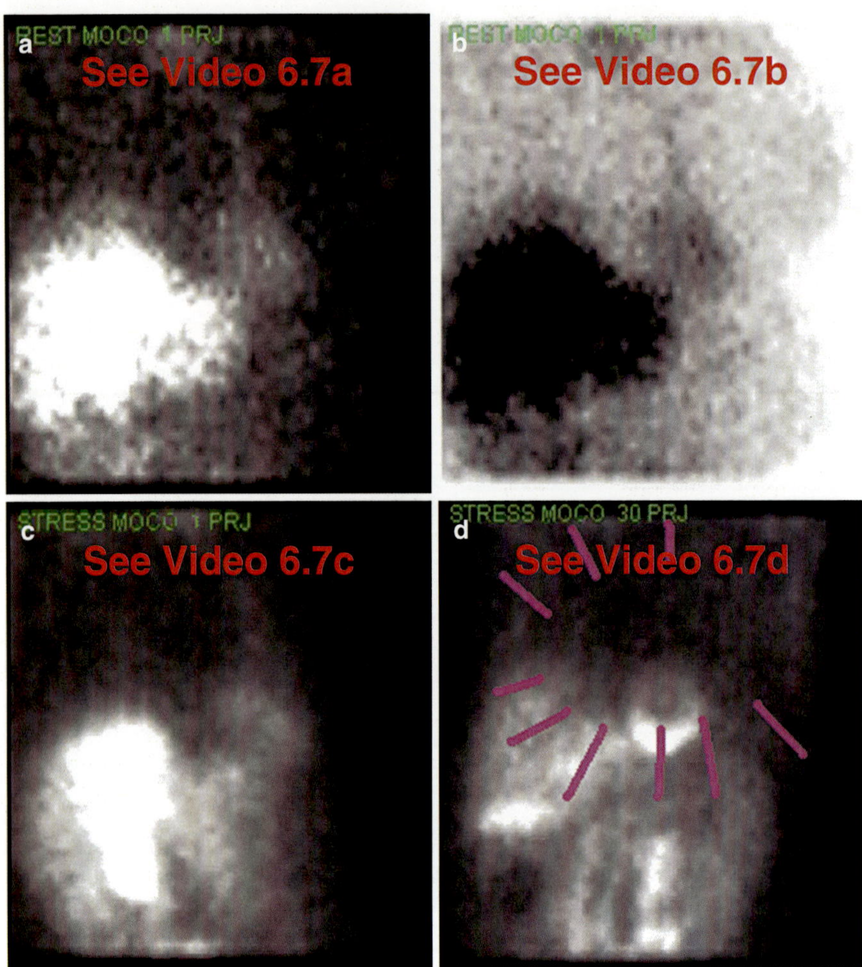

Fig. 6.7 Extreme breast attenuation artifact. This effect is more sharply defined on "white-on-black" gray scale image rendering (compare **a** to **b**, and compare **c** and **d** to **e**). The "cold" fixed anterior wall defect (incorporating the base of the left ventricle and characteristically sparing the apex) on processed SPECT images (**f**) demonstrates normal wall motion and wall thickening on gated SPECT images (**g**), confirming breast attenuation artifact and excluding scar.

(**a**) Rest "white-on-black" raw projection images (Video 6.7a, frame 1), ^{99m}Tc sestamibi. (**b**) Rest "black-on-white" raw projection images (Video 6.7b, frame 1), ^{99m}Tc sestamibi. (**c**) Stress "white-on-black" raw projection images (Video 6.7c, frame 1), ^{99m}Tc sestamibi. (**d**) Stress "white-on-black" raw projection image (Video 6.7d, frame 30), ^{99m}Tc sestamibi, left breast contour (*pink lines*). (**e**) Stress "black-on-white" raw projection images (Video 6.7e, frame 1), ^{99m}Tc sestamibi. (**f**) Stress/rest processed SPECT images (SA, VLA, HLA), fixed anterior wall defect (*yellow ovals* on representative images). (**g**) Stress gated SPECT images (Video 6.7f, frame 1) (SA, VLA, HLA)

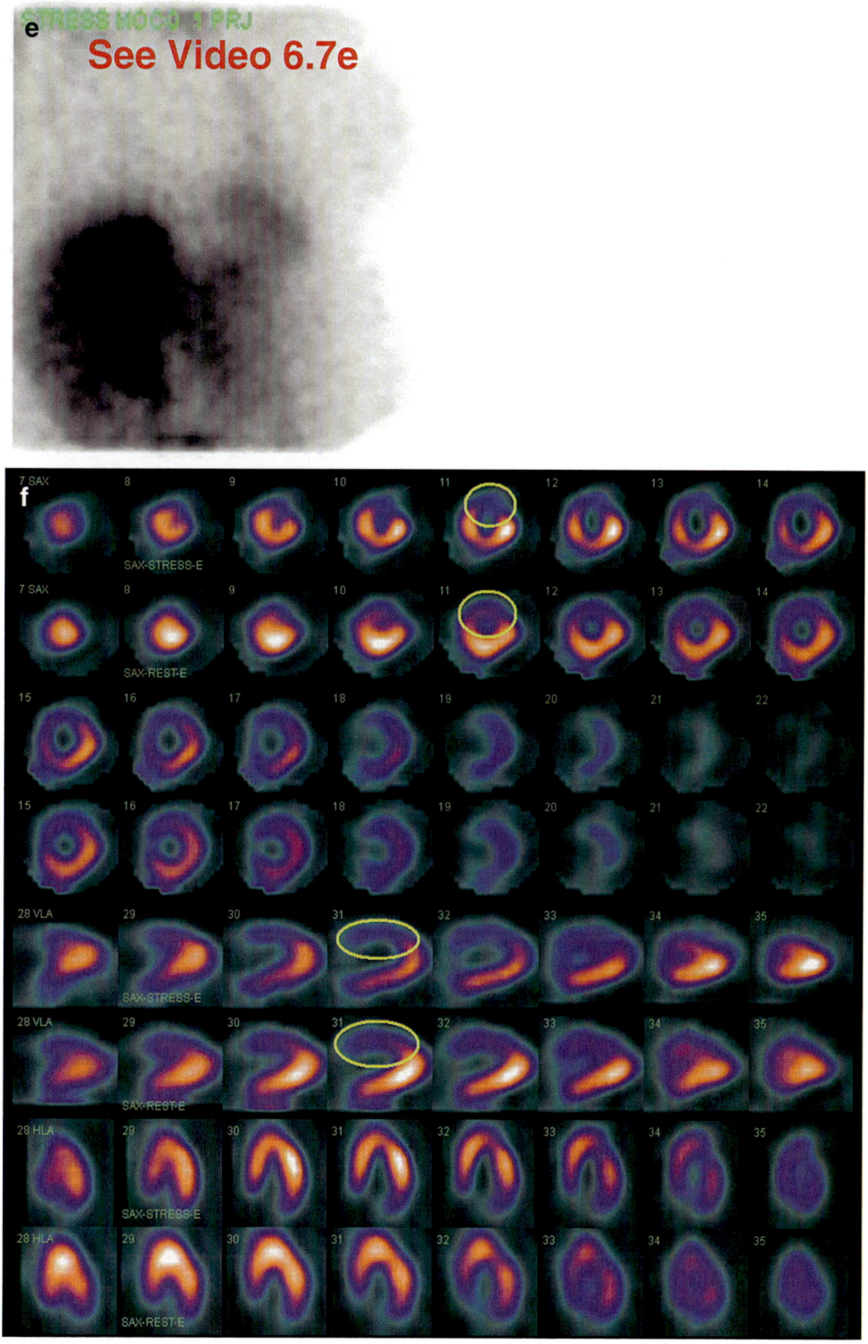

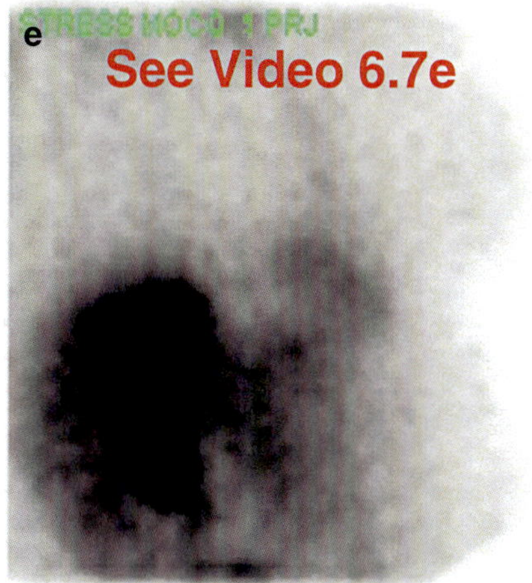

Fig. 6.7 (continued)

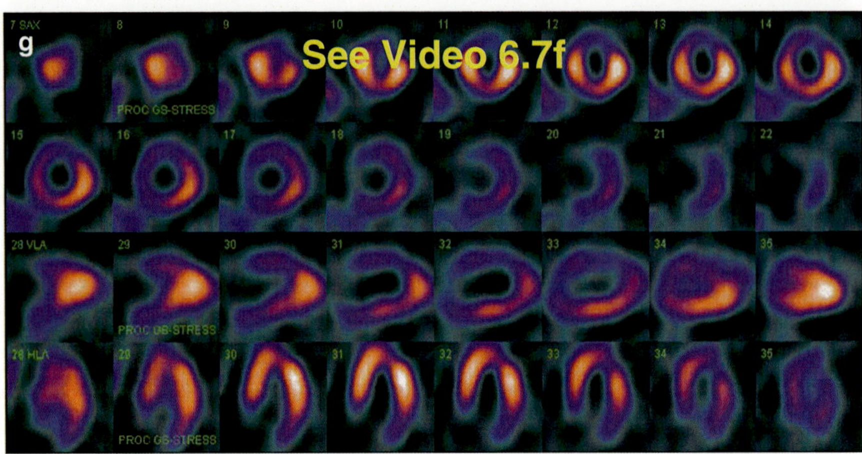

Fig. 6.7 (continued)

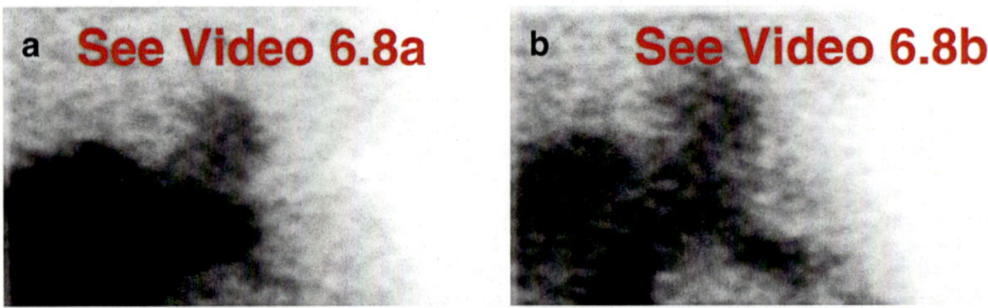

Fig. 6.8 Variable breast position attenuation artifact, two-day protocol. In this morbidly obese female, the difference in the left breast position on a two-day protocol (**a**, **b**) results in a reversible "cold" defect related to attenuation artifact (**c**). Normal wall motion and preserved wall thickening further lowers the likelihood for left ventricular scar (**d**).

(**a**) Day 1: stress raw projection images (Video 6.8a, frame 1), ^{99m}Tc sestamibi. (**b**) Day 2: rest raw projection images (Video 6.8b, frame 1), ^{99m}Tc sestamibi. (**c**) Stress/rest processed SPECT images (SA, HLA, VLA) (without and with AC), defect on selected non-AC vs. AC images (*yellow ovals*). (**d**) Stress and rest gated SPECT images (Video 6.8c, frame 1) (SA, VLA, HLA)

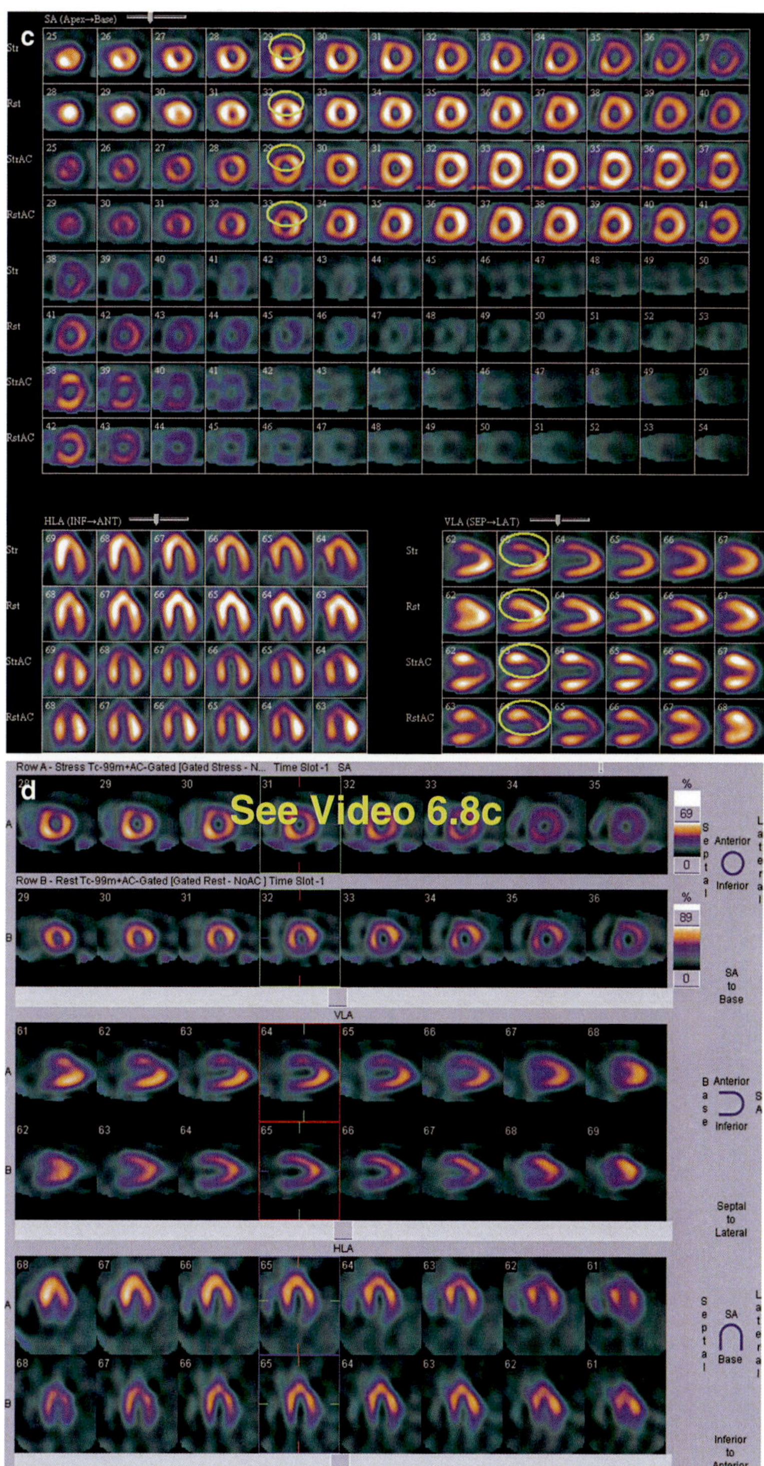

Fig. 6.8 (continued)

Key Points
- Radiopharmaceutical uptake within breast tissue may be symmetric (e.g., lactating breasts, gynecomastia) or asymmetric/focal (e.g., malignancy).
- Breast tissue is often a source of soft-tissue attenuation artifact which can create either fixed or reversible perfusion defects; attention to consistent breast position during rest and stress imaging sessions is important.
- Breast attenuation artifact typically includes the basal anterior wall, has a sharp crescentic border, and may spare the apex unlike the pattern seen with severe LAD coronary artery disease.

Chest Wall

7

During SPECT MPI, there are a myriad of reasons for "hot" and "cold" artifactual and potentially misleading imaging findings related to the chest wall (Table 7.1). Troubleshooting of "hot" and "cold" findings should be undertaken in conjunction with the performing technologist. "Hot" artifacts may be related to contamination on the patient (Fig. 7.1). If the patient's arms are positioned along the chest wall and within the field-of-view, extravasation at the injection site will produce a characteristic focal "hot" region that might create scatter artifact (Fig. 7.2) (Hendel et al. 1999). Nearby radioactive sources emitting photons from another patient or a prepared syringe may be registered on the gamma camera detector during MPI (Fig. 7.3). On review of the raw projection data, blood, injectate, or urine contamination should be superficial, not deep (Hendel et al. 1999). If skin or clothing contamination is suspected, the technologist should ask the patient to wash and change clothing, and the patient should be re-imaged (Gentili et al. 1994; Williams et al. 2003). Analogously, the gamma camera detectors should be routinely checked for contamination and cleaned as necessary before use (Burrell and MacDonald 2006; Chamarthy and Travin 2010; Gedik et al. 2007). Mal-administration of the radiopharmaceutical inadvertently using an arterial instead of a venous access can produce an unusual muscular biodistribution (Afzelius and Henriksen 2008). Radiopharmaceutical-avid brown adipose tissue (BAT) may be present in the supraclavicular regions of the anterior chest wall or in a posterior paraspinal location (Goetze et al. 2008).

Etiologies for "cold" findings range from the uncommon (e.g., soft-tissue masses (Vijayakumar et al. 2005)) to the common (e.g., metallic objects in or on the patient). It is important to remove objects when possible before imaging (Chamarthy and

Electronic supplementary material The online version of this chapter (doi:10.1007/978-3-319-25436-4_7) contains supplementary material, which is available to authorized users.

© Springer International Publishing Switzerland 2017
M.E. Oates, V.L. Sorrell, *Myocardial Perfusion Imaging - Beyond the Left Ventricle: Pathology, Artifacts and Pitfalls in the Chest and Abdomen,* DOI 10.1007/978-3-319-25436-4_7

Table 7.1 Differential diagnosis of "hot" and "cold" imaging findings related to the chest wall

Organ system	"Hot" finding	"Cold" finding	References
Chest wall	Brown adipose tissue Shoulder/upper chest skeletal musculature (due to arterial injection) Contamination (radiopharmaceutical, urine) Cross talk from nearby radioactive source (another patient on treadmill)	Soft-tissue mass Internal metal objects (pacemaker, defibrillator, vascular port) External metal objects (jewelry, chain, coin, keys, belt buckle) Arms by sides (positioning) Cracked crystal Malfunctioning photomultiplier tube	Afzelius and Henriksen (2008) Burrell and MacDonald (2006) Chamarthy & Travin (2010) Gedik et al. (2007) Gentili et al. (1994) Goetze et al. (2008) Hendel et al. (1999) Howarth et al. (1996) Vijayakumar et al. (2005) Williams et al. (2003)

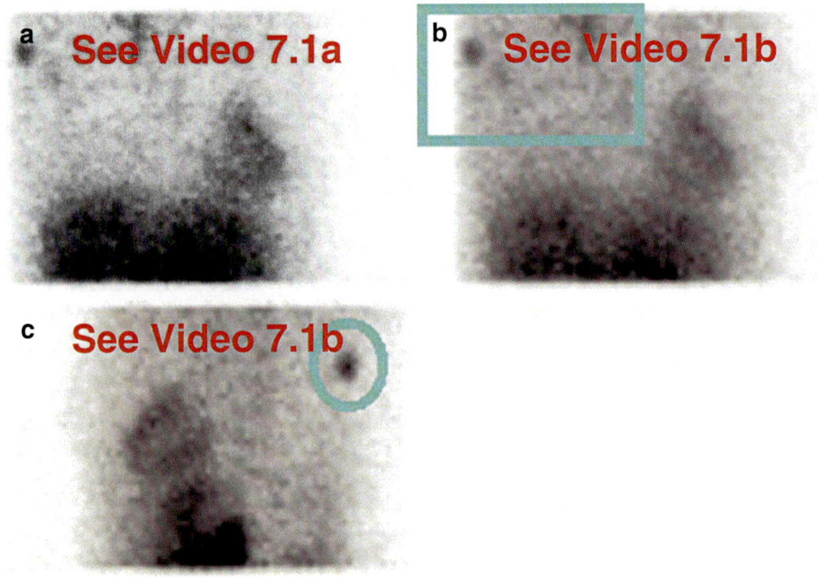

Fig. 7.1 Multifocal superficial "hot" artifacts. Note the multiple "hot spots" around the right shoulder (**a**, **b**) and upper back (**a**, **c**) caused by contamination during radiopharmaceutical administration. All "hot spots" project on the skin surface or clothing (**a**).

(**a**) Stress raw projection images (Video 7.1a, frame 1), [99mTc] sestamibi. (**b**) Stress raw projection image (Video 7.1b, frame 1), [99mTc] sestamibi, multiple droplets and streaks on the right upper chest wall and anterior shoulder (*blue box*). (**c**) Stress raw projection image (Video 7.1b, frame 61), [99mTc] sestamibi, distinctive droplet on the right upper back (*blue circle*)

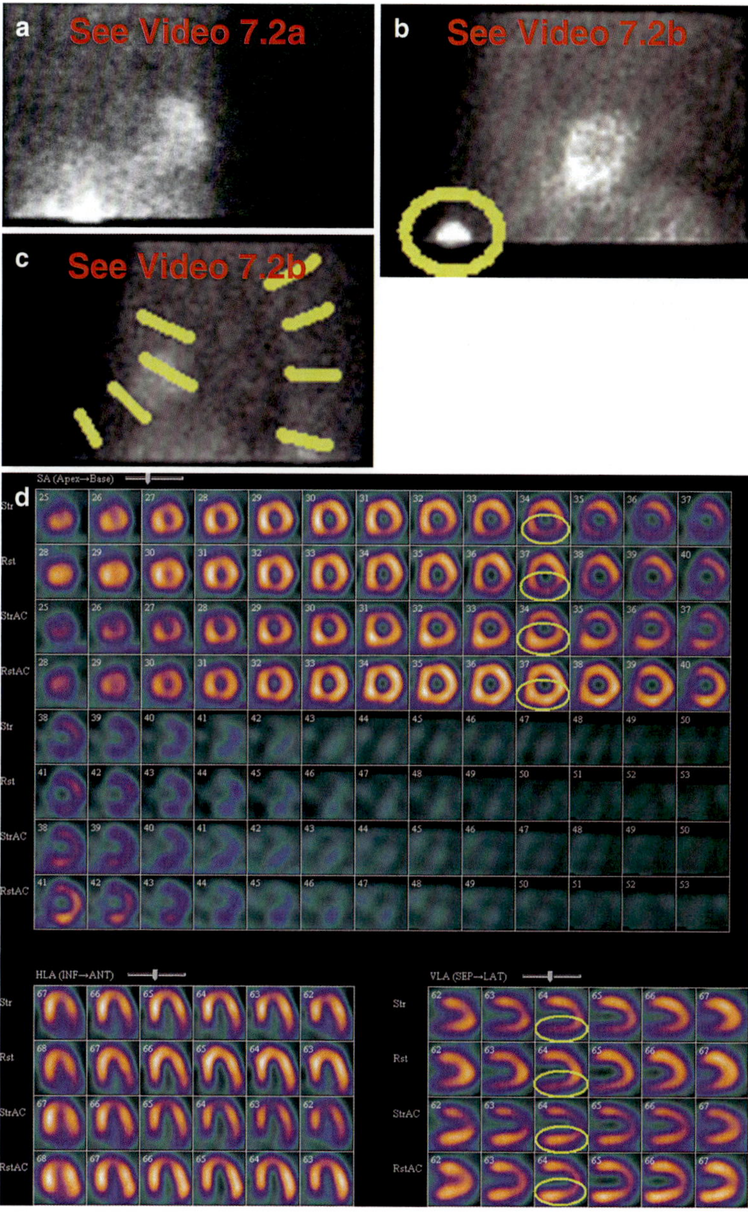

Fig. 7.2 "Hot" right arm and "cold" left arm artifacts. During acquisition, the patient's arms were positioned alongside the chest wall due to inability to keep his arms raised and out of the field-of-view. On the stress raw images (**a**), because the arms are down, the "hot" extravasation at right arm injection site (**b**) and the "cold" left arm (**c**) are apparent. Note that the latter contributes to the fixed inferior-basal wall attenuation artifact (the defect on the non-AC images normalizes with AC) (**d**).

(**a**) Stress raw projection images (Video 7.2a, frame 1), ^{99m}Tc sestamibi. (**b**) Stress raw projection image (Video 7.2b, frame 37), ^{99m}Tc sestamibi, extravasation site, right arm (*yellow oval*). (**c**) Stress raw projection image (Video 7.2b, frame 60), ^{99m}Tc sestamibi, left arm (*yellow lines*). (**d**) Stress/rest processed SPECT images (SA, HLA, VLA) (without and with AC), defect on selected non-AC vs. AC images (*yellow ovals*)

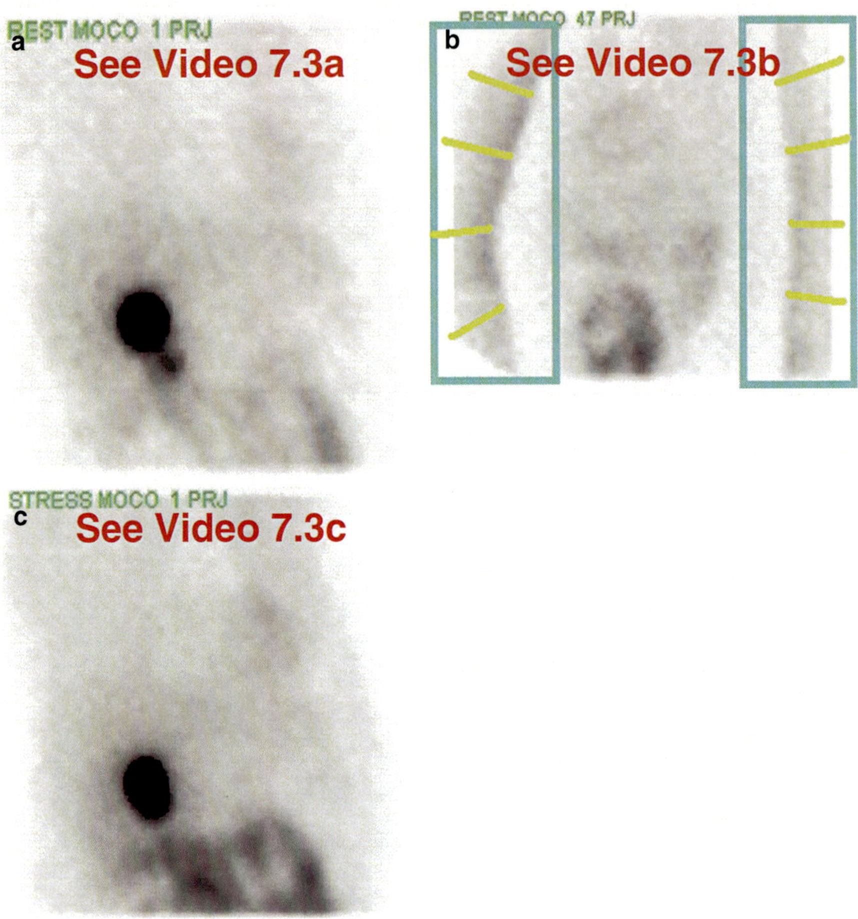

Fig. 7.3 "Hot" cross-talk artifact. Activity from another patient receiving a radiopharmaceutical injection on the treadmill in the next room contributed background counts best seen on frame 47 during this patient's rest acquisition (**a, b**). Given its fleeting nature, it did not affect the processed SPECT data. This artifact is not present on the same-day stress acquisition (**c**). It is important to review both data sets.

(**a**) Rest raw projection images (Video 7.3a, frame 1), ^{99m}Tc sestamibi. (**b**) Rest raw projection image (Video 7.3b, frame 47), ^{99m}Tc sestamibi, an unintended transmission image created by extraneous source (*blue boxes*), patient's body contours (*yellow lines*). (**c**) Stress raw projection images (Video 7.3c, frame 1), ^{99m}Tc sestamibi

Travin 2010; Gedik et al. 2007). Pacemakers, defibrillators, vascular ports, and an increasing number of other implanted devices reside in typical locations in the anterior chest wall and do not change position (Fig. 7.4). Common external culprits include jewelry, belt buckles, coins, and pacemakers/generators (Gentili et al. 1994; Howarth et al. 1996; Joy et al. 2007). These typically have characteristic appearance on the SPECT MPI raw data, but clinical correlation, imaging correlation, and/or

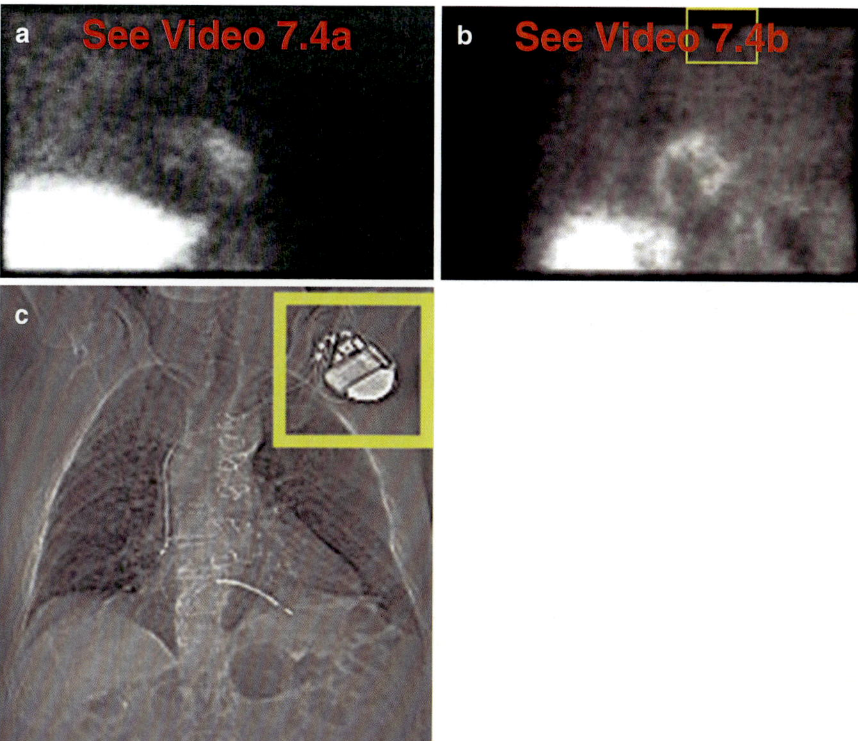

Fig. 7.4 "Cold" pacemaker artifact. The "cold" defect on the anterior chest wall at the top of the field-of-view (**a, b**) corresponds to a pacemaker (**c**). It does not overlie the heart, but should be noted during interpretation.

(**a**) Stress raw projection images (Video 7.4a, frame 1), ^{99m}Tc sestamibi. (**b**) Stress raw projection image (Video 7.4b, frame 35, LAO), ^{99m}Tc sestamibi, pacemaker (*yellow box*). (**c**) CT scout, pacemaker (*yellow box*)

physical examination will be confirmatory; a detailed history or chart review may prove invaluable. Many metallic objects have suggestive shapes, and the resulting "cold" defect may appear on either the anterior (Figs. 7.5 and 7.6) or posterior (Fig. 7.7) chest wall. The patient's arms should be positioned alongside the head and outside the field-of-view. If a patient cannot raise the left arm, it will be positioned alongside the chest wall and will create a characteristic soft-tissue attenuation artifact on the heart (Fig. 7.2). Mechanical or electronic failure in the gamma camera system can lead to distinctive "cold" defects on patient images reinforcing the importance of flood field uniformity testing as a routine quality assurance practice (Hendel et al. 1999).

As a general rule, the written report need not describe patient-related or technical imaging findings related to the chest wall, and personal communication to the referring physician is rarely warranted. However, one could consider mentioning the

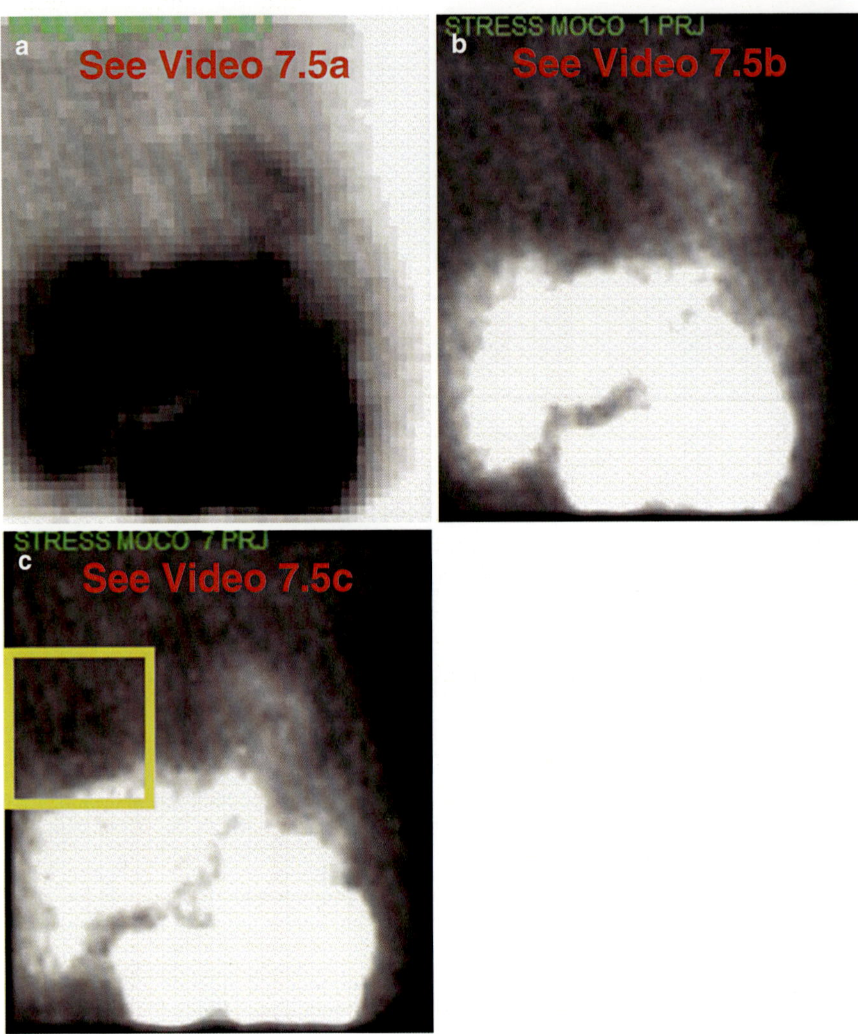

Fig. 7.5 "Cold" Holter monitor artifact. The "cold" defect on the anterior lower right chest wall (**a, b**) corresponds to an external Holter monitor device (**c**). Note how it is easier to appreciate this "cold" finding on the "white-on-black" rendering. It does not overlie the heart and does not impact on MPI quality.

(**a**) Stress "black-on-white" raw projection images (Video 7.5a, frame 1), ^{99m}Tc sestamibi. (**b**) Stress "white-on-black" raw projection images (Video 7.5b, frame 1), ^{99m}Tc sestamibi. (**c**) Stress raw projection image (Video 7.5c, frame 7, RAO), ^{99m}Tc sestamibi, Holter device (*yellow box*)

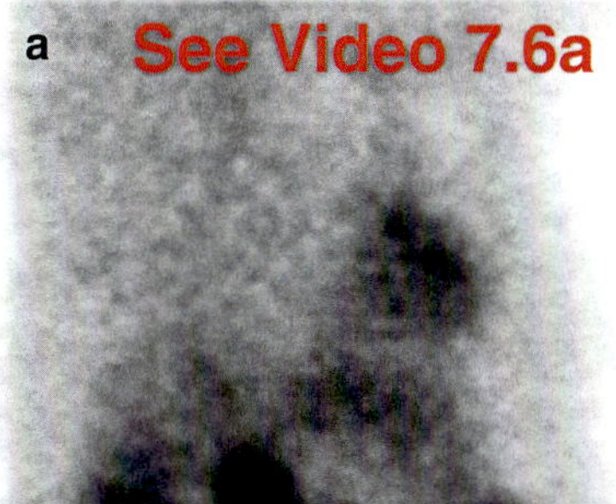

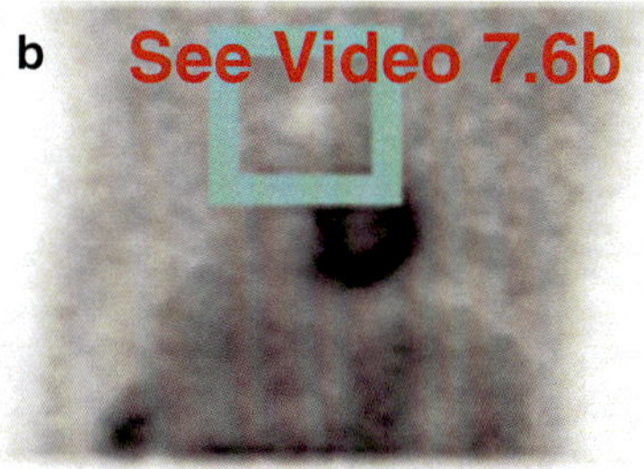

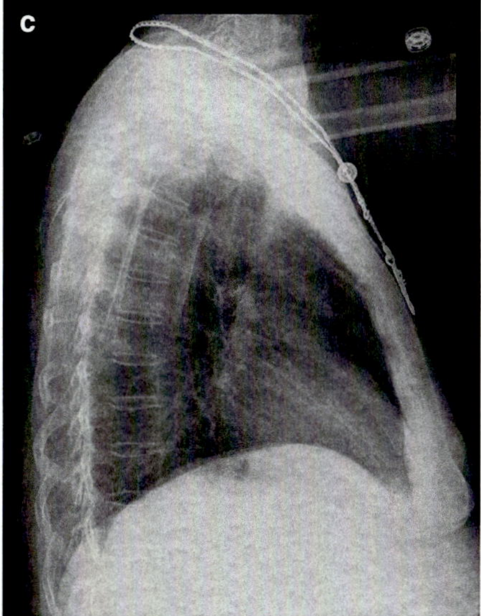

Fig. 7.6 "Cold" necklace artifact. A superficial "cold" defect on the anterior chest wall (**a**, **b**) corresponds to a necklace (**c**); it does not overlie the heart. Note "cold" ascites, a large spleen, and a "hot" stomach, all related to underlying cirrhosis (see Part III, Chaps. 18, 19, 21, and 22).

(**a**) Stress raw projection images (Video 7.6a, frame 1), ^{99m}Tc sestamibi. (**b**) Stress raw projection image (Video 7.6b, frame 27), ^{99m}Tc sestamibi, "cold" necklace (*blue box*). (**c**) Lateral chest radiograph

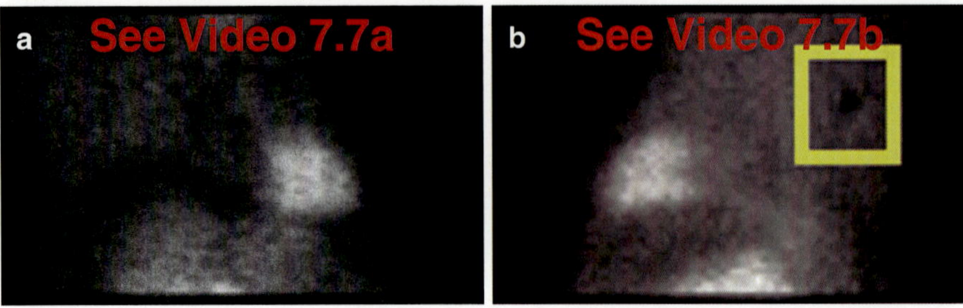

Fig. 7.7 "Cold" necklace artifact. The "cold" defect on the superficial posterior chest wall (**a, b**) corresponds to a necklace that the patient flipped before imaging from its usual position on the anterior chest; some patients prefer not to remove expensive or sentimental jewelry for fear of loss. Note "cold" abdominal ascites (see Part III, Chap. 18).

(**a**) Stress raw projection images (Video 7.7a, frame 1), ^{99m}Tc sestamibi. (**b**) Stress raw projection image (Video 7.7b, frame 60), ^{99m}Tc sestamibi, "cold" necklace (*yellow box*)

findings if only to assist an inexperienced physician or technologist who might review the images remotely. For example, one could state:

> There is a well-defined "cold" focus in the left upper chest wall that corresponds to the patient's implanted pacemaker device. This is an expected finding and does not impact on the interpretation of the SPECT MPI.

Key Points
- "Hot" artifacts affecting the chest wall can result from "contamination" due to radiopharmaceutical extravasation at the injection site, splatter from blood, urine or injectate, or nearby radioactive sources (such as another patient on the treadmill) detected by the gamma camera.
- Brown adipose tissue is avid for MPI radiopharmaceuticals and may be present in the supraclavicular regions.
- "Cold" attenuation artifacts can result from superficial jewelry or implantable devices (e.g., pacemakers), or the patient's arms positioned alongside the chest wall during image acquisition.

Skeleton

8

The field-of-view of SPECT MPI includes red marrow-containing bone such as the sternum, the ribs, the clavicles, the spine, and the upper extremities (Mohr et al. 1996; Williams et al. 2003). While slight skeletal uptake can be normal, many different skeletal conditions might be manifest on SPECT MPI (Table 8.1).

The orientation of the heart relative to the shape of the rib cage may suggest skeletal deformity such as kyphosis, scoliosis, kyphoscoliosis, or pectus carinatum/excavatum (Fig. 8.1). The image reconstruction process generally overcomes such unusual cardiac displacements or distortions. Correlation with physical examination and other imaging can be clarifying.

Although relatively uncommonly apparent on SPECT MPI, incidental benign skeletal conditions will typically appear "hot." They include chronic anemia (Figs. 8.2 and 8.3), fractures (Fig. 8.4), myelofibrosis, and Paget disease (Gowda et al. 2006; Shih et al. 2005). Other nonneoplastic bone lesions include post-sternotomy and osteomyelitis (Chamarthy and Travin 2010; Onsel et al. 1996).

^{99m}Tc sestamibi has been used to gauge the severity of osseous infiltration in Gaucher disease and has been successful in gauging the therapeutic response of malignant bone lesions (Caner et al. 1992; Mariani et al. 2003). On SPECT MPI, malignant conditions—again, uncommonly seen—include primary osteosarcoma, sarcoma, lymphoma, and multiple myeloma as well as metastatic disease involving the sternum, ribs, and spine (Chamarthy and Travin 2010; Fisher et al. 2000; Gowda et al. 2006; Maurea et al. 1995; Soderlund et al. 1997). While most malignant lesions appear "hot," it is prudent to be wary of those (e.g., metastases) that might present as "cold" findings.

Electronic supplementary material The online version of this chapter (doi:10.1007/978-3-319-25436-4_8) contains supplementary material, which is available to authorized users.

© Springer International Publishing Switzerland 2017

M.E. Oates, V.L. Sorrell, *Myocardial Perfusion Imaging - Beyond the Left Ventricle: Pathology, Artifacts and Pitfalls in the Chest and Abdomen,* DOI 10.1007/978-3-319-25436-4_8

Table 8.1 Differential diagnosis of "hot" and "cold" imaging findings related to the skeleton

Organ system	"Hot" finding	"Cold" finding	References
Skeleton	Anemia/thalassemia Fracture/sternotomy Osteomyelitis Gaucher disease Paget disease Myelofibrosis/ myelodysplastic process *Multiple myeloma* *Osteosarcoma/sarcoma* *Neoplasm, metastasis*	*Neoplasm, metastasis*	Caner et al. (1992) Chamarthy and Travin (2010) Fisher et al. (2000) Gowda et al. (2006) Mariani et al. (2003) Maurea et al. (1995) Mohr et al. (1996) Onsel et al. (1996) Shih et al. (2005) Soderlund et al. (1997) Williams et al. (2003)

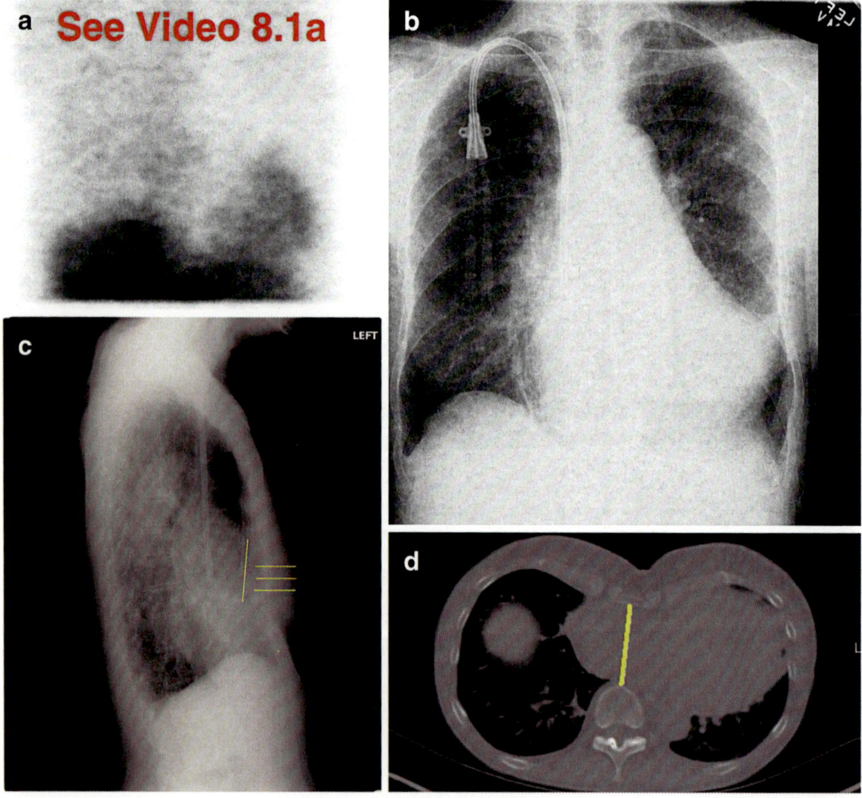

Fig. 8.1 Pectus excavatum deformity. There is displacement of the heart into the left chest (**a**) due to pectus excavatum deformity (**b–d**). Correlation with other imaging (**b–d**) clarifies the MPI findings. The radiographic appearance is characteristic: on the frontal radiograph (**b**), the right heart border is indistinct, the heart displaced to the left, and the ribs more oblique than usual; on the lateral (**c**), the anterior-posterior dimension is narrowed with a concave sternal configuration. These anatomic relationships are well demonstrated by CT scan. The tunneled catheter seen on the radiographs (**b, c**) is used for dialysis.

(**a**) Stress raw projection images (Video 8.1a, frame 1), ^{99m}Tc sestamibi. (**b**) PA chest radiograph. (**c**) Lateral chest radiograph, depressed lower sternum (*yellow lines*). (**d**) CT image through lower chest, depressed lower sternum, and narrow anterior-posterior distance (yellow line)

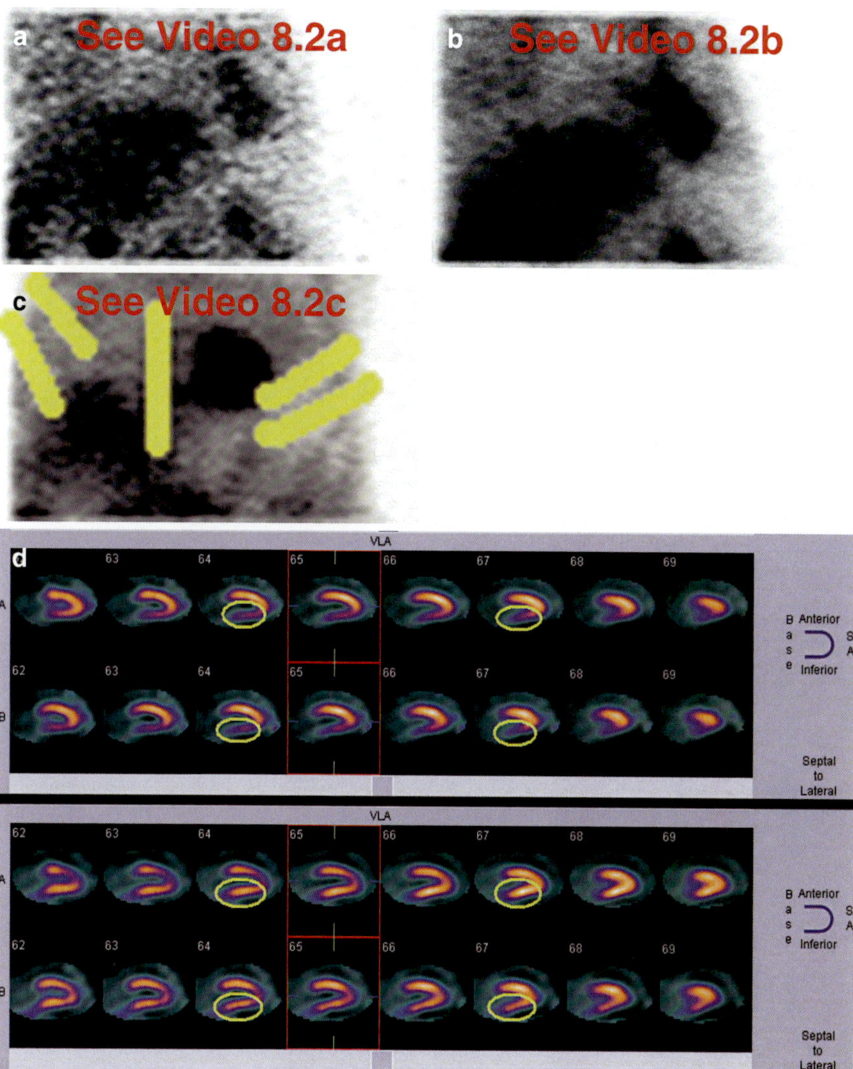

Fig. 8.2 Diffusely "hot" sternum and ribs silhouetted against adjacent "cold" pleural effusions. A 57-year-old male has anemia associated with cirrhosis, bilateral pleural effusions, and ascites. The sternum and ribs are well seen against the pleural effusions (**a–c**). The fixed inferior and inferolateral wall perfusion defects on non-AC images, due to the left pleural effusion and ascites, normalize with attenuation correction (**d**); there is normal wall motion and wall thickening (**e**). Correlative chest radiograph (**f**) shows bibasilar opacification due to left-much-greater-than-right pleural effusions; note the "dense" abdomen due to ascites.

(**a**) Rest raw projection images (Video 8.2a, frame 1), ^{99m}Tc sestamibi. (**b**) Stress raw projection images (Video 8.2b, frame 1), ^{99m}Tc sestamibi. (**c**) Stress raw projection image (Video 8.2c, frame 25), ^{99m}Tc sestamibi, sternum and ribs (*yellow lines*). (**d**) Stress/rest processed SPECT images (VLA) (stress/rest without AC (*top panel*) and stress/rest with AC (*bottom panel*), inferior and inferolateral defects (*yellow ovals* on representative images). (**e**) Stress and rest gated SPECT images (Video 8.2d, frame 1) (SA, VLA, HLA). (**f**) AP portable chest radiograph

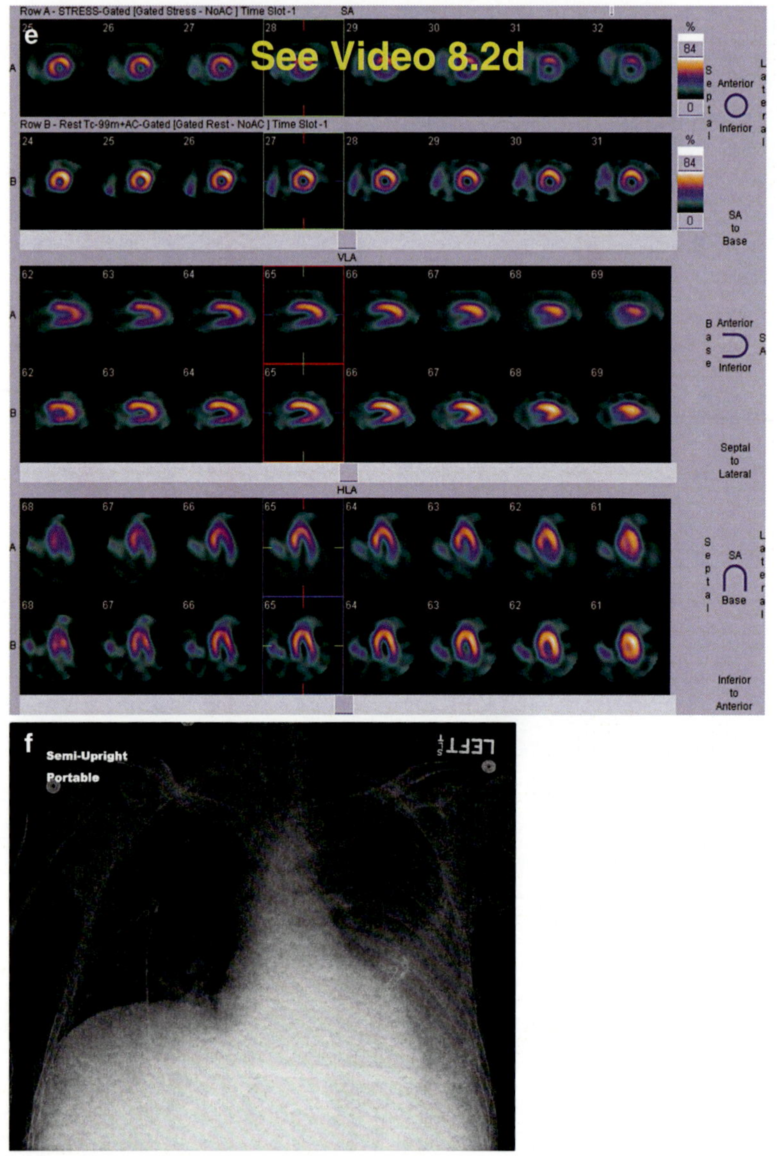

Fig. 8.2 (continued)

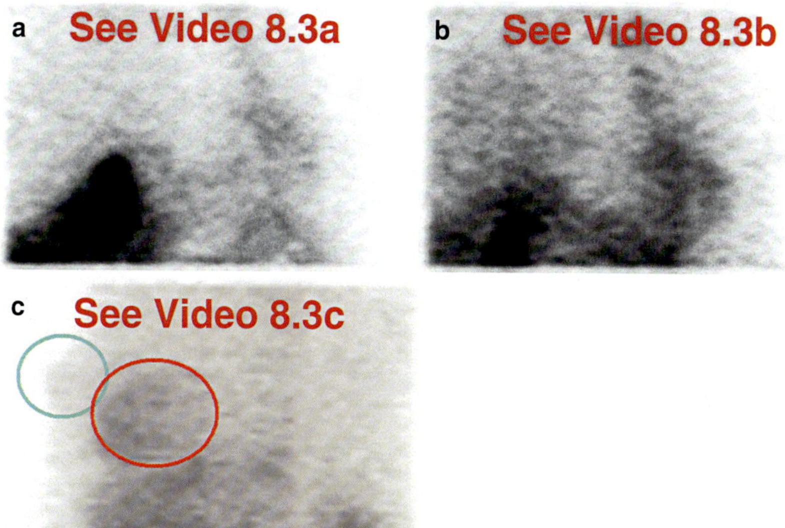

Fig. 8.3 Diffusely "hot" sternum and ribs, unchanged over 1 year. A 43-year-old male has cirrhosis and anemia. The sternum and ribs are diffusely "hot" on both examinations 1 year apart. Note an elongated, "hot," and "high" gallbladder on both examinations; there is subtle peri-areolar uptake on the current examination (**c**) consistent with gynecomastia.

(**a**) Current: stress raw projection images (Video 8.3a, frame 1), ^{99m}Tc sestamibi. (**b**) One year ago: stress raw projection images (Video 8.3b, frame 1), ^{99m}Tc sestamibi. (**c**) Current: stress raw projection image (Video 8.3c, frame 62, LPO), ^{99m}Tc sestamibi, region of the left breast nipple (*blue circle*), left ventricle as landmark (*red oval*)

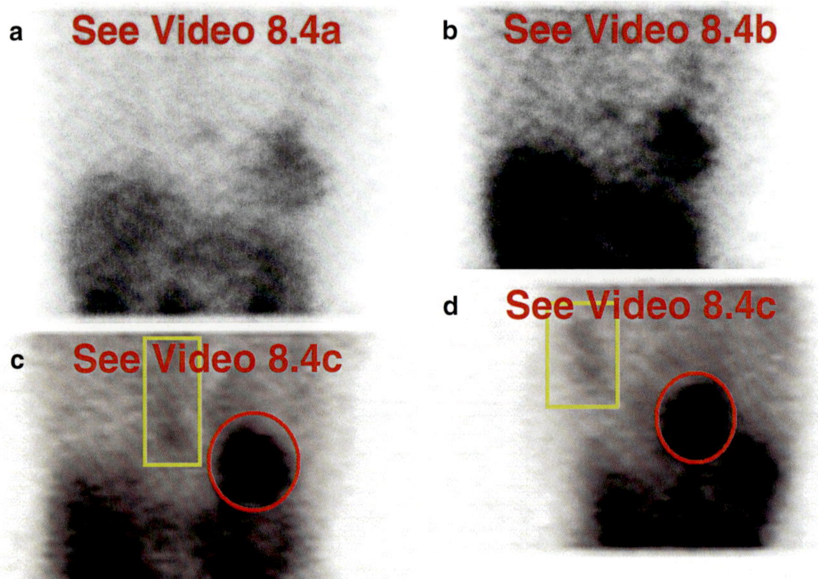

Fig. 8.4 Multifocal "hot" sternum and thoracic vertebrae. Note value of adjusting the contrast settings of the raw data (**a**, **b**) during the review process to uncover subtle findings. An anemic 68-year-old female has osteoporotic compression fractures of the thoracic vertebrae (**a–c, e**) and of the sternum (**a, b, d, f**). Note that the abnormal vertebral uptake is first apparent on the raw projection data in the right anterior oblique/anterior projection (**c**); the abnormal sternum becomes visible as it presents in profile free of overlapping structures later during the cinematic display (**d**). On follow-up imaging 1 year later (**g**), the skeletal uptake is much less intense, consistent with healing fractures; the kyphotic deformity is particularly evident. This patient has cirrhosis and chronic obstructive pulmonary disease; there is no history of coronary artery disease.

(**a**) Stress raw projection images (Video 8.4a, frame 1) at usual contrast setting for the heart, ^{99m}Tc sestamibi. (**b**) Stress raw projection images (Video 8.4b, frame 1) with enhanced contrast setting for skeleton, ^{99m}Tc sestamibi. (**c**) Stress raw projection image (Video 8.4c, frame 10, RAO/Anterior) with enhanced contrast setting for skeleton, ^{99m}Tc sestamibi, vertebral activity (*yellow box*), heart as landmark (*red oval*). (**d**) Stress raw projection image (Video 8.4c, frame 40, steep LAO) with enhanced contrast setting for skeleton, ^{99m}Tc sestamibi, sternal activity (*yellow box*), the heart as landmark (*red oval*). (**e**) Lateral chest radiograph, vertebral compression fractures (*yellow boxes*). (**f**) Axial CT image of chest at mid-sternum, sternal compression fracture (*yellow box*). (**g**) One-year follow-up: stress raw projection images (Video 8.4d, frame 1) with enhanced contrast setting for skeleton, ^{99m}Tc sestamibi

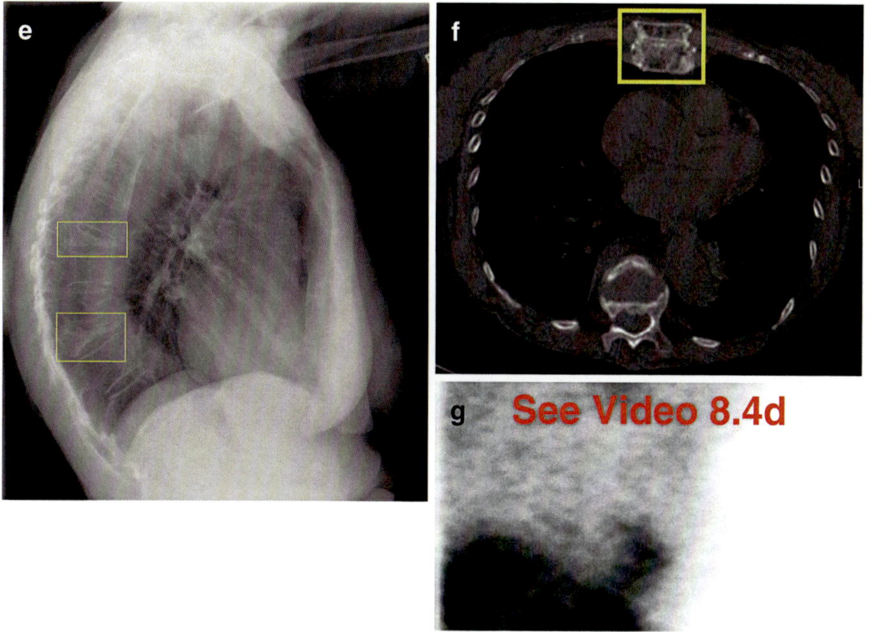

Fig. 8.4 (continued)

Since skeletal activity is relatively uncommon and, when apparent, might signal significant pathology, one should consider reporting it and placing it into the clinical context. For example:

> There is prominent visualization of the skeleton. There are no discrete "hot" or "cold" lesions, rather the skeleton shows diffusely increased uptake. The pattern correlates with the clinical history of chronic anemia, and does not suggest underlying malignancy.

Alternatively, the following report would warrant personal communication to the referring physician:

> Incidentally noted are multiple abnormal foci demonstrating increased uptake ("hot" lesions) and decreased uptake ("cold" lesions) involving the sternum, ribs and spine in a pattern suggesting underlying malignancy with osseous metastases.

Key Points

- The orientation of the heart relative to the shape of the rib cage may suggest a skeletal deformity.
- Abnormal uptake of radiopharmaceutical within the skeleton can be due to chronic anemia, fractures, post-sternotomy, infection, malignancy, and conditions associated with high bone turnover.
- Various skeletal abnormalities may be manifested as "hot" or "cold" findings on SPECT MPI, and some warrant communication to the referring physician.

Pleura

9

The differential diagnosis of pleural findings on MPI is a short list (Table 9.1). Malignant lesions of the pleura can appear "hot" and are uncommonly identified on MPI (Chin et al. 1995; Eftekhari and Gholamrezanezhad 2006). A lung tumor might be associated with a "hot" or "cold" pleural effusion (Eftekhari and Gholamrezanezhad 2006); this topic is covered in more detail in Chap. 10 Lungs.

Pleural effusions, whether benign or malignant, are usually "cold" and are readily identified on MPI raw projection data (Chamarthy and Travin 2010; Gedik et al. 2007). They may be unilateral or bilateral and vary in volume from small to quite large (Shih et al. 2002). For SPECT MPI, the patient is positioned supine or semirecumbent, depending on the gamma camera system; and free pleural fluid will settle posteriorly. Right-sided pleural effusions are more difficult to appreciate unless they are large (Figs. 9.1 and 9.2). Left-sided pleural effusions are more readily apparent because the field-of-view extends more posteriorly around the left hemithorax, providing a more complete survey (Figs. 9.3 and 9.4). Left pleural effusions may be problematic because they may create attenuation artifact in the processed cardiac images with the inferior wall typically affected. Readers need to be aware of this potential source of artifact at the time of image interpretation. It is a good practice to access correlative imaging whenever available (Figs. 9.1, 9.2, 9.3, and 9.4) (Williams et al. 2003). Pleural effusions may be associated with abdominal ascites (Figs. 9.1, 9.3, and 9.4); this topic is covered in Chap. 18 Peritoneum (Joy et al. 2007).

The written report could include wording along the lines of:

The projection data demonstrate a large left pleural effusion (correlated with same-day chest radiography). There is a fixed inferior wall defect that normalizes with attenuation-correction; thus, it is related to attenuation artifact from the pleural effusion and does not represent a scar.

Electronic supplementary material The online version of this chapter (doi:10.1007/978-3-319-25436-4_9) contains supplementary material, which is available to authorized users.

© Springer International Publishing Switzerland 2017
M.E. Oates, V.L. Sorrell, *Myocardial Perfusion Imaging - Beyond the Left Ventricle: Pathology, Artifacts and Pitfalls in the Chest and Abdomen*,
DOI 10.1007/978-3-319-25436-4_9

Table 9.1 Differential diagnosis of "hot" and "cold" imaging findings related to the pleura

Organ system	"Hot" finding	"Cold" finding	References
Pleura	*Neoplasm, malignant/ mesothelioma* *Pleural effusion, malignant*	Pleural effusion, benign *Pleural effusion, malignant*	Chamarthy and Travin (2010) Chin et al. (1995) Eftekhari and Gholamrezanezhad (2006) Gedik et al. (2007) Joy et al. (2007) Shih et al. (2002) Williams et al. (2003)

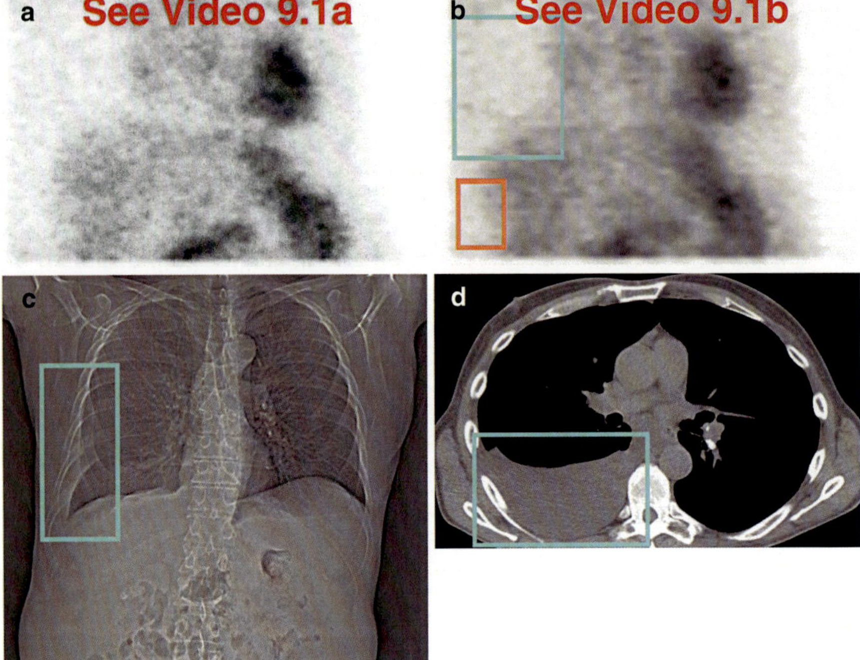

Fig. 9.1 "Cold" right pleural effusion confirmed by other imaging. There is a "cold" region in the right lower hemithorax (**a**, **b**) that corresponds to a pleural effusion radiographically (**c**, **d**). There is no left pleural effusion (**c**, **d**). An isolated right pleural effusion typically does not affect the processed SPECT images; however, it may be clinically significant. Note a relative elevation of the left hemidiaphragm with "cold" ascites beneath it (**a**, **e**, **f**).

(**a**) Stress raw projection images (Video 9.1a, frame 1), ^{99m}Tc sestamibi. (**b**) Stress raw projection image (Video 9.1b, frame 3), ^{99m}Tc sestamibi, "cold" pleural fluid (*blue box*), "cold" abdominal ascites (*orange box*). (**c**) Frontal chest radiograph, right pleural fluid (*blue box*). (**d**) CT at level of lower chest, right pleural fluid (*blue box*). (**e**) Stress raw projection image (Video 9.1b, frame 48), ^{99m}Tc sestamibi, "cold" ascites outlining the elevated left hemidiaphragm (orange lines). (**f**) CT at the level of upper abdomen, perihepatic and perisplenic ascites (*orange boxes*)

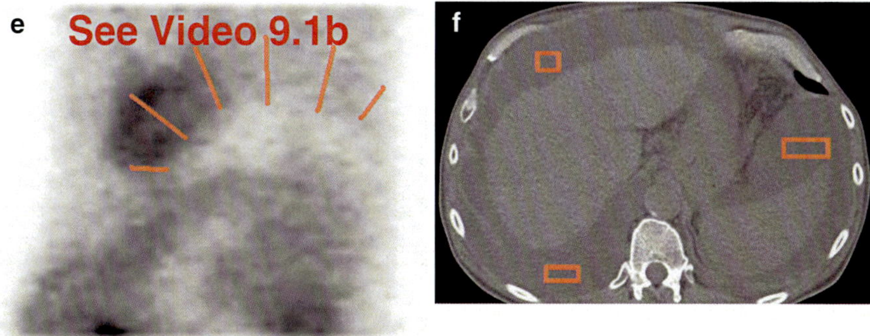

Fig. 9.1 (continued)

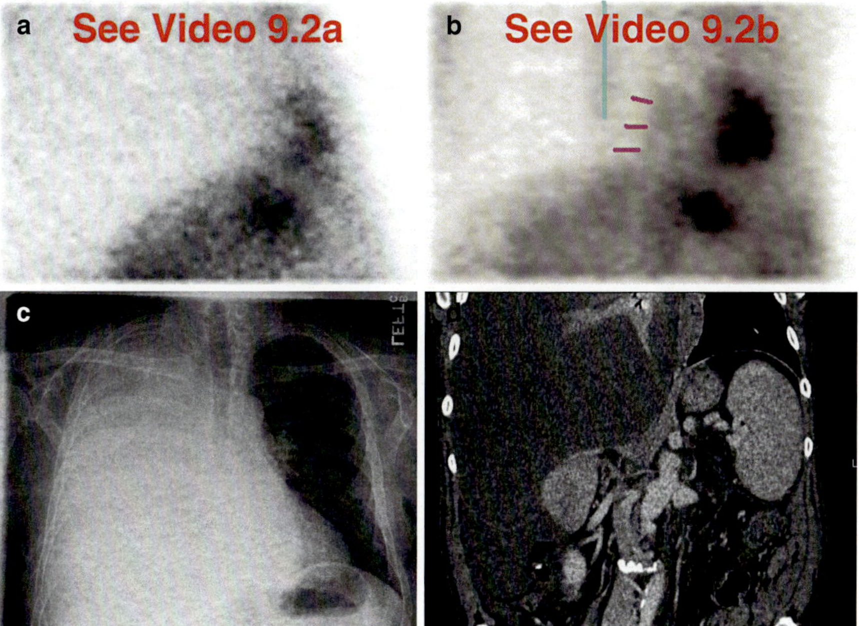

Fig. 9.2 Very large "cold" right pleural effusion creating mass effect on the heart. There is a very large "cold" right pleural effusion (**a, b**). The mass effect shifts the heart into the left hemithorax (**b**). Chest radiography (**c**) defines its size. This 58-year-old male has cirrhosis. There is neither left pleural effusion nor significant perisplenic ascites on same-day CT scan (**d**). MPI is normal (**e**).

(**a**) Stress raw projection images (Video 9.2a, frame 1), ^{99m}Tc sestamibi. (**b**) Stress raw projection image (Video 9.2b, frame 1), ^{99m}Tc sestamibi, sternum (*blue line*) as a midline reference point, right heart border (*pink lines*) shifted to left of midline. (**c**) PA chest radiograph. (**d**) Coronal CT of lower chest and abdomen at level of the kidneys and spleen. (**e**) Stress/rest processed SPECT images (SA, HLA, VLA) (without and with AC)

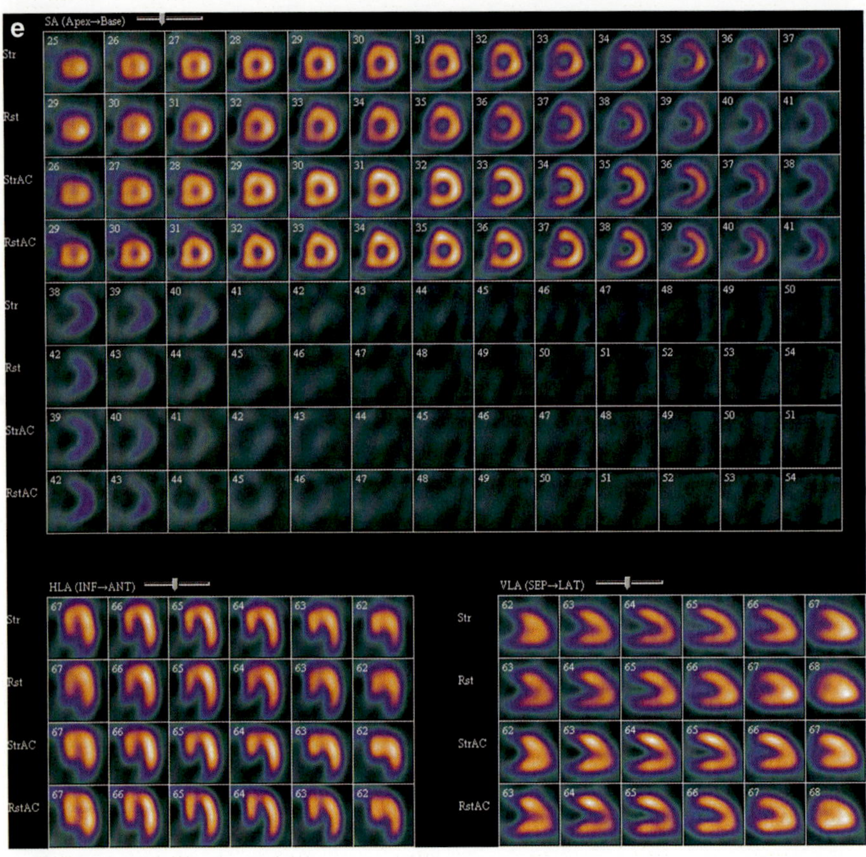

Fig. 9.2 (continued)

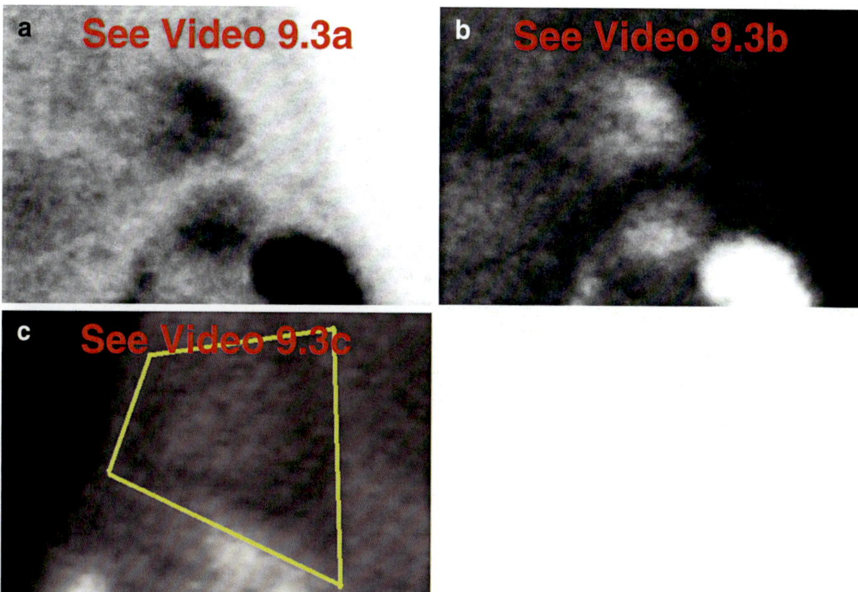

Fig. 9.3 Large "cold" left pleural effusion creating attenuation artifact. The large "cold" left pleural effusion (**a–c**) creates lateral, inferior, and basal attenuation-related defects on processed images that normalize on attenuation-correction images (**d**), confirming an artifactual cause. Note that adjusting the color table from "black-on-white" (**a**) to "white-on-black" (**b, c**) when reviewing the raw data can enhance visualization of "cold" findings. There is a subtle, small, "cold" pleural effusion at the right lung base (**a, b**). Radiography (**e, f**) confirms the pleural effusions, left much larger than right. Note the protuberant abdomen containing "cold" ascites below the hemidiaphragms (**a, b**).

(**a**) Stress "black-on-white" raw projection images (Video 9.3a, frame 1), ^{99m}Tc sestamibi. (**b**) Stress "white-on-black" raw projection images (Video 9.3b, frame 1), ^{99m}Tc sestamibi. (**c**) Stress "white-on-black" raw projection image (Video 9.3c, frame 61), ^{99m}Tc sestamibi, "cold" fluid overlies the entire heart on lateral-most images (*yellow polygon*). (**d**) Stress/rest processed SPECT images (SA, HLA, VLA) (without and with AC), inferior and basal fixed defect normalizes with AC (*yellow ovals* on representative SA and VLA images) and lateral wall attenuation effect also normalizes with AC (*blue boxes* on representative HLA images). (**e**) PA chest radiograph. (**f**) Lateral chest radiograph

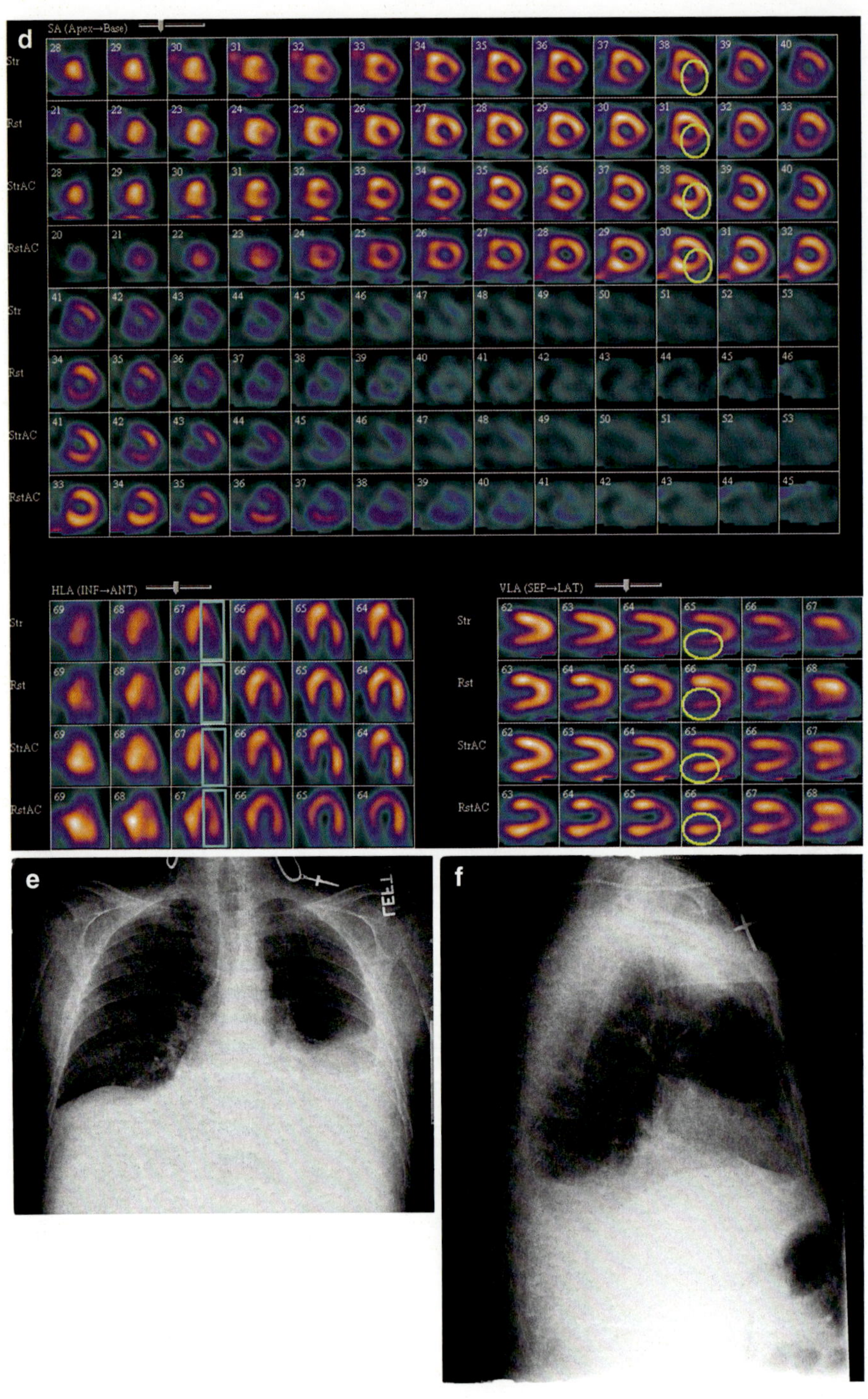

Fig. 9.3 (continued)

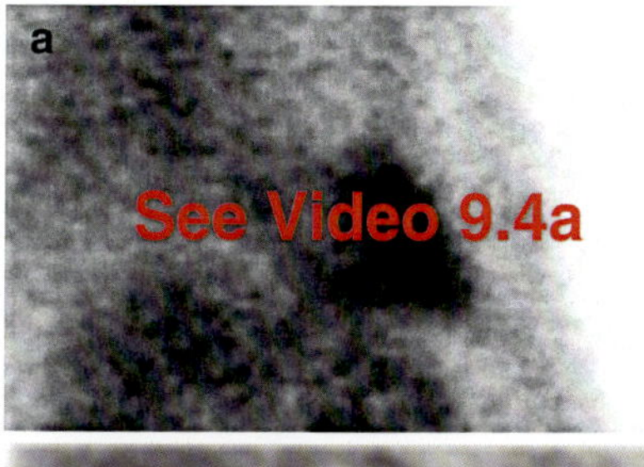

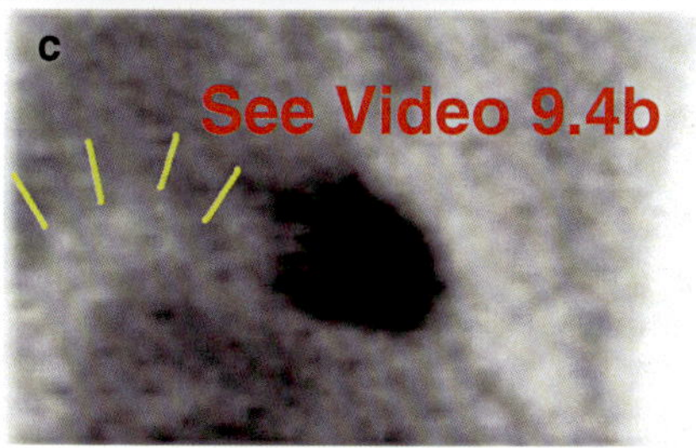

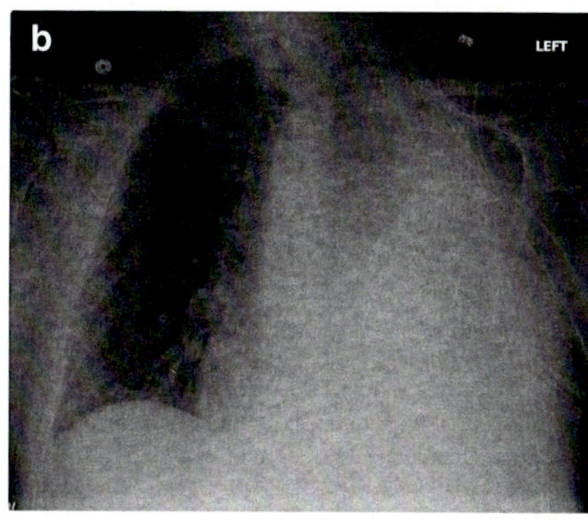

Fig. 9.4 Large "cold" left pleural effusion. The large "cold" left hemithorax (**a**) corresponds to a pleural effusion (**b**). Confirmatory chest radiograph (**b**) demonstrates the rightward cardiomediastinal shift due to mass effect from the large pleural effusion; specifically, there is tracheal deviation to the right and the right heart border is displaced into the right lower hemithorax. The minimal diffuse right pulmonary activity is normal (**a, c**). Note "cold" ascites below the elevated right hemidiaphragm (**c**).

(**a**) Stress raw projection images (Video 9.4a, frame 1), ^{99m}Tc sestamibi. (**b**) PA chest radiograph. (**c**) Stress raw projection image (Video 9.4b, frame 20), ^{99m}Tc sestamibi, right hemidiaphragm (*yellow lines*) with "cold" ascites underneath

Key Points
- Pleural effusions are usually "cold."
- Right-sided pleural effusions are difficult to appreciate unless large; left-sided pleural effusions are more easily seen.
- Pleural effusions can be a source of attenuation artifact, typically affecting the inferior wall if left-sided.
- Correlative imaging aids interpretation.

Lungs

10

There are many causes of diffuse and focal "hot" and "cold" lungs on SPECT MPI (Table 10.1). Left ventricular dysfunction may be associated with diffusely increased lung uptake (Fig. 10.1) (Chamarthy and Travin 2010; Hendel et al. 1999; Mohr et al. 1996; Shih et al. 2002). Various benign pulmonary conditions, including infectious, occupational, and granulomatous processes (tuberculosis, sarcoidosis), may show diffusely or focally increased uptake of MPI radiopharmaceuticals (Aras et al. 2003; Chin et al. 1995; Gedik et al. 2007). Avidity may reflect disease activity in tuberculosis (Onsel et al. 1996).

Through various mechanisms and local factors, primary and metastatic lung neoplasms accumulate MPI radiopharmaceuticals (Bom et al. 1998; Takekawa et al. 1999). Certain primary lung malignancies may be less avid for ^{99m}Tc sestamibi compared to ^{201}Tl chloride (Nishiyama et al. 1997). Focal increased uptake in the lung may signal unknown lung cancer (Fig. 10.2) (Aras et al. 2003; Chin et al. 1995; Hendel et al. 1999; Shih et al. 2002). "Whole-field-of-view reconstruction" of the projection data set from Tc-99m sestamibi SPECT MPI has revealed a carcinoid tumor located behind the heart (Reyhan et al. 2004).

Some findings in the lungs may be more prominent on the rest raw data compared to the stress data, emphasizing the importance of reviewing the stress and rest raw data side-by-side to improve visualization and detection of subtle abnormalities (Seo et al. 2005). A lung tumor might be associated with a "cold" or "hot" pleural effusion (Eftekhari and Gholamrezanezhad 2006). Many of these unexpected noncardiac findings require personal communication with the referring physician and inclusion in the written report, for example:

Electronic supplementary material The online version of this chapter (doi:10.1007/978-3-319-25436-4_10) contains supplementary material, which is available to authorized users.

© Springer International Publishing Switzerland 2017
M.E. Oates, V.L. Sorrell, *Myocardial Perfusion Imaging - Beyond the Left Ventricle: Pathology, Artifacts and Pitfalls in the Chest and Abdomen*,
DOI 10.1007/978-3-319-25436-4_10

Table 10.1 Differential diagnosis of "hot" and "cold" imaging findings related to the lungs

Organ system	"Hot" finding	"Cold" finding	References
Lungs	*Congestive heart failure (diffuse pattern)* Interstitial lung disease Smoking Atelectasis Hematoma Pneumonia Fibrosing alveolitis Actinomycosis Granulomatous disease (sarcoidosis/ tuberculosis) *Neoplasm, primary malignant (lung carcinoma, carcinoid)* *Neoplasm, metastasis* Lymphangitic carcinomatosis	Hyperinflation/emphysema Pneumonectomy/elevated right hemidiaphragm Elevated left hemidiaphragm	Aras et al. (2003) Bom et al. (1998) Chamarthy and Travin (2010) Chin et al. (1995) Eftekhari and Gholamrezanezhad (2006) Gedik et al. (2007) Hendel et al. (1999) Mohr et al. (1996) Nishiyama et al. (1997) Onsel et al. (1996) Reyhan et al. (2004) Seo et al. (2005) Shih et al. (2002) Takekawa et al. (1999)

Fig. 10.1 Congestive heart failure. An 86-year-old male with known coronary artery disease complains of shortness of breath and fatigue. MPI shows diffusely "hot" lungs (**a–c**), an enlarged right ventricular cavity and prominent right ventricular myocardial wall (**a, b, d**), a minimally enlarged left ventricular cavity (**a, b, e**), and depressed left ventricular function with global hypokinesis and LVEF of 40 % (**f**). The inferolateral-basal wall perfusion defect is more pronounced on rest images and normalizes with AC, suggesting diaphragmatic attenuation artifact (**e**). Cardiomegaly, a small right pleural effusion, and increased lung markings are evident on chest radiography (**g**). Echocardiography demonstrated concordant findings: left ventricular cavity enlargement, reduced function (LVEF of 30–40 %), and a slightly dilated right ventricle with reduced systolic function.

(**a**) Rest raw projection images (Video 10.1a, frame 1), ^{99m}Tc sestamibi. (**b**) Stress raw projection images (Video 10.1b, frame 1), ^{99m}Tc sestamibi. (**c**) Stress raw projection image (Video 10.1c, frame 14), ^{99m}Tc sestamibi, lung activity (*pink boxes*). (**d**) Stress raw projection image (Video 10.1c, frame 43), ^{99m}Tc sestamibi, right ventricle (*blue lines*). (**e**) Stress/rest processed SPECT images (without and with AC) (SA, HLA, VLA), inferolateral-basal defect most pronounced on non-AC rest images normalizes on AC (*yellow ovals* on representative SA images, *yellow boxes* on representative HLA and VLA images). (**f**) Stress and rest gated SPECT images (Video 10.1d, frame 1) (SA, VLA, HLA). (**g**) PA chest radiograph

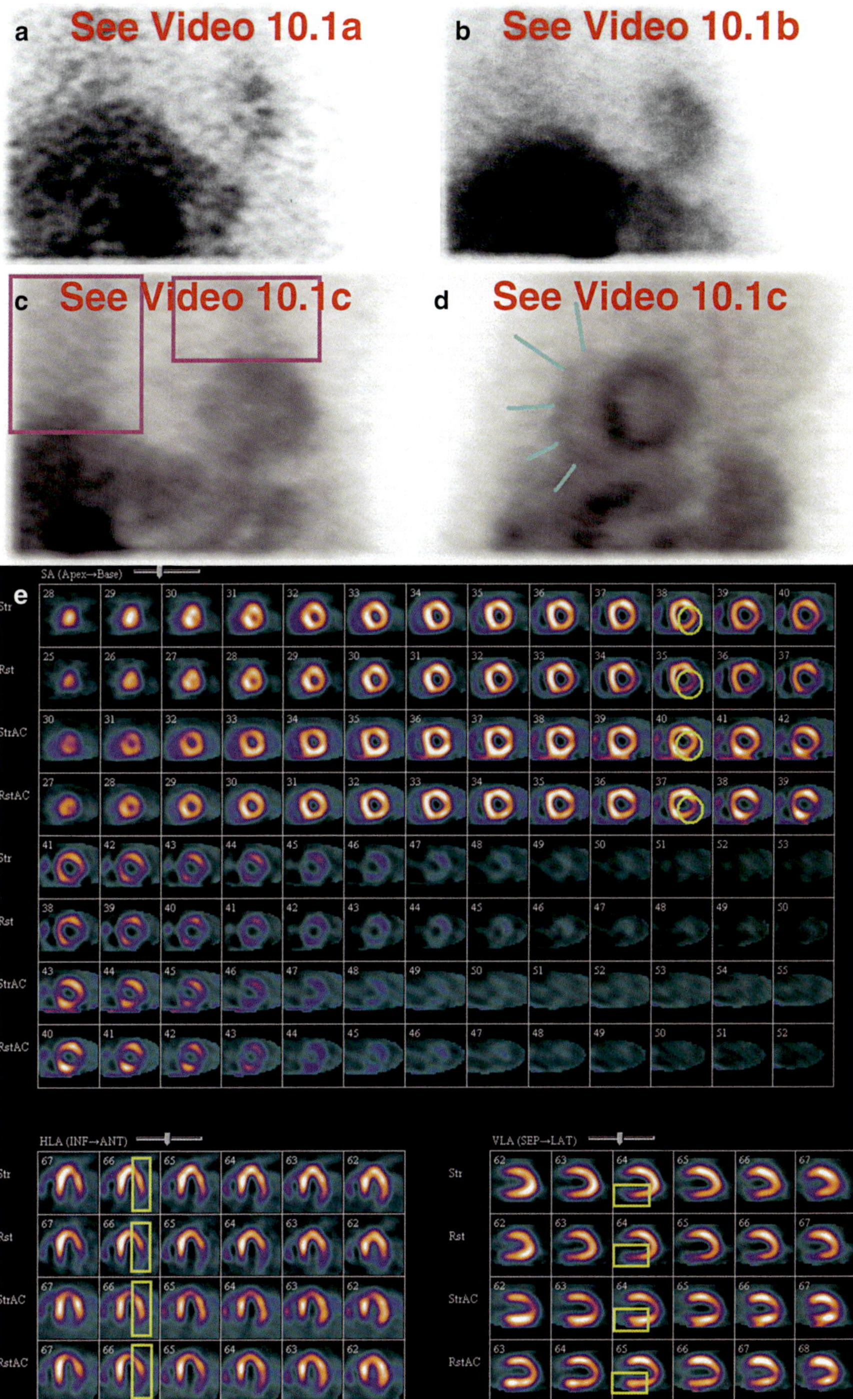
a See Video 10.1a
b See Video 10.1b
c See Video 10.1c
d See Video 10.1c

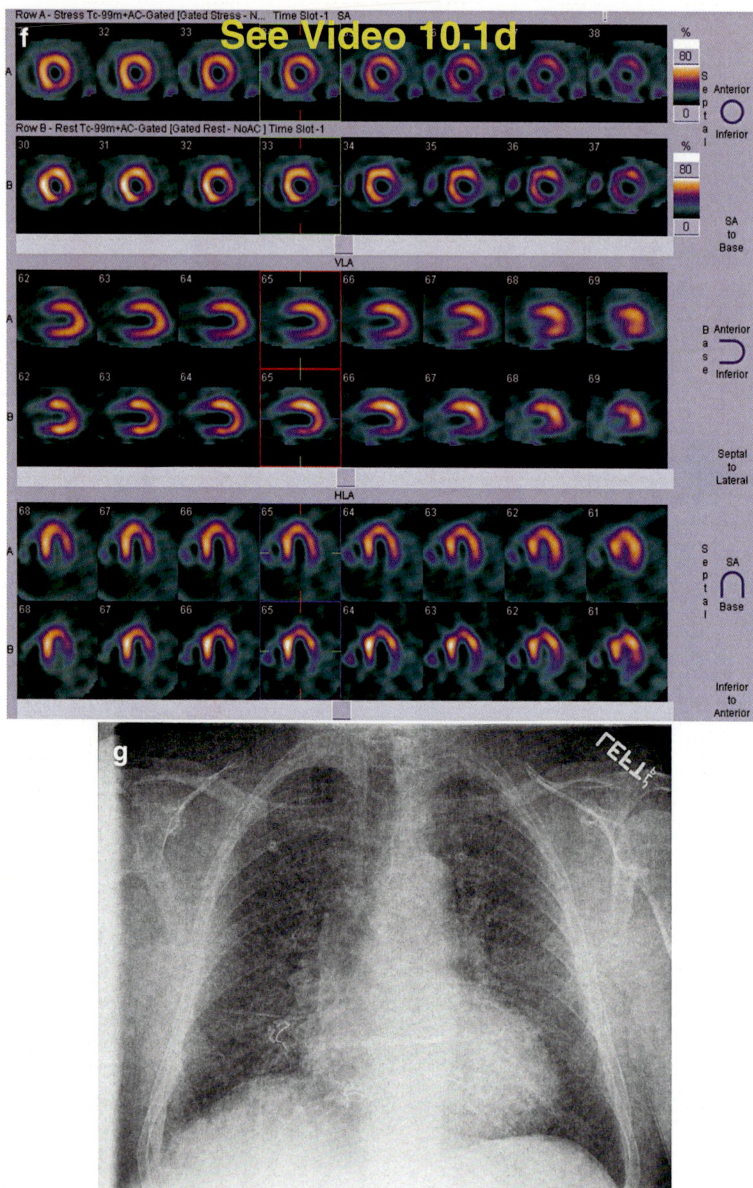

Fig. 10.1 (continued)

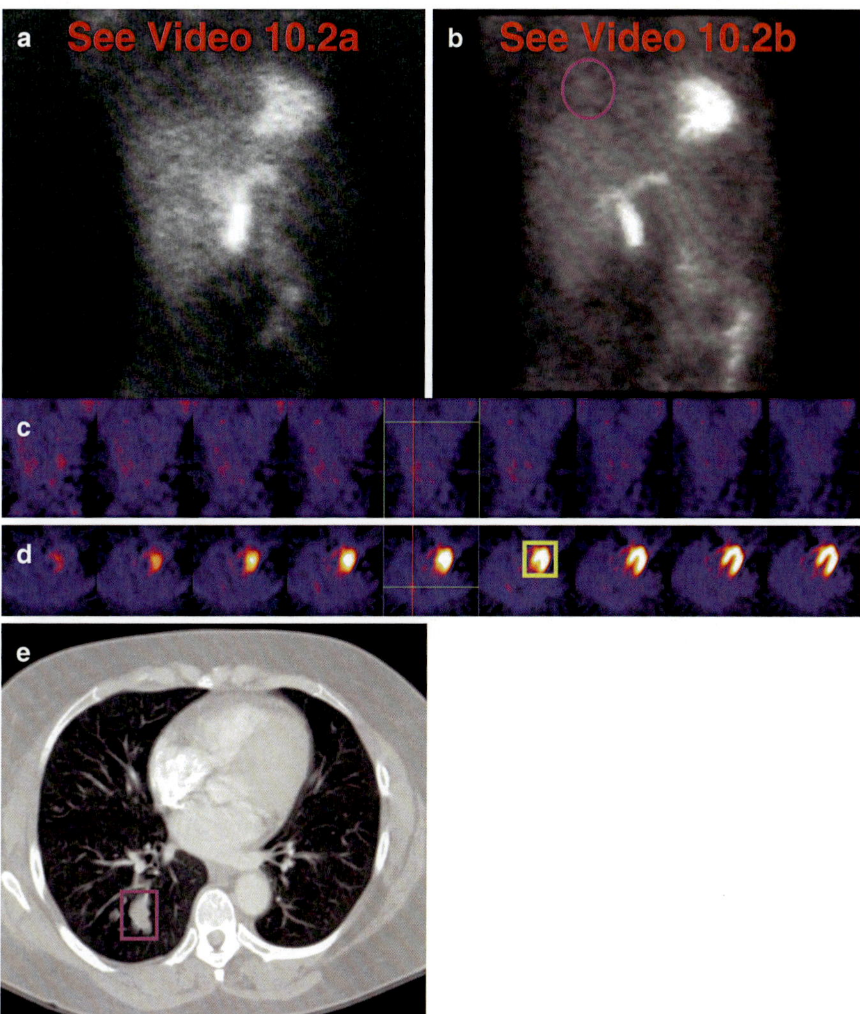

Fig. 10.2 Lung cancer. A 60-year-old female has a focal "hot" lesion in the posterior right lung (**a–d**) that corresponds to a discrete nodular mass on CT (**e**).

(**a**) Stress raw projection images (Video 10.2a, frame 1), ^{99m}Tc tetrofosmin. (**b**) Stress raw projection image (Video 10.2b, frame 13), ^{99m}Tc tetrofosmin, lesion (*pink oval*). (**c**) Stress "whole-field-of-view" processed SPECT images, coronal from anterior to posterior, lesion (crosshairs in middle image). (**d**) Stress "whole-field-of-view" processed SPECT images, axial from superior to inferior, lesion (crosshairs in middle image), heart for reference (*yellow box*). (**e**) CT image through the lower lungs, lesion (*pink box*)

There is a discrete, well-defined focus of abnormal radioactivity in the left lung base that may warrant further diagnostic investigation; primary malignancy is included in the differential diagnosis.

Many pulmonary conditions show diffusely decreased activity and appear relatively "cold." Hyperinflated, emphysematous lungs may be accompanied by significant associated findings (Figs. 10.3, 10.4, and 10.5). Specific pulmonary conditions include cystic fibrosis (Fig. 10.6) and postoperative changes affecting one lung (Fig. 10.7) (Fig. 10.8). The scintigraphic pattern is often nonspecific; correlation with medical and surgical history can help narrow the differential diagnosis as to the etiology and its significance in the particular clinical context under review.

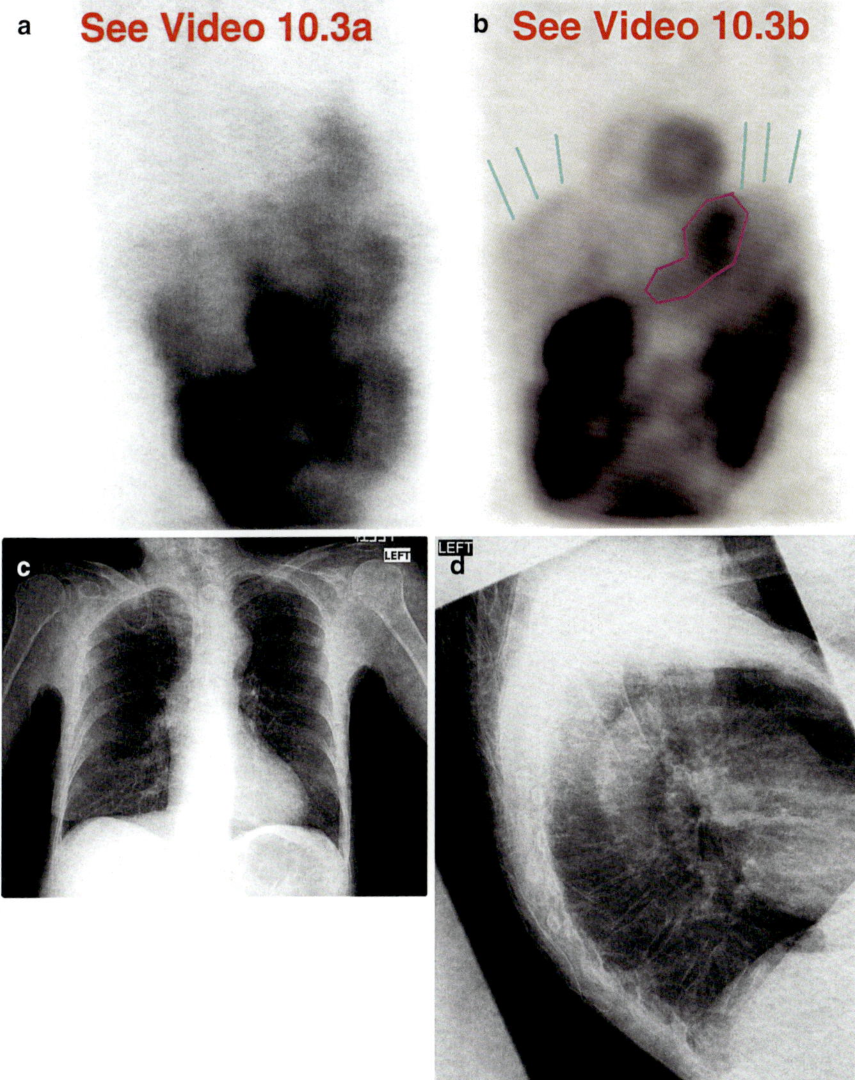

Fig. 10.3 Emphysema. There are hyperexpanded "cold" lungs with flattened diaphragms (**a–d**). Note that the flattened liver dome serves as a reference marker for the right hemidiaphragm (**a, b**). The stomach (seen here, **b**) and the spleen, which are variably visible on MPI, can estimate the position of the left hemidiaphragm. On radiography, the lateral view demonstrates the flattened diaphragms particularly well; note kyphosis and loss of height of two mid-thoracic vertebrae (**d**).

(**a**) Stress raw projection images (Video 10.3a, frame 1), ^{99m}Tc sestamibi. (**b**) Stress raw projection image (Video 10.3b, frame 28), ^{99m}Tc sestamibi, hemidiaphragms (*blue lines*), gastric activity (*pink polygon*). (**c**) PA chest radiograph. (**d**) Lateral chest radiograph

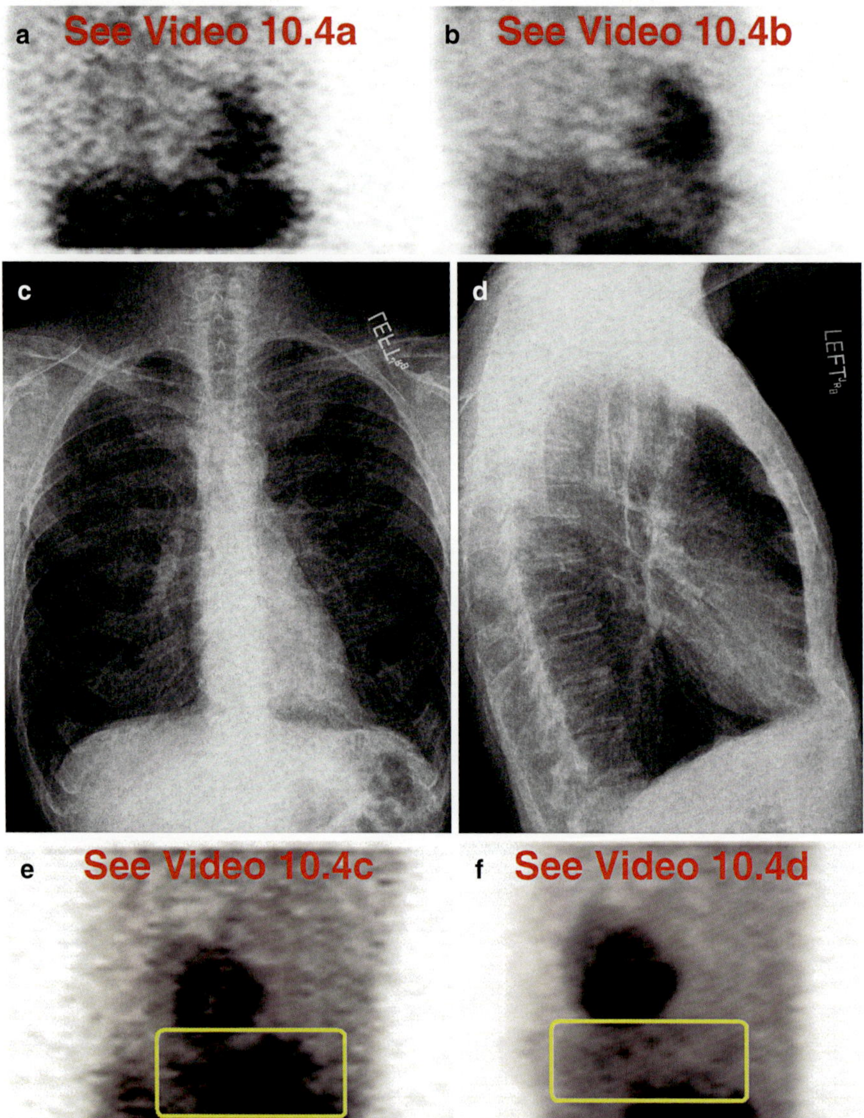

Fig. 10.4 Hyperinflation due to chronic obstructive pulmonary disease. The lungs are hyperinflated and diaphragms flattened on the MPI (**a**, **b**) and chest radiographs (**c**, **d**). The stomach appears "hot" due to duodenogastric bile reflux on the rest raw images (**a**, **e**); after water ingestion, it has cleared and appears "cold" on the stress raw images (**b**, **e**). The stomach serves as a convenient marker of the relatively low and flattened left hemidiaphragm. The "hot" gastric lumen on the rest images (**a**) does not affect the nearby myocardium on the processed SPECT (**g**) or the gated SPECT images (**h**).

(**a**) Rest raw projection images (Video 10.4a, frame 1), ^{99m}Tc sestamibi. (**b**) Stress raw projection images (Video 10.4b, frame 1), ^{99m}Tc sestamibi. (**c**) PA chest radiograph. (**d**) Lateral chest radiograph. (**e**) Rest raw projection image (Video 10.4c, frame 41), ^{99m}Tc sestamibi, stomach (*yellow box*). (**f**) Stress raw projection image (Video 10.4d, frame 46), ^{99m}Tc sestamibi, stomach (*yellow box*). (**g**) Stress/rest processed SPECT images (SA, VLA, HLA) (without and with AC). (**h**) Stress and rest gated SPECT images (Video 10.4e, frame 1) (SA, HLA, VLA)

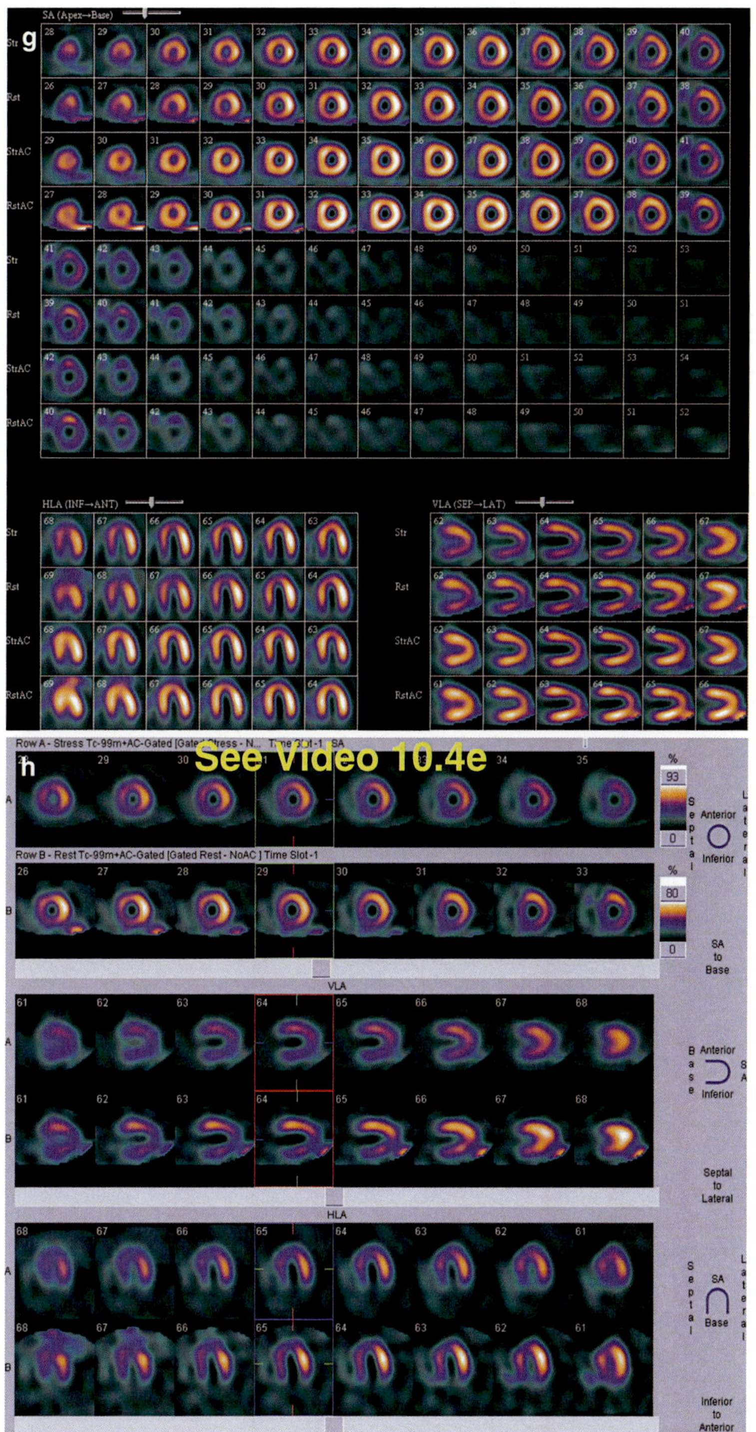

Fig. 10.4 (continued)

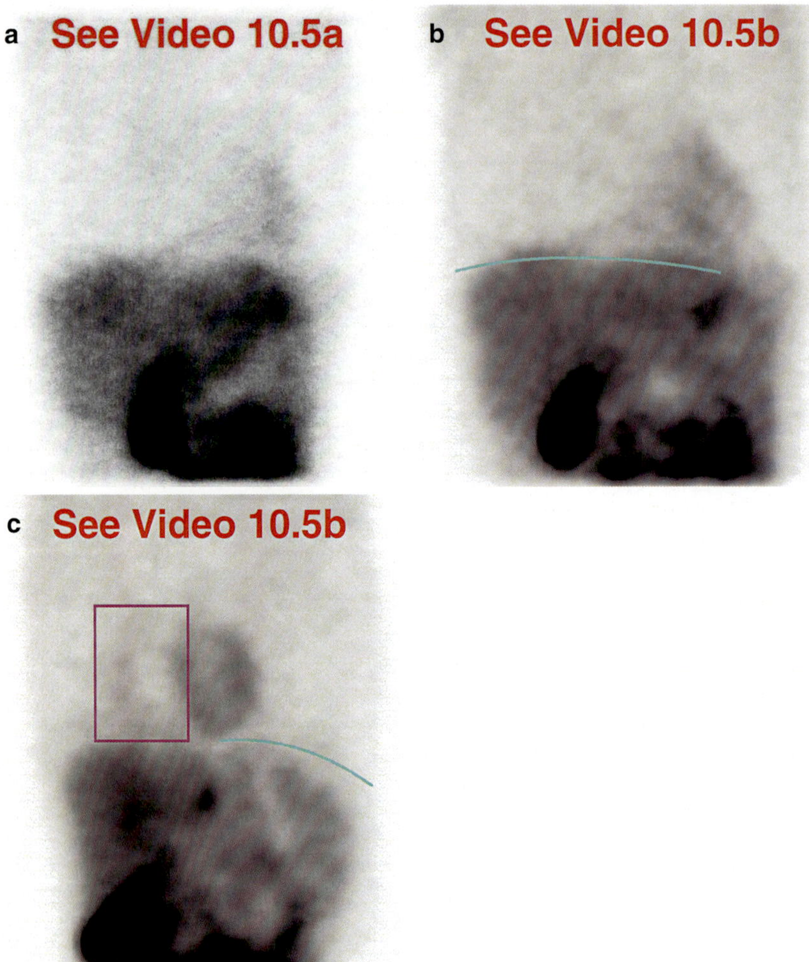

Fig. 10.5 Flattened liver dome due to emphysema with enlarged right ventricle (pulmonary hypertension). The right hemidiaphragm is displaced inferiorly and flattened; the liver dome is a landmark for the diaphragm (**a**, **b**). The left hemidiaphragm is also flattened (**c**). Note the enlarged right ventricle in the setting of pulmonary hypertension (**a**, **c**).

(**a**) Stress raw projection images (Video 10.5a, frame 1), ^{99m}Tc sestamibi. (**b**) Stress raw projection image (Video 10.5b, frame 8), ^{99m}Tc sestamibi, flattened right hemidiaphragm (*blue arc*). (**c**) Stress raw projection image (Video 10.5b, frame 34), ^{99m}Tc sestamibi, enlarged right ventricle (*pink box*), flattened left hemidiaphragm (*blue arc*)

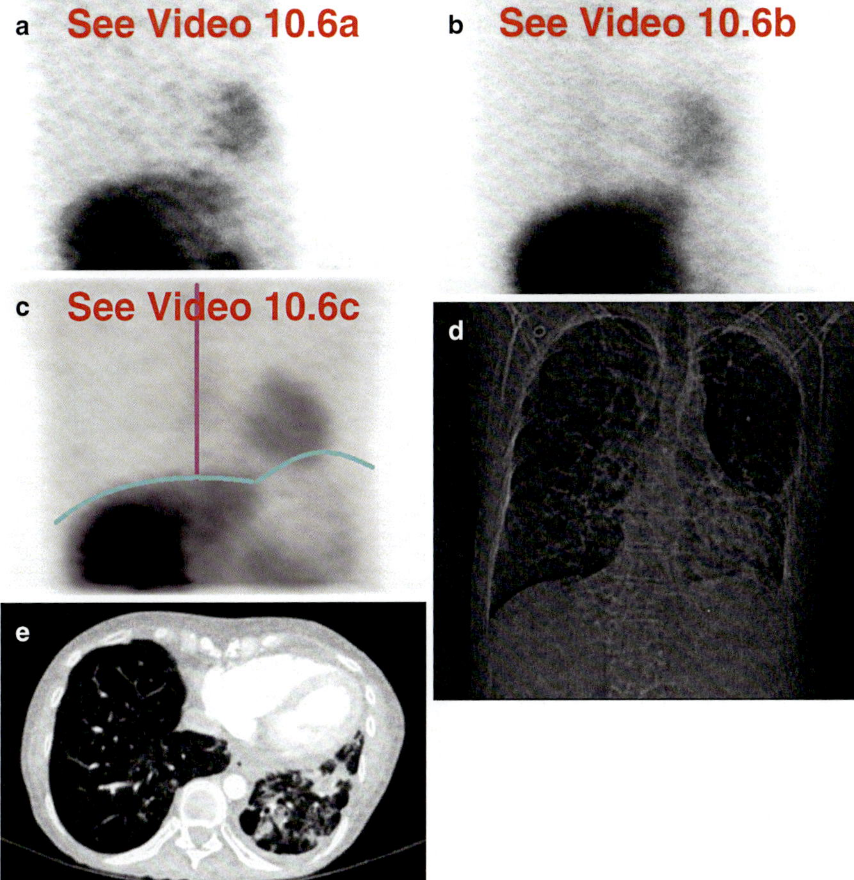

Fig. 10.6 Hyperexpanded right lung and hypoexpanded left lung. A 51-year-old female has cystic fibrosis (**a, b**). Note that the heart is positioned more to the left of midline than usual and the hemidiaphragms are at different levels, left higher than right (**c**). Differential diagnosis includes left pneumothorax, atelectasis/lobar collapse, and lower lobe lobectomy. Correlation with chest CT (**d**) reveals marked asymmetry of chronically diseased lungs with significant expansion on the right and volume loss on the left, resulting in mediastinal shift to the left (**e**). Note that the heart lies almost entirely in the left chest (**e**). Incidentally, the stomach appears "hot" on rest raw images (**a**), but "cold" after ingestion of fluids before stress imaging (**b**).

(**a**) Rest raw projection images (Video 10.6a, frame 1), ^{99m}Tc sestamibi. (**b**) Stress raw projection images (Video 10.6b, frame 1), ^{99m}Tc sestamibi. (**c**) Stress raw projection image (Video 10.6c, frame 19), ^{99m}Tc sestamibi, midline reference (*pink line*), hemidiaphragms (*blue lines*). (**d**) Scout chest CT. (**e**) CT image through the heart and lower lungs

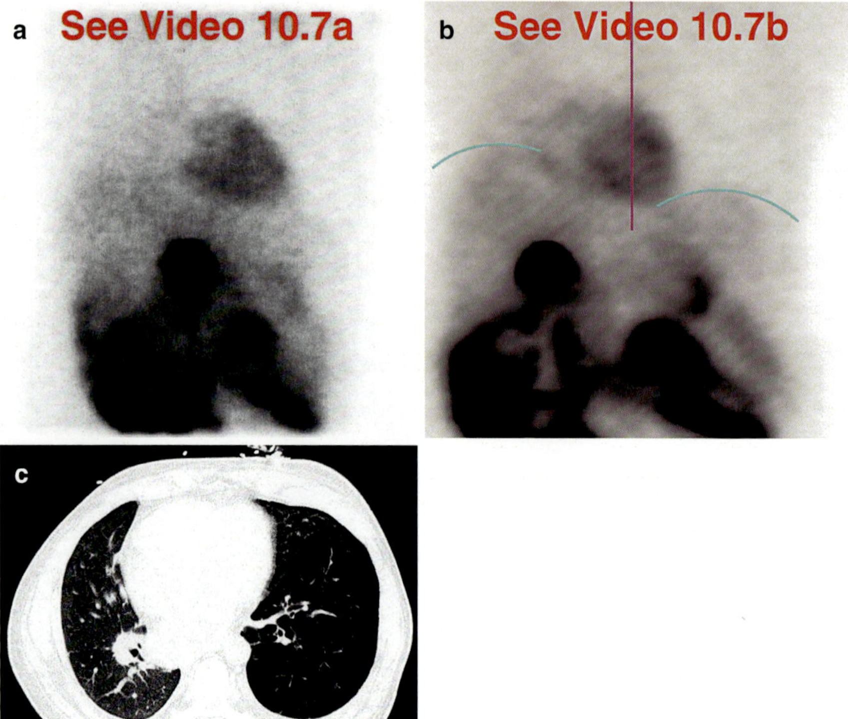

Fig. 10.7 Relatively "cold" and hyperexpanded native left lung with more normal "low-level" activity in smaller transplanted right lung. The left lung appears "cold" and expanded, and the right appears to have the usual activity and appears smaller (**a**, **b**). Note the marked mediastinal shift to the right (**a**, **b**), confirmed by the CT scan (**c**); much of the heart lies to the right of midline. The hemidiaphragms are at strikingly different levels, right higher than left (**a**, **b**). The prominent right ventricle (**a**) reflects pulmonary hypertension related to chronic lung disease.

(**a**) Stress raw projection images (Video 10.7a, frame 1), ^{99m}Tc sestamibi. (**b**) Stress raw projection image (Video 10.7b, frame 15), ^{99m}Tc sestamibi, approximated midline (*pink line*), hemidiaphragms (*blue lines*). (**c**) CT image of lungs

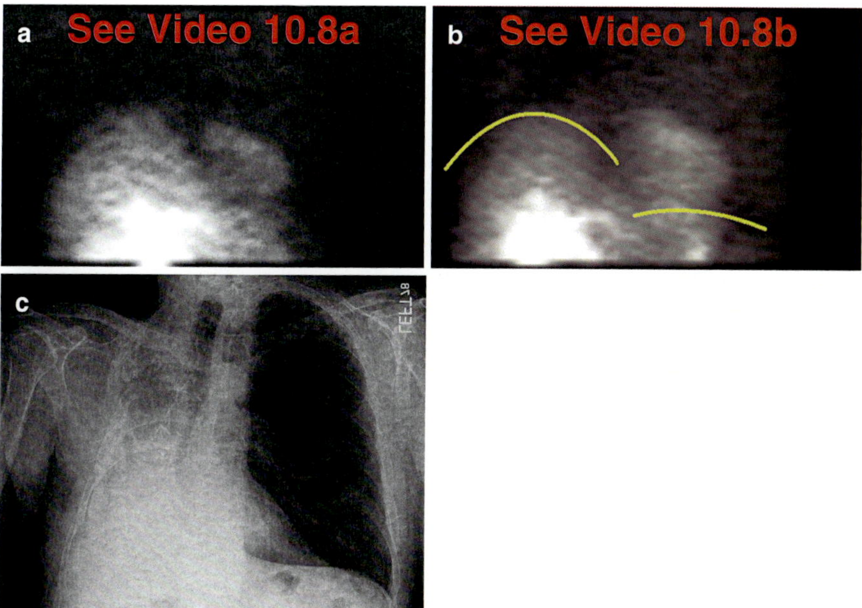

Fig. 10.8 Right pneumonectomy. The right pneumonectomy is manifested by a "cold" right hemithorax with marked mediastinal shift to the right (**a**, **b**). Note the elevated liver dome as a sign of reduced volume on the right (**b**). Radiographic correlation (**c**) confirms postoperative changes (e.g., surgical clips, rib resection/fractures, opacification of hemithorax, tracheal deviation to the right) as the etiology for the findings on MPI. Reviewing all of the pertinent images, ideally on side-by-side computer screens, is a useful technique for confident interpretation of unusual findings. The MPI report can place the findings in their proper context.

(**a**) Stress "white-on-black" raw projection images (Video 10.8a, frame 1), ^{99m}Tc sestamibi. (**b**) Stress "white-on-black" raw projection image (Video 10.8b, frame 12), ^{99m}Tc sestamibi, hemidiaphragms (*yellow lines*). (**c**) PA chest radiograph

Key Points
- Radiopharmaceutical localization within the lungs may be diffuse or focal.
- Diffuse uptake may be associated with LV dysfunction and severe multivessel CAD.
- Neoplastic and inflammatory lung conditions may demonstrate focal avidity for MPI radiopharmaceuticals; these findings should be correlated with other imaging, reported, and communicated to the referring physician.
- Hyperinflated lungs, as seen in emphysema, appear relatively "cold," are associated with flattened diaphragms and increased anterior-posterior dimension, and are generally easy to recognize, especially when correlated with conventional radiography or CT.

Mediastinum

Table 11.1 outlines benign and malignant conditions affecting the mediastinum that may be detected during review of MPI projection data (Seo et al. 2005). The most common in routine clinical practice is hiatal hernia. Hiatal hernias are created when a portion of the stomach invaginates through the esophageal hiatal opening in the diaphragm and transiently or permanently resides above the diaphragm. Hiatal hernias can be quite large, and in those cases, most of the stomach becomes intrathoracic in location (Fig. 11.1). On SPECT MPI, hiatal hernias may appear "hot" when containing refluxed bile or "cold" when containing nonradioactive fluid or food (Burrell and MacDonald 2006; Chamarthy and Travin 2010; Gedik et al. 2007; Raza et al. 2005a; Slavin et al. 1998). "Hot" or "cold" hiatal hernias can be problematic because processing artifacts commonly lead to misinterpretation; thus, recognition of this common condition may be critical for proper reporting. Correlation with other imaging and clinical history is often essential.

In the anterior mediastinum, thymoma, a potentially malignant neoplasm arising from the thymus, may be quite avid for MPI radiopharmaceuticals (Bhambhvani et al. 2010a, b; Chadika et al. 2005; Chamarthy and Travin 2010; Gedik et al. 2007; Hawkins et al. 2007; Vijayakumar et al. 2005). One case report demonstrated synchronous primary tumors in the breast and thymus (García-Talavera et al. 2013). In the middle mediastinum, benign and malignant hilar masses may be found and typically appear "hot." Esophageal cancer is "hot" (Watanabe et al. 1997). Benign masses include "hot" mediastinal lymph nodes affected by sarcoidosis (Gedik et al. 2007). Mediastinal masses may be of thyroid or parathyroid origin; these are discussed in Chaps. 4 and 5. "Whole-field-of-view reconstruction" facilitates localization and permits anatomic correlation (Fig. 11.2). In the posterior mediastinum,

Electronic supplementary material The online version of this chapter (doi:10.1007/978-3-319-25436-4_11) contains supplementary material, which is available to authorized users.

© Springer International Publishing Switzerland 2017
M.E. Oates, V.L. Sorrell, *Myocardial Perfusion Imaging - Beyond the Left Ventricle: Pathology, Artifacts and Pitfalls in the Chest and Abdomen,* DOI 10.1007/978-3-319-25436-4_11

Table 11.1 Differential diagnosis of "hot" and "cold" imaging findings related to the mediastinum

Organ system	"Hot" finding	"Cold" finding	References
Mediastinum	Gastroesophageal reflux Hiatal hernia (refluxed duodenogastric bile) *Neoplasm, primary malignant (esophageal cancer, lymphoma, thymoma)* Extramedullary hematopoiesis (paravertebral masses)	Cyst Dilated esophagus fluid- or food-filled hiatal hernia	Bhambhvani et al. (2010a, b) Burrell and MacDonald (2006) Chadika et al. (2005) Chamarthy and Travin (2010) García-Talavera et al. (2013) Gedik et al. (2007) Hawkins et al. (2007) Niederkohr et al. (2009) Raza et al. (2005a) Seo et al. (2005) Slavin et al. (1998) Vijayakumar et al. (2005) Watanabe et al. (1997)

large "hot" paraspinal masses represented extramedullary hematopoiesis in a patient with thalassemia (Niederkohr et al. 2009).

As a general rule, mediastinal findings should be included in the SPECT MPI report. For example:

> There is an intense focus of abnormal radiotracer uptake in the anterior mediastinum; differential diagnosis includes malignancy. This finding likely correlates with the known thymoma; according to the patient, surgical resection is planned.

If the lesion is unknown, personal communication with the referring physician is appropriate.

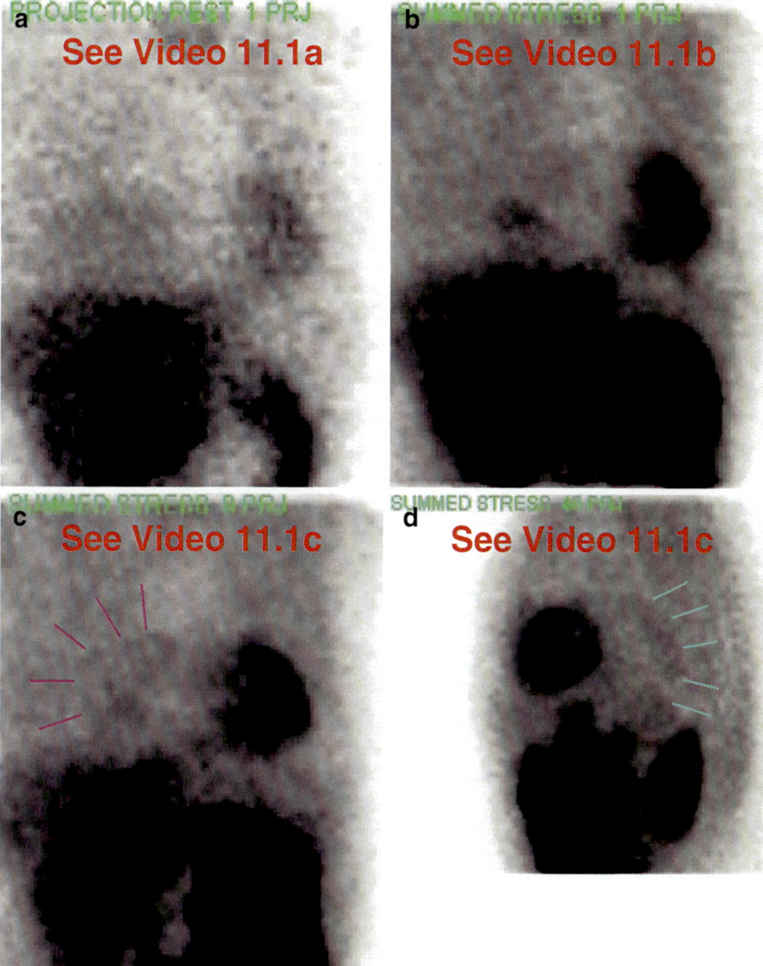

Fig. 11.1 Huge hiatal hernia/intrathoracic stomach. In the thorax, there is a striking abnormality: lateral to the right side of the heart and behind the left side of the heart, there are large mixed "hot" and "cold" regions (**a–d**). Two selected contrast-adjusted stress images (**c, d**) orient the viewer to the locations of the abnormalities to best advantage. Re-reviewing the rest and stress raw images (**a, b**) with attention to these regions facilitates perception of the swirling radioactivity, suggesting duodenogastric reflux into the large herniated stomach. By radiography, there is a corresponding huge hiatal hernia/intrathoracic stomach behind and to the right of the heart (**e, f**). Note the normal thyroid gland at the top of the field-of-view on the rest raw images (**a**). MPI (**g, h**) shows a small-to-medium-sized, moderately severe, fixed anteroseptal-apical defect. There is normal LV function, regional wall motion, and wall thickening. The perfusion defect is likely artifactual in nature. LVEF is 64 %. RV function is normal (**h**).

(**a**) Rest raw projection images (Video 11.1a, frame 1), at usual contrast setting for the heart, ^{99m}Tc sestamibi. (**b**) Stress raw projection images (Video 11.1b, frame 1) contrast-adjusted for intrathoracic abnormality, ^{99m}Tc sestamibi. (**c**) Stress raw projection image (Video 11.1c, frame 8), ^{99m}Tc sestamibi, activity lateral to the right heart (*pink lines*). (**d**) Stress raw projection image (Video 11.1c, frame 46), ^{99m}Tc sestamibi, activity behind the left heart (*blue lines*).

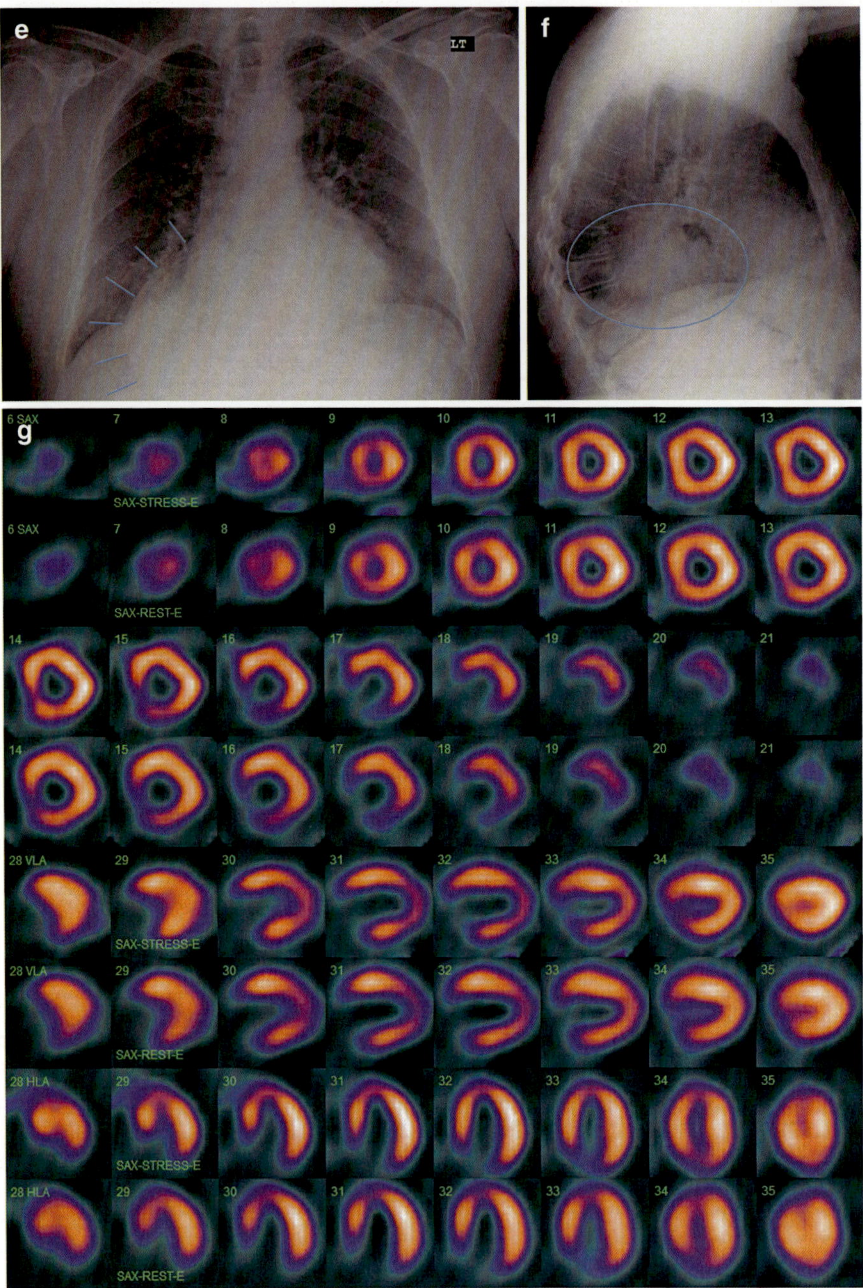

Fig. 11.1 (continued) (**e**) PA chest radiograph, right lateral margin of hiatal hernia (*blue lines*). (**f**) Lateral chest radiograph, approximate position of hiatal hernia containing gas (*blue oval*). (**g**) Stress/rest processed SPECT images (SA, HLA, VLA). (**h**) Stress gated SPECT images (Video 11.1d, frame 1) (SA, HLA, VLA)

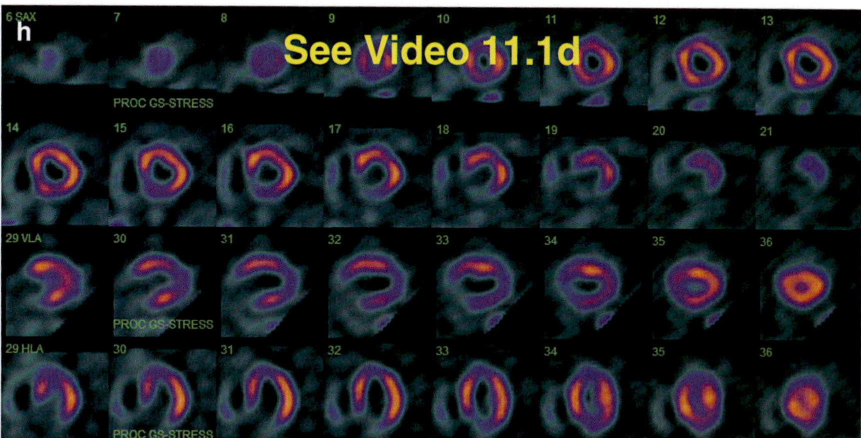

Fig. 11.1 (continued)

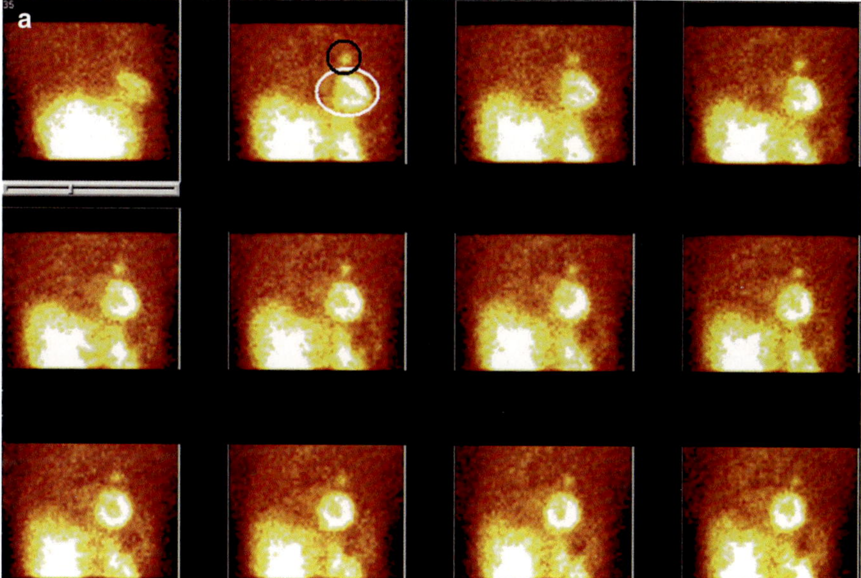

Fig. 11.2 Hilar mass. A discrete "hot" lesion is clearly identified in the left hilum just cephalad to the heart (**a–c**). It corresponds to a hilar fullness on CT (**d**) and was presumptively diagnosed as a pathologic lymph node in the immunocompromised patient. Its location did not interfere with cardiac processing or interpretation.

(**a**) Selected sequential stress raw projection planar images, anterior to LAO projections, ^{99m}Tc tetrofosmin, "hot" focal lesion (*black circle*), heart for reference landmark (*white oval*) on first planar image in series.

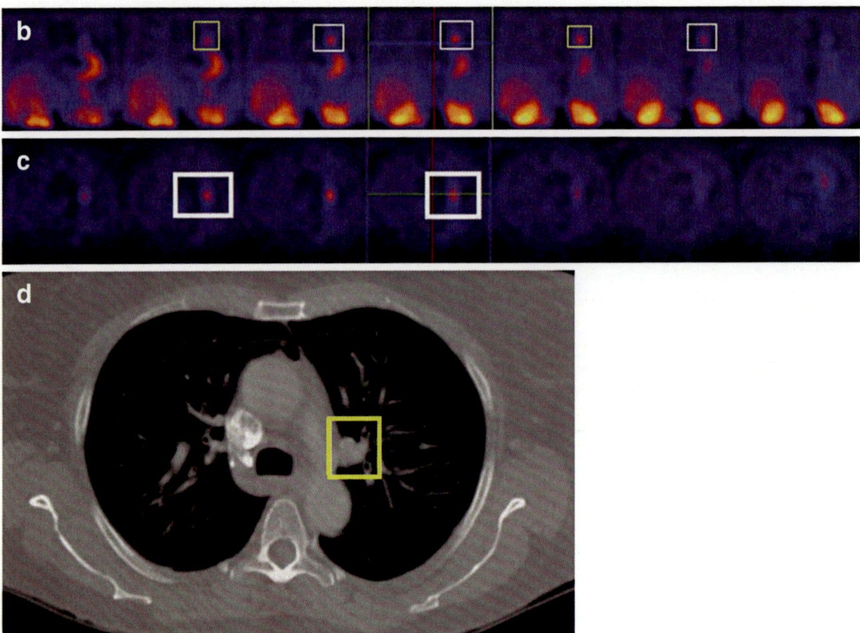

Fig. 11.2 (continued) (**b**) Stress "whole-field-of-view" reconstructed SPECT images, coronal from anterior to posterior, "hot" focal lesion (*white boxes* on representative images); the lesion is cephalad to the heart. (**c**) Stress "whole-field-of-view" reconstructed SPECT images, axial from superior to inferior, "hot" focal lesion (*white boxes* on representative images); the lesion is cephalad to the heart. (**d**) CT image of chest at level of hilum and corresponding to (**c**), left hilar fullness (*yellow box*)

Key Points
- The most common mediastinal condition detected on MPI projection data is hiatal hernia.
- Hiatal hernias may be "hot" when containing refluxed bile or "cold" when containing nonradioactive fluid or food, and can be a source of SPECT MPI artifact given proximity to the heart.
- Malignant mediastinal masses (e.g., thymoma) typically appear "hot."

Myocardium and Pericardium 12

Uncommonly, SPECT MPI can reveal abnormalities or normal variants related to the myocardium and pericardium (Table 12.1). Malignant myocardial and pericardial masses often appear as focal "hot" lesions (Chamarthy and Travin 2010; Kasi et al. 2002).

A pericardial effusion typically appears "cold" and mimics a "halo" around the heart (Fig. 12.1) (Williams et al. 2003). It is important to recognize effusions, which may be large, circumferential, or loculated and may be unknown to the physician or patient. They are a potential cause for a typical patient's clinical presentation (e.g., chest pain, dyspnea). As such, they should be noted in the MPI report, and personal communication may be warranted. A typical report would state something along the lines of:

There is a "cold" region around the heart. This suggests a sizeable pericardial effusion. Consider echocardiography.

Table 12.1 Differential diagnosis of "hot" and "cold" imaging findings related to the myocardium and pericardium

Organ system	"Hot" finding	"Cold" finding	References
Myocardium and pericardium	*Myocardial mass* *Pericardial mass*	*Pericardial effusion*	Chamarthy and Travin (2010) Kasi et al. (2002) Williams et al. (2003)

Electronic supplementary material The online version of this chapter (doi:10.1007/978-3-319-25436-4_12) contains supplementary material, which is available to authorized users.

© Springer International Publishing Switzerland 2017
M.E. Oates, V.L. Sorrell, *Myocardial Perfusion Imaging - Beyond the Left Ventricle: Pathology, Artifacts and Pitfalls in the Chest and Abdomen*,
DOI 10.1007/978-3-319-25436-4_12

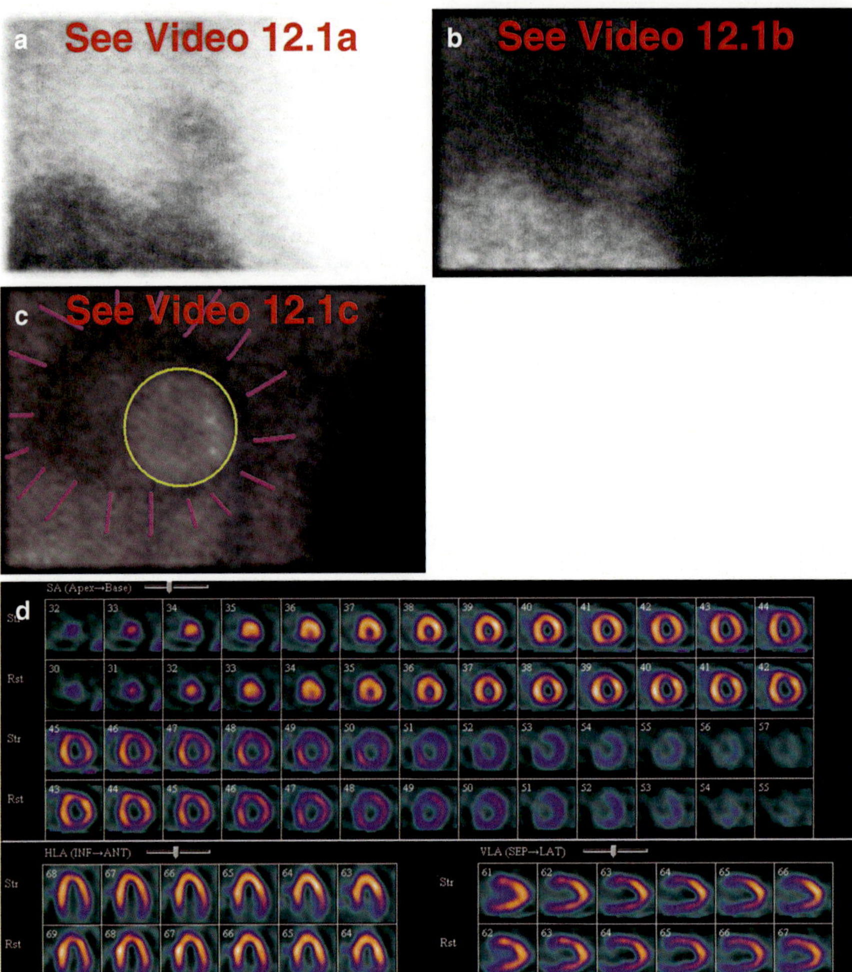

Fig. 12.1 Pericardial effusion. The circumferential "cold" region around the ventricles (**a–c**) corresponds to a large pericardial effusion. Note how visualization of the "cold" fluid is enhanced by using alternative color tables (compare **a**, **b**). On the processed SPECT images (**d**) and gated SPECT images (**e**), there is a well-defined "cold" band adjacent to the lateral left ventricular wall: note how the "cold" pericardial fluid compares to the "cold" center of the ventricles containing fluid (blood). Despite the pericardial effusion, no specific attenuation effect is apparent.

(**a**) Stress "black-on-white" raw projection images (Video 12.1a, frame 1), ^{99m}Tc sestamibi. (**b**) Stress "white-on-black" raw projection images (Video 12.1b, frame 1), ^{99m}Tc sestamibi. (**c**) Stress "white-on-black" raw projection image (Video 12.1c, frame 26), ^{99m}Tc sestamibi, pericardial fluid (*pink lines*), left ventricular myocardium (*yellow circle*) for reference. (**d**) Stress/rest processed SPECT images (SA, HLA, VLA). (**e**) Stress gated SPECT images (Video 12.1d, frame 1) (SA, VLA, HLA)

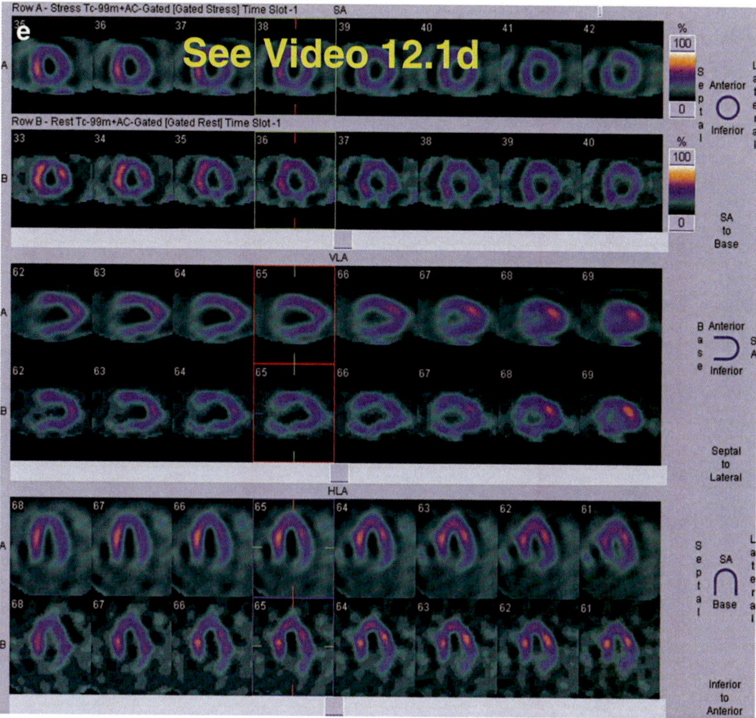

Fig. 12.1 (continued)

Key Points

- A pericardial effusion often appears as a "cold halo" surrounding the heart.
- Visualization of a pericardial effusion should prompt personal communication with the referring physician and be included in the report.

Right Atrium and Right Ventricle

13

SPECT MPI can reveal abnormalities or normal variants related to the right side of the heart (Table 13.1). Not uncommonly, focal, often intense, radiopharmaceutical localization is seen in the region of the right atrium (Fig. 13.1). This represents uptake in the right auricular appendage which contains mitochondrial-rich myocardial tissue. This is a normal finding and should not be misinterpreted as a mediastinal mass (Mlikotic and Mishkin 2000; Mohr et al. 1996). Another benign etiology for a similar appearance is brown adipose tissue (BAT) which is avid for the MPI radiopharmaceuticals. Correlation with SPECT/CT is helpful in clinching the diagnosis by demonstrating the associated fat density (Goetze et al. 2008).

The right ventricular free wall may appear "thicker" ("hotter") and is commonly associated with primary or secondary pulmonary hypertension and right ventricular hypertrophy (Fig. 13.2) (Chamarthy and Travin 2010). In these cases, the ventricular septum is relatively "flat," creating a "D-shaped" left ventricular cavity. After exercise stress, prominent right ventricular uptake may signal right ventricular strain and left heart failure due to multivessel coronary artery disease (Williams and Schneider 1999).

Electronic supplementary material The online version of this chapter (doi:10.1007/978-3-319-25436-4_13) contains supplementary material, which is available to authorized users.

© Springer International Publishing Switzerland 2017
M.E. Oates, V.L. Sorrell, *Myocardial Perfusion Imaging - Beyond the Left Ventricle: Pathology, Artifacts and Pitfalls in the Chest and Abdomen,* DOI 10.1007/978-3-319-25436-4_13

Table 13.1 Differential diagnosis of "hot" and "cold" imaging findings related to the right atrium and right ventricle

Organ system	"Hot" finding	"Cold" finding	References
Right atrium and right ventricle	Prominent right ventricular wall (coronary artery disease, valvular disease, pulmonary hypertension) Brown adipose tissue Prominent right auricular appendage *Neoplasm, primary or metastatic*	Enlarged atria	Chamarthy and Travin (2010) Goetze et al. (2008) Mlikotic and Mishkin (2000) Mohr et al. (1996) Williams and Schneider (1999) Wosnitzer et al. (2012)

A dilated right atrium and/or the right ventricle may appear "cold." Dilatation of the right heart may be isolated or may be associated with dilatation of the left heart (Fig. 13.3) (Wosnitzer et al. 2012). Causes for right heart dilatation include valvular disease, cardiac shunts or cardiomyopathy (Chamarthy and Travin 2010).

Isolated abnormalities of the right heart should be recognized and may be directly responsible for the patient's symptoms. Thus, SPECT MPI reports should mention the right-sided cardiac abnormalities whenever they are present, potentially significant, and certainly when they represent a new diagnosis. Suggested language includes:

The right ventricle appears enlarged and the free wall appears thickened. In view of the patient's chronic pulmonary disease, this constellation of findings suggests pulmonary hypertension.

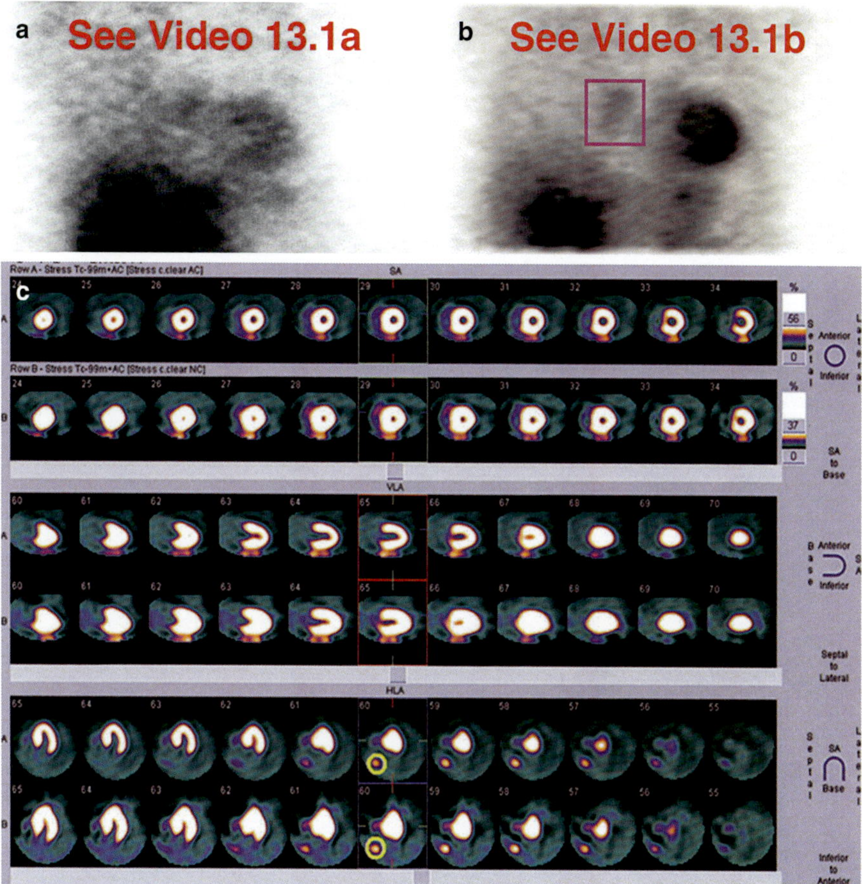

Fig. 13.1 Right auricular appendage. Focal activity in the region of the right atrium (**a–e**) is a normal variant.

(**a**) Stress raw projection images (Video 13.1a, frame 1), ^{99m}Tc sestamibi. (**b**) Stress raw projection image (Video 13.1b, frame 20), ^{99m}Tc sestamibi, right auricular appendage (*pink box*). (**c**) Stress/rest processed SPECT images (SA, VLA, HLA), right auricular appendage (HLA, *yellow ovals*). (**d**) Stress and rest gated SPECT images (Video 13.1c, frame 1) (SA, VLA, HLA). (**e**) Stress and rest gated SPECT image (Video 13.1d, frame 1) (SA, VLA, HLA), right auricular appendage (HLA, *yellow ovals*)

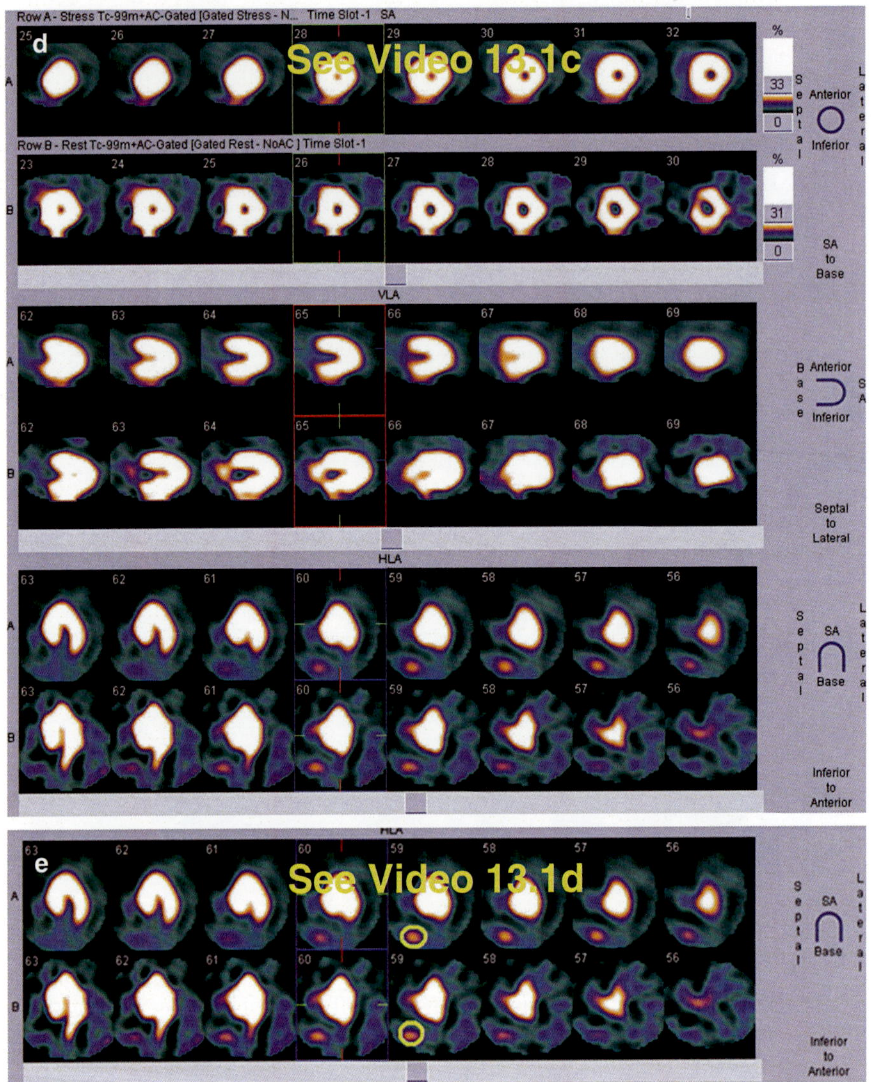

Fig. 13.1 (continued)

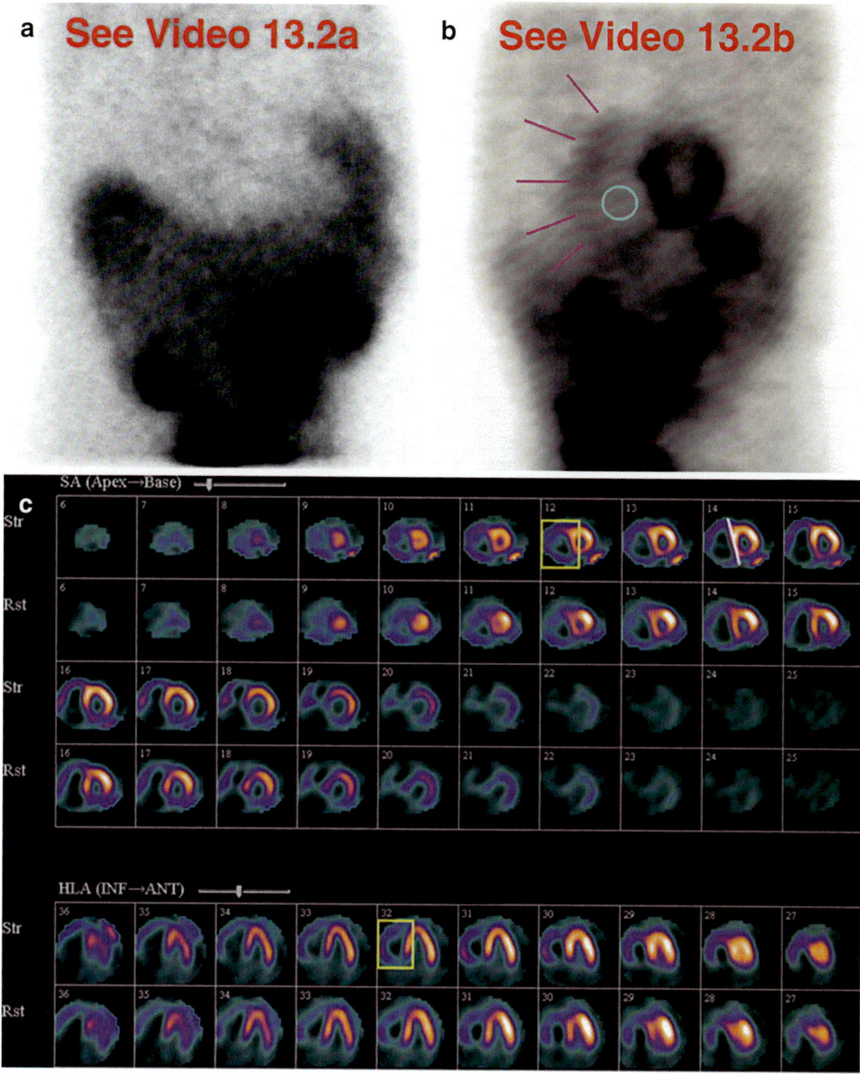

Fig. 13.2 Pulmonary hypertension and emphysema. An 84-year-old male has an enlarged right ventricular cavity and a thickened free wall (**a–c**). The enlarged "cold" right atrium adjacent to the right ventricle can be appreciated on the raw data (**a**). Note the flattened septum (**c**) giving rise to a D-shaped left ventricle, a characteristic finding of pulmonary arterial hypertension and cor pulmonale. Visually depressed right ventricular function (**d**) correlates with slightly reduced RV function by echocardiography.

(**a**) Stress raw projection images (Video 13.2a, frame 1), ^{99m}Tc sestamibi. (**b**) Stress raw projection image (Video 13.2b, frame 38), ^{99m}Tc sestamibi, right ventricular myocardial wall (*pink lines*), right ventricular cavity (*blue circle*). (**c**) Stress/rest processed SPECT images (SA, HLA), enlarged right ventricular cavity (*yellow boxes* on representative SA and HLA images), flattened septum (*white line* on representative SA image). (**d**) Stress gated SPECT images (Video 13.2c, frame 1) (SA, VLA, HLA)

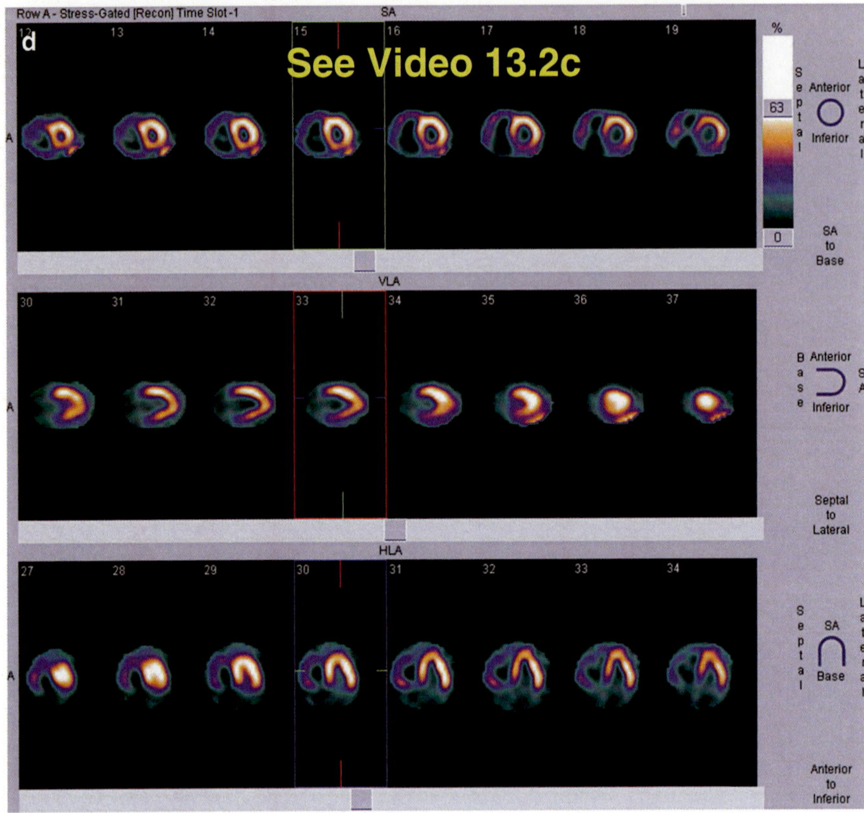

Fig. 13.2 (continued)

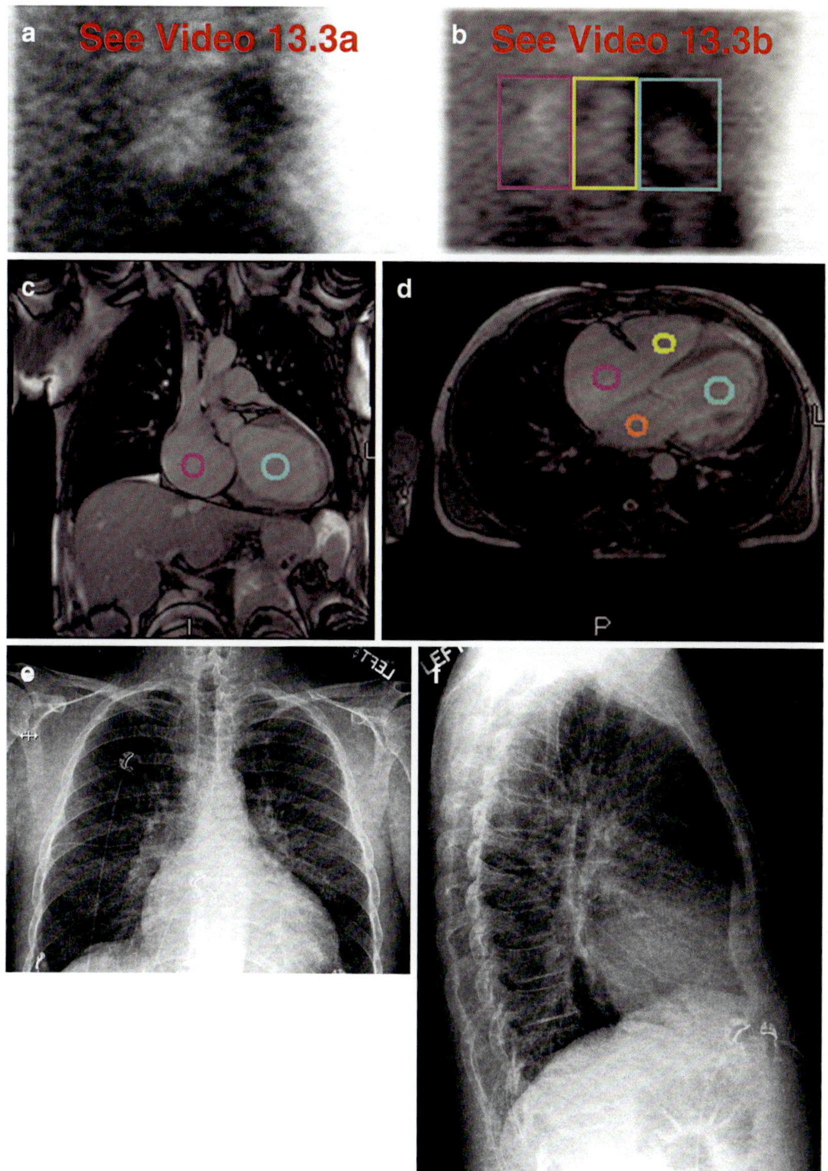

Fig. 13.3 Enlarged right atrium and right ventricle. The enlarged right heart is associated with an enlarged left atrium and left ventricle (four chamber enlargement) (**a–d**). Diffusely "hot" lungs (**a**) correlate with increased lung markings and cardiomegaly radiographically (**e, f**). Left ventricular function is markedly depressed (LVEF of 10 %).

(**a**) Stress raw projection images (Video 13.3a, frame 1), ^{99m}Tc sestamibi. (**b**) Stress raw projection image (Video 13.3b, frame 23), ^{99m}Tc sestamibi, right atrium (*pink box*), right ventricle (*yellow box*), left ventricle (*blue box*). (**c**) Coronal MRI of heart, dilated right atrium (*pink circle*), dilated left ventricle (*blue circle*). (**d**) Axial MRI of heart, dilatation of all four cardiac chambers, right atrium (*pink circle*), right ventricle (*yellow circle*), left atrium (*orange circle*), left ventricle (*blue circle*). (**e**) PA chest radiograph. (**f**) Lateral chest radiograph

Key Points
- Uptake of SPECT MPI radiopharmaceuticals within the thin-walled right atrium itself, and more focally within the right auricular appendage, is normal.
- Avid uptake within the right ventricular free wall, particularly when associated with a flattened septum and D-shaped left ventricle, is consistent with pulmonary hypertension and RV hypertrophy.
- Prominent uptake within the right ventricular myocardium *after* exercise stress could signify RV strain and left heart failure due to severe multivessel CAD.

There are several etiologies for abnormal findings related to the peripheral or central vascular system in the chest (Table 14.1). Extravasation may occur during intravenous injection of the radiopharmaceutical. Depending on the amount extravasated, the radiopharmaceutical may be picked up by the lymphatics and deposited in the regional lymph node basin, typically the axilla after an injection in the upper extremity (Fig. 14.1). When extravasation is suspected, it might be prudent to image the injection site to ensure complete intravascular delivery of the radiopharmaceutical. An incomplete injection, particularly during the stress portion of the examination, may result in spuriously normal-appearing (false-negative) myocardial perfusion due to an inadequate ratio of administered activity relative to the earlier rest injection (Burrell and MacDonald 2006; Chamarthy and Travin 2010; Gedik et al. 2007; Gentili et al. 1994; Howarth et al. 1996; Strauss et al. 2008). Extreme extravasations can cause scatter artifact, reiterating the importance of raising the patient's arms out of the field-of-view. Additionally, other maneuvers such as shielding can be employed when appropriate.

Implanted ports may be used for radiopharmaceutical administration (Fig. 14.2) and should not be confused with contamination artifact (Burrell and MacDonald 2006). Flushing catheters well can eliminate or reduce retention of the radiopharmaceutical and is important because "hot" ports overlying the heart can be problematic for image reconstruction (Burrell and MacDonald 2006). Radiopharmaceuticals may be retained in indwelling central catheters in the superior vena cava (Shih et al. 2002; Tallaj and Iskandrian 2000). Even when using antecubital venous access, it is well known that ^{201}Tl chloride and the ^{99m}Tc MPI radiopharmaceuticals can be retained in the large central veins, despite flushing (Howarth et al. 1996). These

Electronic supplementary material The online version of this chapter (doi:10.1007/978-3-319-25436-4_14) contains supplementary material, which is available to authorized users.

© Springer International Publishing Switzerland 2017
M.E. Oates, V.L. Sorrell, *Myocardial Perfusion Imaging - Beyond the Left Ventricle: Pathology, Artifacts and Pitfalls in the Chest and Abdomen,* DOI 10.1007/978-3-319-25436-4_14

Table 14.1 Differential diagnosis of "hot" and "cold" imaging findings related to the vascular system

Organ system	"Hot" finding	"Cold" finding	References
Vascular system	Contamination during injection Extravasation at injection site Retention in central veins Retention in central venous catheters/ports Pulmonary arterial wall	Dilated pulmonary arteries	Aras et al. (2003) Burrell and MacDonald (2006) Chamarthy and Travin (2010) Gedik et al. (2007) Gentili et al. (1994) Howarth et al. (1996) Shih et al. (2002) Strauss et al. (2008) Tallaj and Iskandrian (2000)

Fig. 14.1 Marked radiopharmaceutical extravasation at right arm injection site with visualization of right axillary lymph node. This occurred during the rest portion of the one-day rest/stress MPI protocol (**a–c**). The patient's right arm was positioned alongside the right chest wall for imaging. Note the significant "streaky" scatter effect onto the patient's right chest wall and abdomen (**a**). The injection site can be more clearly defined by adjusting the contrast settings during review (**b, c**). The extravasation is still evident on the later stress imaging (**d, e, f**). Although it can be appreciated on the rest raw data (**a**), the right axillary lymph node is more clearly defined with time (**e**). The scatter effect is still present, although somewhat mitigated (**f**). However disconcerting on the raw data (**a, d**), there is no significant detrimental effect on the processed SPECT images (**g**) nor the gated SPECT images (**h**), and the examination is reportable. There is a small, mild, fixed inferior-lateral-basal defect, probably artifactual. If the extravasation had occurred during the stress test, the MPI would have been compromised because the desired 3:1 ratio of stress-to-rest administered activity would not have been achieved. A 50-year-old male is on dialysis for diabetes-related end-stage renal disease, has hypertension, and had coronary artery bypass surgery (CABG).

(**a**) Rest raw projection images at usual contrast setting to view heart (Video 14.1a, frame 1), ^{99m}Tc sestamibi. (**b**) Rest raw projection image (Video 14.1b, frame 20) adjusted to show relative intensity of injection site to heart, ^{99m}Tc sestamibi, injection site (*blue box*), heart (*pink box*), gallbladder as reference point (*yellow box*). (**c**) Rest raw projection image (Video 14.1b, frame 20) adjusted to show focality of very "hot" injection site (*blue box*) in right arm without blooming artifact, ^{99m}Tc sestamibi. (**d**) Stress raw projection images at usual contrast setting to view heart (Video 14.1c, frame 1), ^{99m}Tc sestamibi. (**e**) Stress raw projection images at usual contrast setting to view heart (Video 14.1d, frame 9), ^{99m}Tc sestamibi, right axillary uptake (*blue box*). (**f**) Stress raw projection image (Video 14.1d, frame 16) at usual contrast setting to view heart, ^{99m}Tc sestamibi, injection site (*blue box*), scatter artifact (*red box*). (**g**) Stress/rest processed SPECT images (SA, HLA, VLA). (**h**) Stress gated SPECT images (Video 14.1e, frame 1) (SA, VLA, HLA)

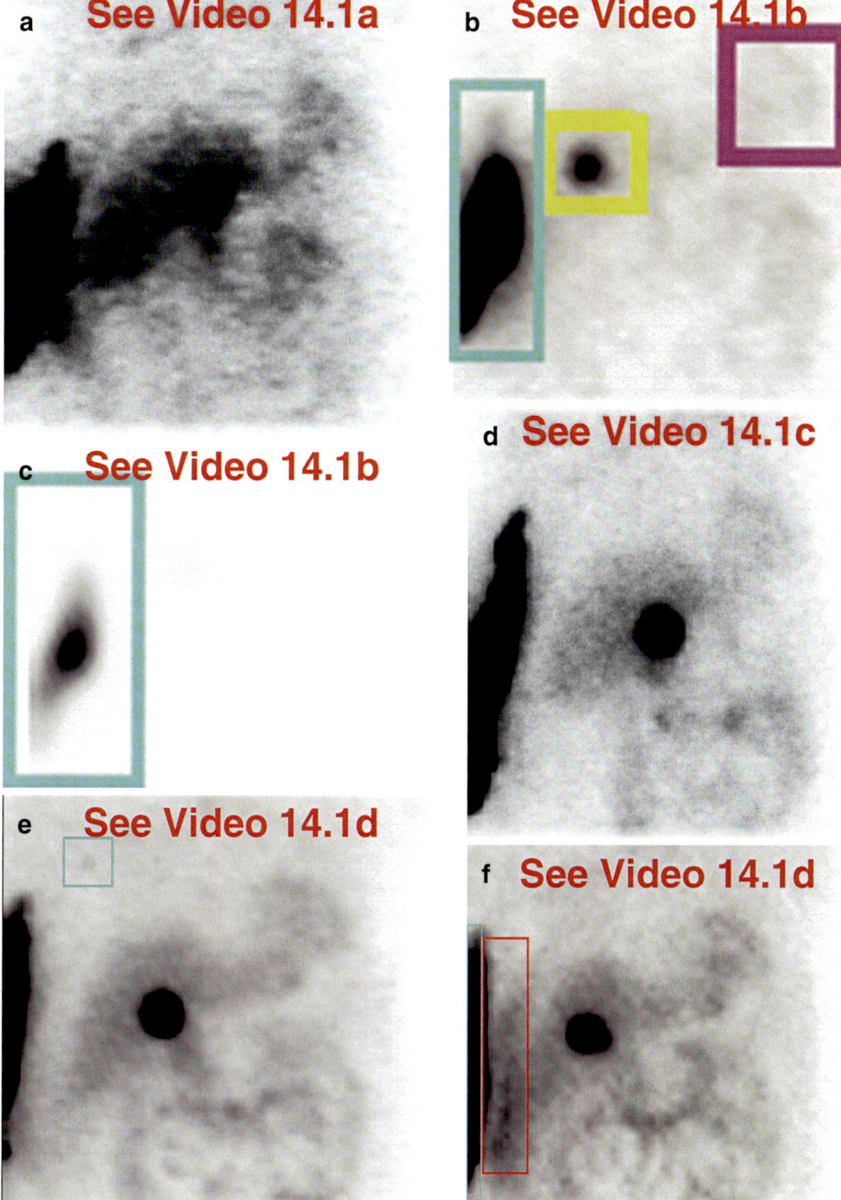
a See Video 14.1a
b See Video 14.1b
c See Video 14.1b
d See Video 14.1c
e See Video 14.1d
f See Video 14.1d

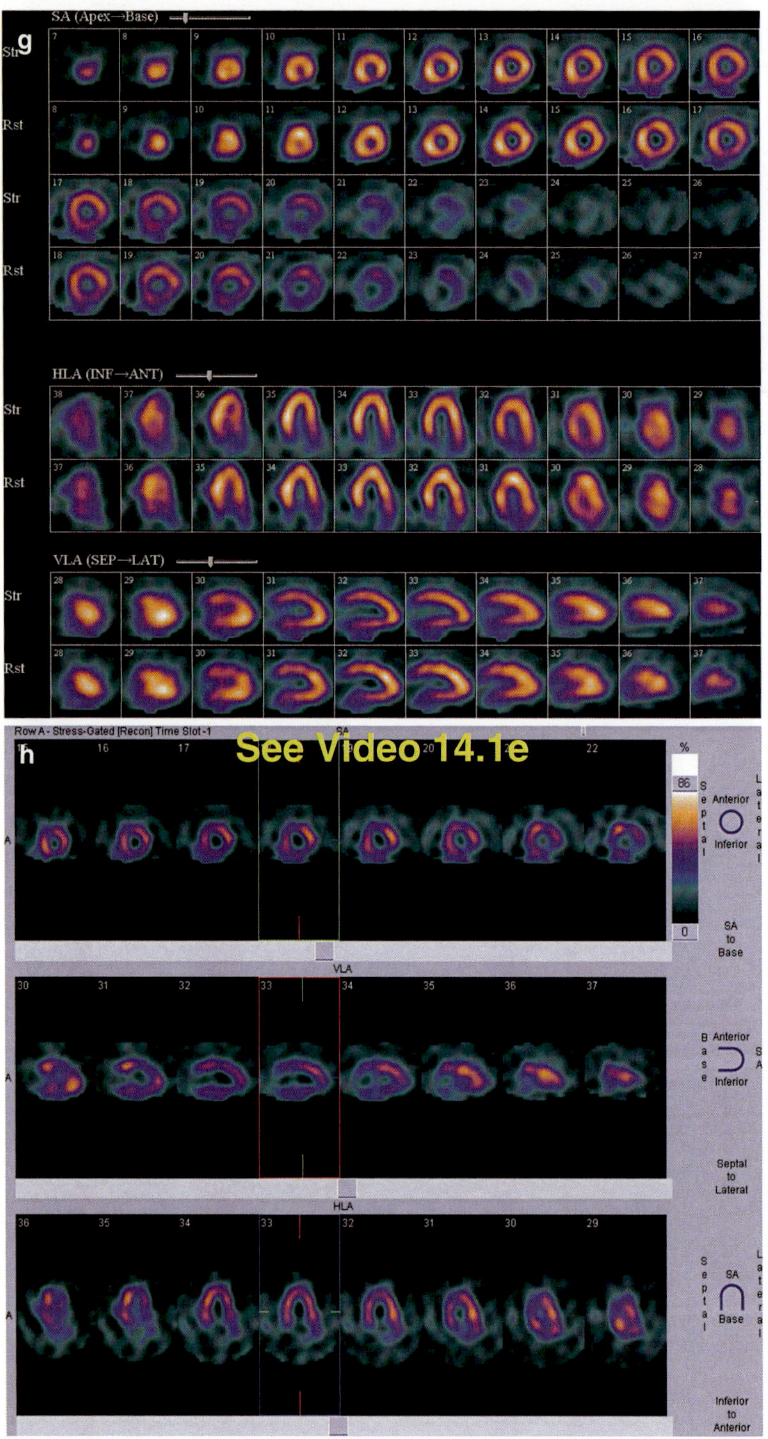

Fig. 14.1 (continued)

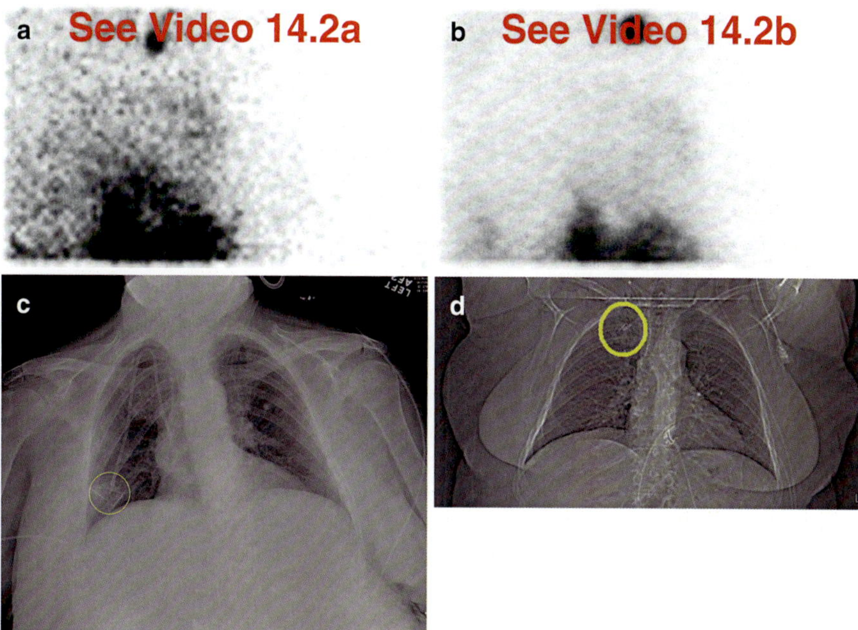

Fig. 14.2 Right chest port used for rest and stress injections, one-day protocol. This patient was receiving chemotherapy for a brain tumor. Note how the relative intensity of the discrete, round, "hot" focus at the top of the field-of-view to the right of midline changes between the initial rest injection (**a**) and the subsequent stress injection (**b**). This is due to administering three times as much radiopharmaceutical during stress compared to rest when following a one-day rest/stress protocol. For confirmation, the chest radiograph (**c**) demonstrates the implanted port, but its position is variable as shown on the scout CT of the chest (**d**); the latter more closely approximates the patient's position during image acquisition. As a standard practice, the technologists should record the site of radiopharmaceutical administration.

(**a**) Rest raw projection images (Video 14.2a, frame 1), ^{99m}Tc sestamibi. (**b**) Stress raw projection images (Video 14.2b, frame 1), ^{99m}Tc sestamibi. (**c**) AP portable chest radiograph with arms down, right-sided port (*yellow circle*). (**d**) Scout CT image of the chest with arms up (same position as MPI), right-sided port (*yellow oval*)

potential findings highlight the importance of knowing the injection site at the time of interpretation.

Apparent localized uptake in the right pulmonary arterial wall has been reported (Aras et al. 2003; Gedik et al. 2007). Markedly dilated pulmonary arteries, for example, in association with pulmonary hypertension, can appear "cold" and can be prominent (Gedik et al. 2007).

As a general approach, these technical issues need not be reported unless they are of potential clinical significance and warrant further investigation. Thus, one should explain visualization of axillary lymph nodes (refer to Chap. 15) and should qualify the examination if most of the radiopharmaceutical extravasated, rendering the scintigraphic results suspect. For the latter, a sample report could read:

Due to significant extravascular infiltration during the stress portion of the examination, the MPI is inconclusive. The patient has been rescheduled for the nuclear stress test. The rest portion of the examination need not be repeated.

Communication with the referring physician might be in order.

Key Points
- Knowledge of the injection site and the adequacy of the injection are helpful at the time of image interpretation.
- Extravasation of radiopharmaceutical can result in an incomplete intravascular injection which, in turn, can lead to a false-negative interpretation of SPECT MPI.
- Lymphatic uptake and deposition within regional lymph nodes (usually axillary) can occur after a significant extravasation.
- Implanted IV ports or central venous catheters can be used for radiopharmaceutical administration and can be a source of "hot" artifacts on the final images even if well-flushed.

Lymphatic System

15

Table 15.1 lists benign and malignant conditions affecting the lymphatic system that may be seen during SPECT MPI. Axillary lymph nodes may be visualized, particularly if the arms are positioned "up." As discussed in Chap. 14, extravasated injections result in lymphatic clearing with deposition in the axillary lymph nodes (Figs. 15.1 and 15.2) (Chamarthy and Travin 2010; Gedik et al. 2007; Gentili et al. 1994; Shih et al. 2002; Williams et al. 2003). At times, the lymphatic channels can be visualized as "hot" lines (Shih et al. 1999). Verifying extravasation is important so as not to casually attribute malignant uptake incorrectly to a benign reason.

Differential diagnosis of "hot" lymph nodes in the axilla includes malignant disease such as lymphoma or metastatic disease from ipsilateral breast cancer (Mlikotic and Mishkin 2000; Shih et al. 2002; Taillefer et al. 1995, 1998; Waxman 1997). Other lymphatic conditions include active granulomatous diseases such as untreated sarcoidosis; treated sarcoidosis does not show radiopharmaceutical avidity (Aktolun et al. 1994). On occasion, diseased lymph nodes may also be seen in the hilum, mediastinum, or supraclavicular regions (Aktolun and Bayhan 1994; Gedik et al. 2007; Williams et al. 2003).

Visualization of axillary lymph nodes might merit mention in the MPI report and may warrant personal communication with the referring physician. For example:

> Incidentally noted is abnormal radiopharmaceutical uptake by the left axillary lymph nodes. Given that the radiopharmaceutical was administered in the right arm [or, that the patient has a history of left breast cancer], this finding raises concern for nodal pathology. This finding should be investigated. Differential diagnosis includes malignancy.

Electronic supplementary material The online version of this chapter (doi:10.1007/978-3-319-25436-4_15) contains supplementary material, which is available to authorized users.

© Springer International Publishing Switzerland 2017
M.E. Oates, V.L. Sorrell, *Myocardial Perfusion Imaging - Beyond the Left Ventricle: Pathology, Artifacts and Pitfalls in the Chest and Abdomen,* DOI 10.1007/978-3-319-25436-4_15

Table 15.1 Differential diagnosis of "hot" and "cold" imaging findings related to the lymphatic system

Organ system	"Hot" finding	"Cold" finding	References
Lymphatic system	Sarcoidosis *Neoplasm, metastasis (e.g., breast carcinoma)* Lymphoma Venous extravasation resulting in visualization of axillary lymph node(s)	Necrotic lymph node(s) *Neoplasm, metastasis*	Aktolun et al. (1994) Aktolun and Bayhan (1994) Chamarthy and Travin (2010) Gedik et al. (2007) Gentili et al. (1994) Mlikotic and Mishkin (2000) Shih et al. (2002) Shih et al. (1999) Taillefer et al. (1995) Taillefer et al. (1998) Waxman (1997) Williams et al. (2003)

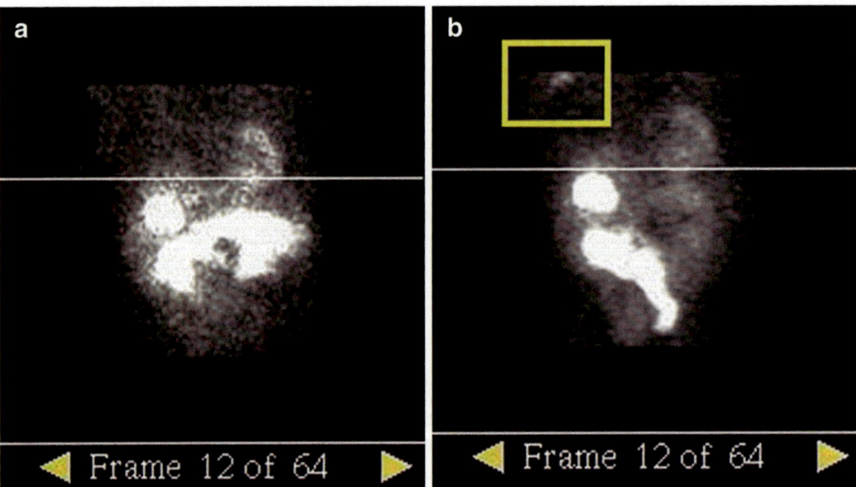

Fig. 15.1 Right axillary lymph node visualization. The right axilla appears normal on rest imaging (**a**). Extravasation at the right arm injection site during the stress test resulted in lymphatic uptake on stress imaging (**b**). Note how the right arm is raised on both acquisitions, permitting a clear view of the right axilla on the more right anterior oblique projections. Conversely, the left axilla is generally seen to better advantage on the more left anterior oblique projections (see Fig. 15.2).

(**a**) Rest raw projection image, RAO, ^{99m}Tc tetrofosmin, inferior aspect of the heart (*white line*). (**b**) Stress raw projection image, RAO, ^{99m}Tc tetrofosmin, right axillary lymph node (*yellow box*)

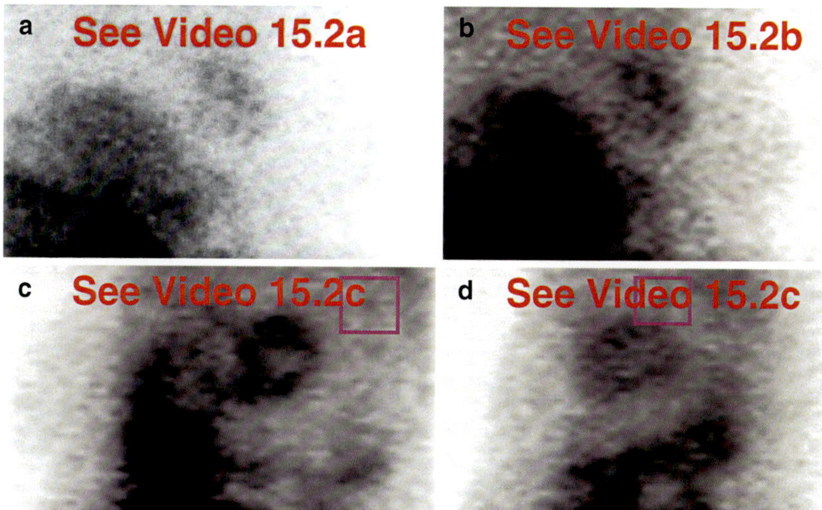

Fig. 15.2 Left axillary lymph node, subtle. Extravasation that occurred at the left arm injection site (left arm raised and out of field-of-view) led to regional lymphatic visualization. The focus is subtle on usual contrast setting to evaluate the heart and is better appreciated after contrast-adjusted rendering (**b, c, d**). This example underscores the value of manipulating the image contrast settings during the review process. Note the relatively "cold" breast tissue. Mammography and breast ultrasonography did not reveal breast cancer or axillary lymphadenopathy in this 77-year-old female.

(**a**) Stress raw projection images at usual setting for the heart (Video 15.2a, frame 1), ^{99m}Tc sestamibi. (**b**) Stress raw projection image with enhanced contrast intensity for soft tissues (Video 15.2b, frame 1), ^{99m}Tc sestamibi. (**c**) Stress raw projection image with enhanced contrast intensity for soft tissues (Video 15.2c, frame 37, LAO), ^{99m}Tc sestamibi, left axillary lymph node (*pink box*). (**d**) Stress raw projection image with enhanced contrast intensity for soft tissues (Video 15.2c, frame 51, left lateral), ^{99m}Tc sestamibi, left axillary lymph node (*pink box*)

> **Key Points**
> - Incomplete intravascular injection due to extravasation can result in lymphatic clearance with deposition in regional lymph nodes, usually axillary.
> - Verifying extravasation is important so as to not incorrectly attribute visualization of one or more lymph nodes to underlying pathology.
> - Otherwise, "hot" lymph nodes could signify malignancy or active granulomatous disease.

Diaphragm

16

The diaphragm is a large flat muscle that divides the chest and abdomen. Various conditions that affect the diaphragm may be identified on SPECT MPI raw projection image data (Table 16.1). The position of the hemidiaphragms should be noted during review. The left hemidiaphragm is a common vexing source of artifact on the reconstructed SPECT images.

When fluid is present on both sides of the diaphragm (as in pleural effusion with ascites), the hemidiaphragm(s) may be visualized as a soft-tissue structure outlined by surrounding "cold" fluid (Fig. 16.1). A high right hemidiaphragm may lead to a processing artifact when the liver is "hot" and adjacent to the heart (Burrell and MacDonald 2006). Normally, the dome of the liver has a smooth and curvilinear margin; surgical changes to the right hemidiaphragm may result in an irregular contour at the dome of the liver (Fig. 16.2). A high left hemidiaphragm may have "hot" stomach or small intestine, or even spleen or large intestine, immediately subjacent to it, leading to well-known problematic "hot" and/or "cold" processing artifacts in the inferior and inferior-lateral myocardium (Pitman et al. 2005). Eventration of the left hemidiaphragm leads to elevation into the chest with displacement of abdominal contents alongside the heart (see Fig. 22.5). Diaphragmatic hernias contain abdominal contents, including the stomach and small intestine (Chamarthy and Travin 2010; Gedik et al. 2007).

Electronic supplementary material The online version of this chapter (doi:10.1007/978-3-319-25436-4_16) contains supplementary material, which is available to authorized users.

© Springer International Publishing Switzerland 2017
M.E. Oates, V.L. Sorrell, *Myocardial Perfusion Imaging - Beyond the Left Ventricle: Pathology, Artifacts and Pitfalls in the Chest and Abdomen*, DOI 10.1007/978-3-319-25436-4_16

Table 16.1 Differential diagnosis of "hot" and "cold" imaging findings related to the diaphragm

Organ system	"Hot" finding	"Cold" finding	References
Diaphragm	Elevated liver (due to right-sided eventration) Elevated bile-containing stomach (due to left-sided eventration) Herniated small or large intestine	Muscular diaphragm (causes inferior wall attenuation artifact)	Burrell and MacDonald (2006) Chamarthy and Travin (2010) Friedman et al. (1989) Gedik et al. (2007) Hendel et al. (1999) Howarth et al. (1996) Pitman et al. (2005)

Most commonly, the inferior myocardial wall may be subjected to attenuation artifact related to the left hemidiaphragm (Fig. 16.3); this effect is particularly apparent in muscular males when imaged in the supine position. The prone position has been used to mitigate this long-recognized diaphragmatic attenuation effect (Howarth et al. 1996; Pitman et al. 2005). An alternative approach is use of attenuation correction systems; normalization of the inferior wall on the AC images supports diaphragmatic attenuation artifact rather than scar as the explanation for a fixed perfusion defect. In these cases, the inferior wall will demonstrate normal wall motion and wall thickening on gated SPECT images.

Normally, patients are quietly breathing during SPECT MPI acquisition. Coughing, talking, sleeping and snoring, and hiccups cause erratic diaphragmatic motion, which can produce characteristic motion artifact on the processed images (Fig. 16.4) (Hendel et al. 1999; Pitman et al. 2005). This is reminiscent of "upward creep" that used to be seen commonly with single-detector gamma camera systems and the use of ^{201}Tl chloride as the radiopharmaceutical (Friedman et al. 1989).

Correlation with other imaging is often helpful to define the position of the hemidiaphragms. The MPI report may need to qualify an inferior wall defect as potentially artifactual; for example, it could state:

There is a large, moderately severe, fixed inferior wall perfusion defect. On review of the raw projection data, the left hemidiaphragm appears to overlap the inferior wall. Correlation with the same-day upright chest radiograph shows a slightly elevated left hemidiaphragm. On gated SPECT images, the inferior wall has normal wall motion and wall thickening. Thus, the inferior wall perfusion defect is most likely artifactual and not representative of a true perfusion defect related to coronary artery disease.

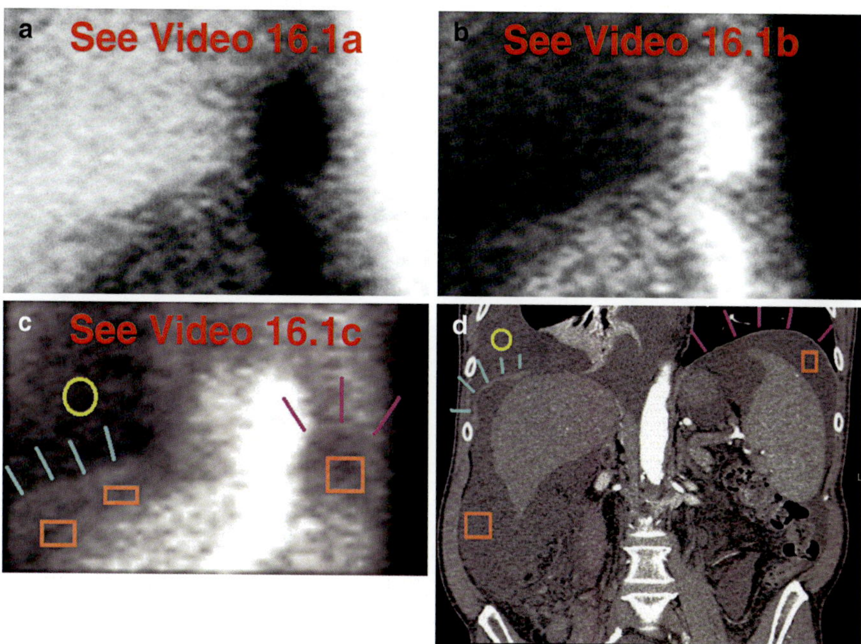

Fig. 16.1 Visualization of the right hemidiaphragm. A 61-year-old male awaits liver transplant. The right hemidiaphragm is outlined superiorly by a right pleural effusion and inferiorly by abdominal ascites (**a–d**). Right basilar atelectasis is seen (**d**). Note how the ascites and the *left* hemidiaphragm create a typical attenuation artifact in the inferior-basal wall (**e**).

(**a**) Stress "black-on-white" raw projection images (Video 16.1a, frame 1), ^{99m}Tc sestamibi. (**b**) Stress "white-on-black" raw projection images (Video 16.1b, frame 1), ^{99m}Tc sestamibi. (**c**) Stress "white-on-black" raw projection image (Video 16.1c, frame 20), ^{99m}Tc sestamibi, right pleural effusion (*yellow circle*), perihepatic and perisplenic ascites (*orange boxes*), right hemidiaphragm (*blue lines*), left hemidiaphragm (*pink lines*). (**d**) Coronal CT image at level of posterior lower chest/upper abdomen, right pleural effusion (*yellow circle*), perihepatic and perisplenic ascites (*orange boxes*), right hemidiaphragm (*blue lines*), left hemidiaphragm (*pink lines*). (**e**) Stress/rest processed SPECT images (SA, HLA, VLA), fixed inferior-basal defect normalizes on AC (*yellow ovals* and *yellow boxes* on representative SA and VLA images, respectively)

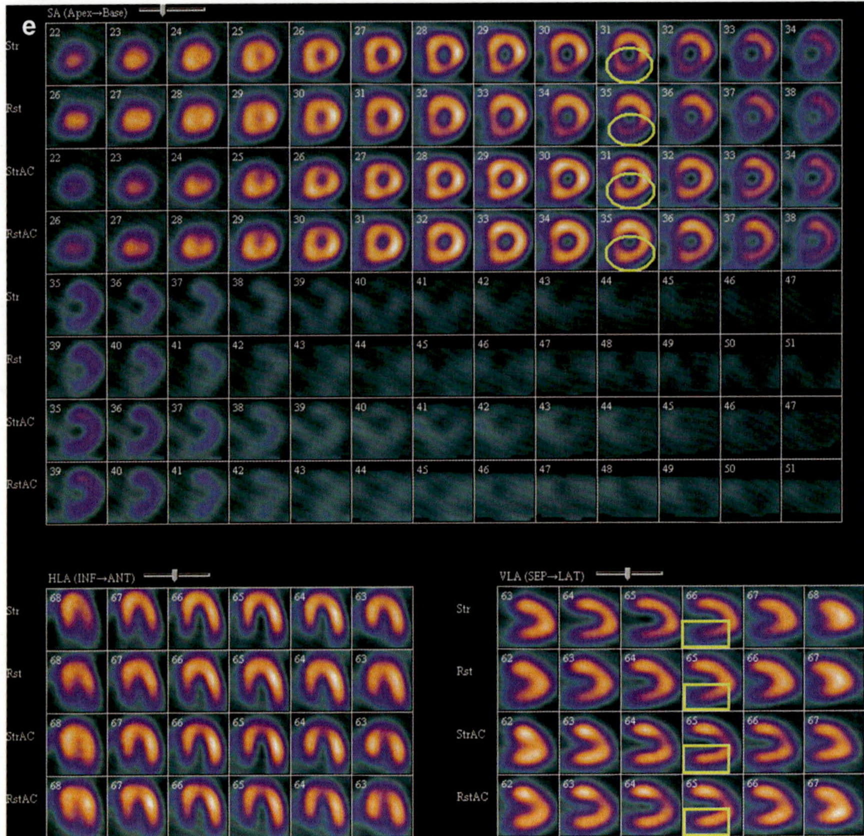

Fig. 16.1 (continued)

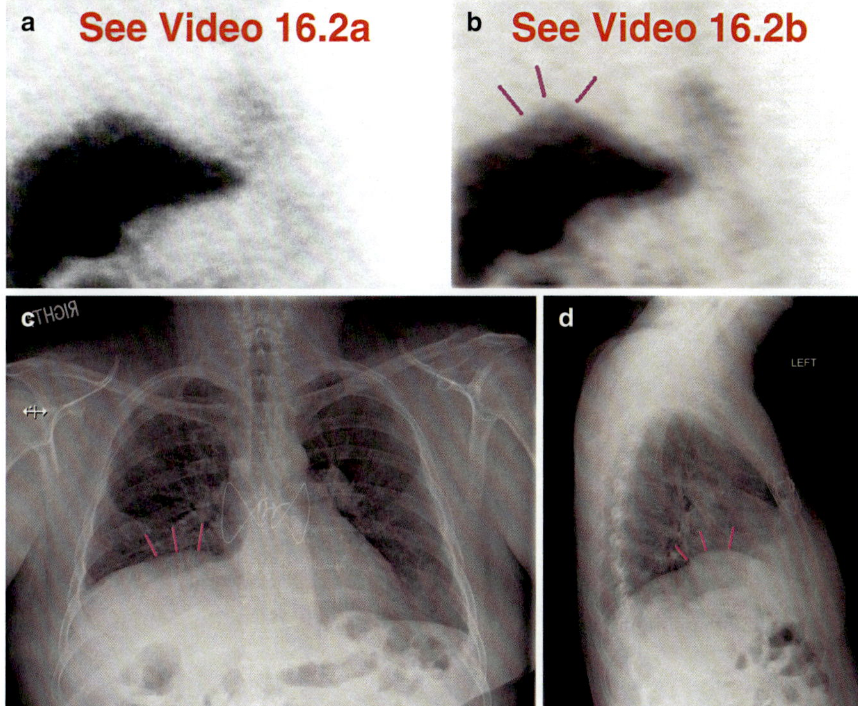

Fig. 16.2 Postoperative deformity of right hemidiaphragm. This patient underwent plication for diaphragmatic paralysis and paradoxical respiratory motion following double lung transplant for coal-miner's pneumoconiosis. The right hemidiaphragm (defined by the liver dome) appears deformed (**a**, **b**). Radiographically, it appears tented (**c**, **d**).

(**a**) Stress raw projection images (Video 16.2a, frame 1), ^{99m}Tc sestamibi. (**b**) Stress raw projection image (Video 16.2b, frame 3), ^{99m}Tc sestamibi, deformity (*pink lines*). (**c**) PA chest radiograph, deformity (*pink lines*). (**d**) Lateral chest radiograph, deformity (*pink lines*)

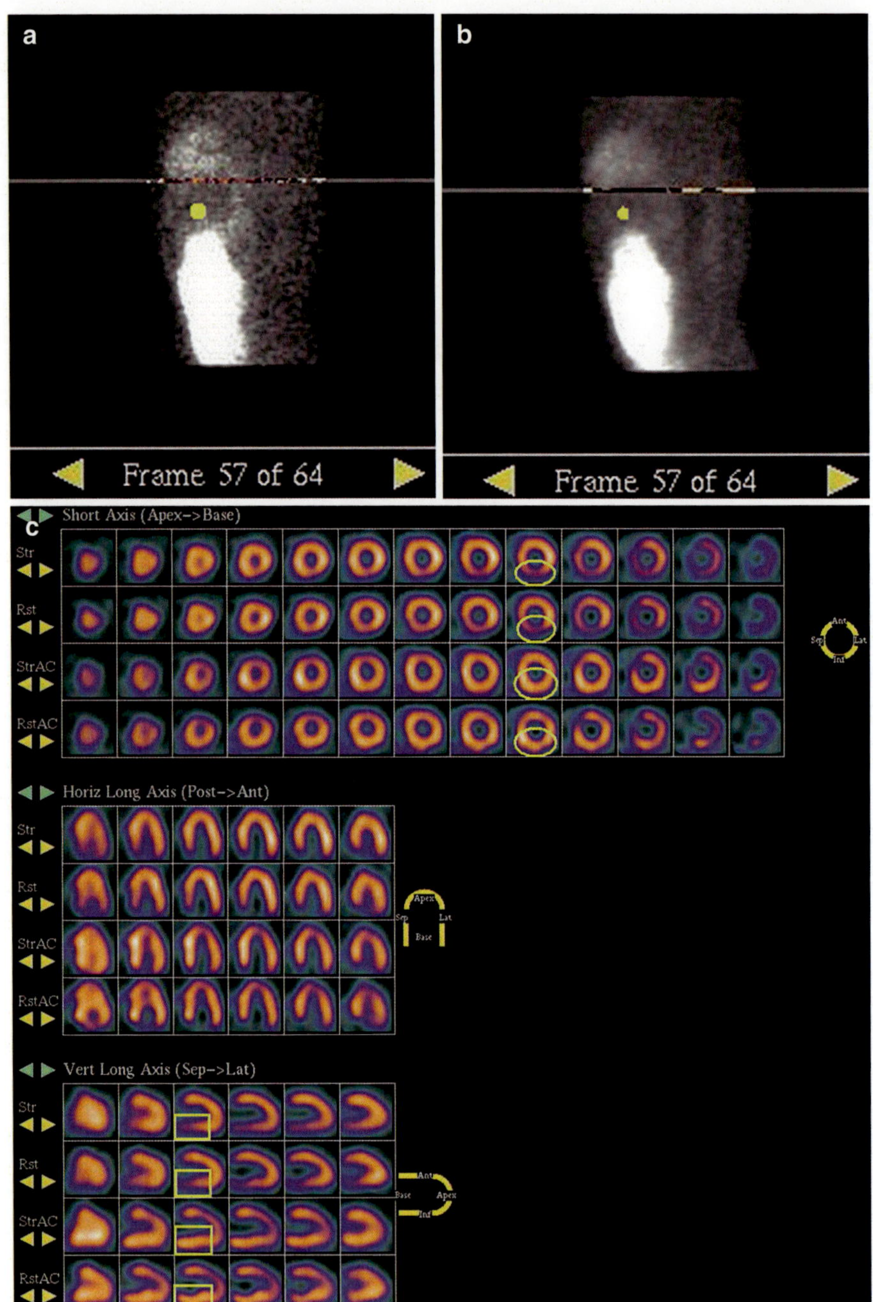
a
Frame 57 of 64
b
Frame 57 of 64
c
Short Axis (Apex->Base)
Str
Rst
StrAC
RstAC
Ant
Sep
Lat
Inf
Horiz Long Axis (Post->Ant)
Str
Rst
StrAC
RstAC
Apex
Sep
Lat
Base
Vert Long Axis (Sep->Lat)
Str
Rst
StrAC
RstAC
Ant
Base
Apex
Inf

Fig. 16.3 Diaphragmatic attenuation artifact of inferior and inferior-basal wall. For ease of review, the position of the left hemidiaphragm can be demarcated by a line on the images; note the subjacent "cold" stomach as a landmark (**a, b**). There is a characteristic fixed perfusion defect on stress and rest non-AC images that normalizes completely on AC images (**c**). Compare this approach of reviewing the raw projection data in static format to using the more desirable cinematic display (as in Figs. 16.1 and 16.2).

(**a**) Rest raw projection image, ^{99m}Tc sestamibi, left hemidiaphragm (*white line*), fluid-filled "cold" stomach (*yellow dot*). (**b**) Stress raw projection image, ^{99m}Tc sestamibi, left hemidiaphragm (*white line*), fluid-filled "cold" stomach (*yellow dot*). (**c**) Stress/rest processed SPECT images (SA, HLA, VLA), fixed inferior and inferior-basal defect normalizes on AC (*yellow ovals* and *yellow boxes* on representative SA and VLA images, respectively)

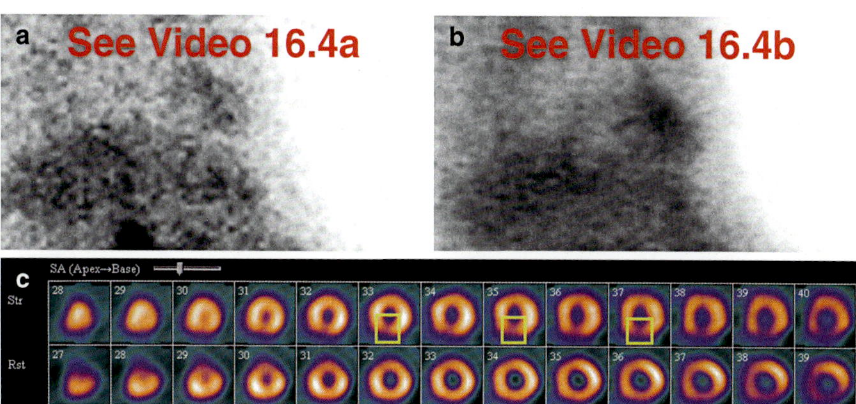

Fig. 16.4 Intractable hiccups. This patient was breathing normally during the rest acquisition (**a**), but developed intractable hiccups during the stress acquisition (**b**). Despite the hiccups, there is only a modest effect on the quality of the processed SPECT images (**c**): compare slightly blurry stress images to sharp rest images. Note a small, likely artifactual reversible defect in the inferior wall (**c**).

(**a**) Rest raw projection images (Video 16.4a, frame 1), ^{99m}Tc sestamibi. (**b**) Stress raw projection images (Video 16.4b, frame 1), ^{99m}Tc sestamibi. (**c**) Stress/rest processed SPECT images (SA), inferior wall defect (*yellow boxes*) on selected stress images

Key Points
- Elevation of the left or right hemidiaphragms due to postsurgical changes in anatomical relationships, diaphragmatic eventration, or congenital anatomic variations can result in "hot" and/or "cold" processing artifacts.
- A high right hemidiaphragm can cause processing artifacts affecting the septal, apical, and inferior myocardial wall segments.
- A high left hemidiaphragm can cause similar artifacts affecting the inferior and inferolateral myocardial wall segments.
- Cinematic evaluation of the raw projection images is helpful in detecting erratic diaphragmatic motion due to hiccups, talking, laughing, coughing, or snoring.

Part III

The Abdomen ("Below the Diaphragm")

17

As in Chap. 7, "cold" imaging findings related to the abdominal wall occur much more commonly than do "hot" findings. Table 17.1 lists these potential sources of "hot" and "cold" findings on SPECT MPI. Technical- or patient-related "hot" artifacts are caused by contamination that occurs during or after radiopharmaceutical administration or from excreted urinary activity (Fig. 17.1) (Burrell and MacDonald 2006).

"Cold" patient-related artifacts may be superimposed over the abdomen and they should be removed before imaging whenever possible. The patient's arms should be raised or, if that is not possible, positioned alongside the body; ideally, the arms should be superimposed on the body only when the patient is unable to cooperate (Fig. 17.2). Some "cold" artifacts are medical-related and removable such as telemetry monitors, while others are related to a gamma camera system damage or malfunction such as a cracked crystal or a non-functioning photomultiplier tube (Burrell and MacDonald 2006; Chamarthy and Travin 2010; Hendel et al. 1999). The latter require immediate recognition and call to the service engineer for replacement or repair to prevent recurrent artifacts.

The report need not mention the abdominal wall artifact unless deemed significant. Here is an example:

> The patient's left arm could not be raised during imaging because of limited mobility. However, the examination is of diagnostic quality.

Electronic supplementary material The online version of this chapter (doi:10.1007/978-3-319-25436-4_17) contains supplementary material, which is available to authorized users.

© Springer International Publishing Switzerland 2017
M.E. Oates, V.L. Sorrell, *Myocardial Perfusion Imaging - Beyond the Left Ventricle: Pathology, Artifacts and Pitfalls in the Chest and Abdomen,* DOI 10.1007/978-3-319-25436-4_17

Table 17.1 Differential diagnosis of "hot" and "cold" imaging findings related to the abdominal wall

Organ system	"Hot" finding	"Cold" finding	References
Abdominal Wall	Contamination (radiopharmaceutical, urine)	Internal metal objects (implanted devices) External metal objects (jewelry, coin, key, belt buckle) Arms by sides and superimposed on abdominal wall (positioning) Cracked crystal Malfunctioning photomultiplier tube	Burrell and MacDonald (2006) Chamarthy and Travin (2010) Hendel et al. (1999)

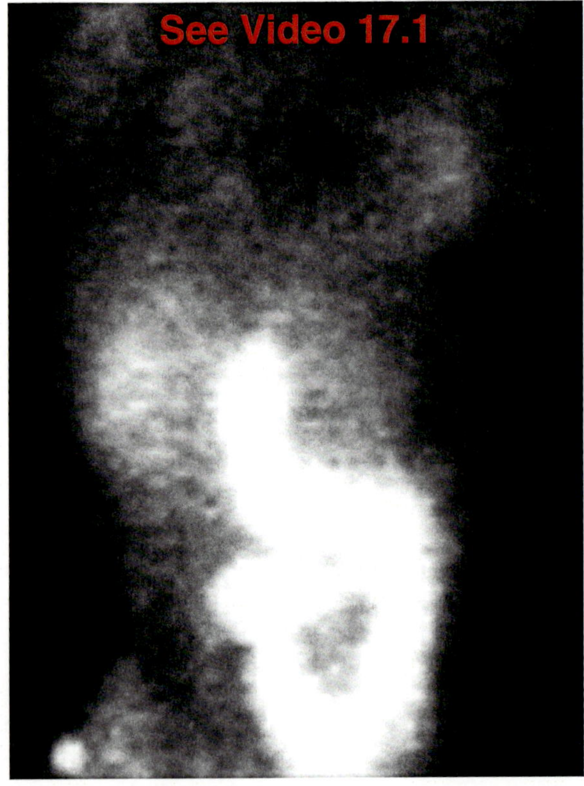

Fig. 17.1 "Hot" radiopharmaceutical or radioactive urine droplet. There is a discrete, intense, round, "hot" focus that lies outside the right lower abdominal wall. Likely culprits include contamination on a sheet/blanket covering the patient during imaging or on her clothing/skin. Note to reader: this is the same cinematic image shown in Fig. 6.2—did you notice this incidental finding when reviewing that case? Stress raw projection images (Video 17.1a, frame 1), ^{99m}Tc sestamibi

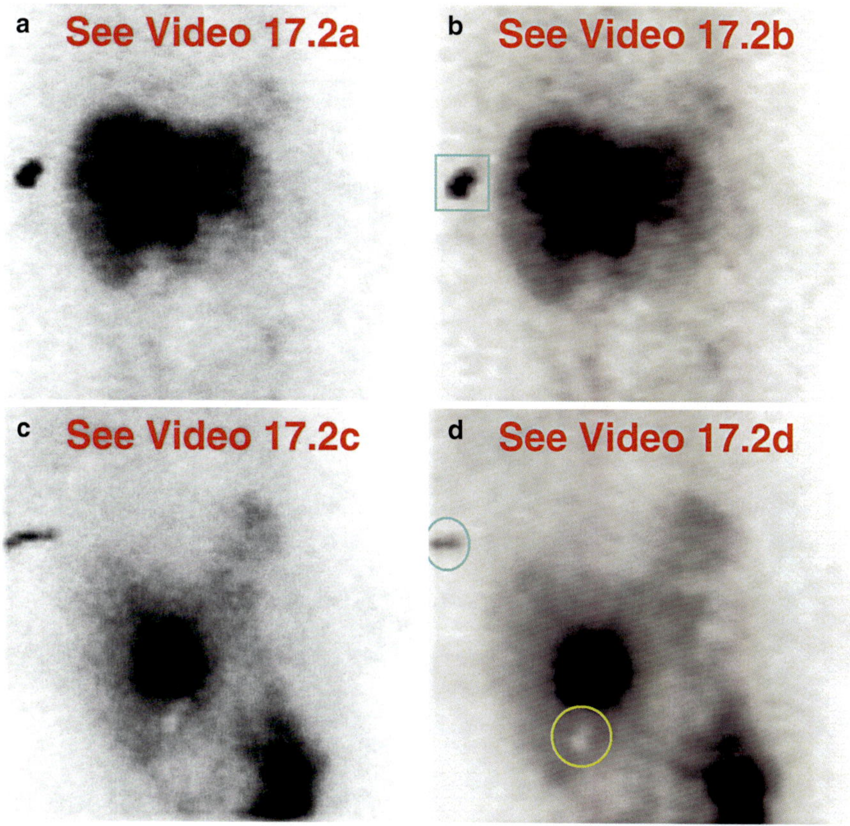

Fig. 17.2 Constellation of "hot" and "cold" findings. There is a "hot" injection site in the right antecubital fossa (**a–d**). The arms and rings on the fingers of the right hand appear "cold" (**a, c, d, e**). A 57-year-old female could not raise her arms due to severe rheumatoid arthritis; consequently, her arms are positioned along her sides with her hands across her upper abdominal wall. Sandwiched between the heart and the detectors, her left arm is a potential source of attenuation artifact. The SPECT data (**f**) show a mild, fixed inferior and inferolateral defect that demonstrates normal wall motion and wall thickening on gated SPECT (**g**). This represents a minimal artifactual effect. Note that there is a "dead zone" on the stress raw data (**c**); this acquisition artifact occasionally occurs when one of the detectors cannot get close enough to the patient.

(**a**) Rest raw projection images (Video 17.2a, frame 1), ^{99m}Tc sestamibi. (**b**) Rest raw projection images (Video 17.2b, frame 1), ^{99m}Tc sestamibi, "hot" injection site (*blue circle*). (**c**) Stress raw projection images (Video 17.2c, frame 1), ^{99m}Tc sestamibi. (**d**) Stress raw projection image (Video 17.2d, frame 4), ^{99m}Tc sestamibi, "cold" rings on right hand (*yellow circle*), "hot" injection site (*blue oval*). (**e**) Stress raw projection image (Video 17.2d, frame 59), ^{99m}Tc sestamibi, left arm (*inside pink lines*). (**f**) Stress/rest processed SPECT images (SA, VLA, HLA), mild, fixed inferior and inferolateral defect (*yellow boxes* on representative VLA and HLA images). (**g**) Stress gated SPECT images (Video 17.2e, frame 1) (SA, VLA, HLA)

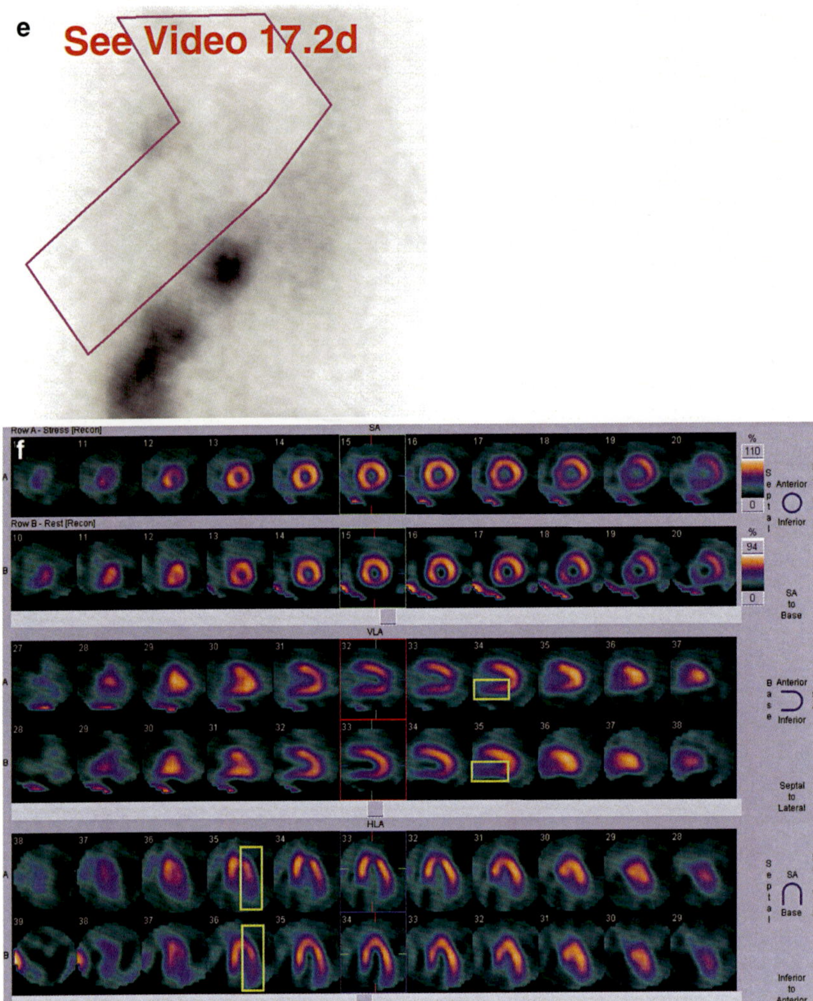

Fig. 17.2 (continued)

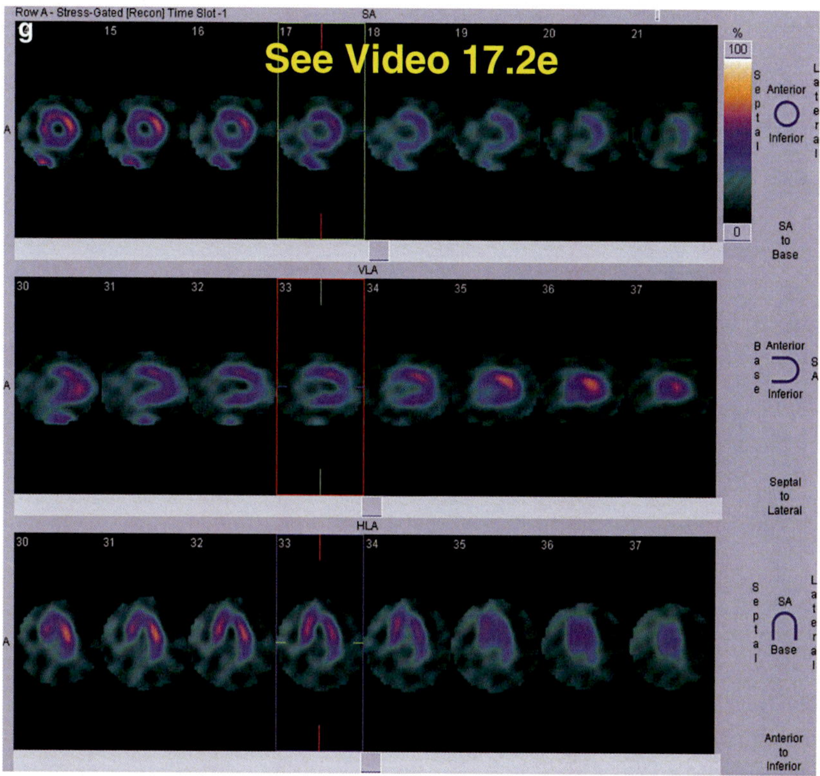

Fig. 17.2 (continued)

Key Points
- "Hot" artifacts affecting the abdominal wall are mostly related to radio-pharmaceutical or radioactive urine contamination.
- "Cold" artifacts are generally patient-related or due to gamma camera damage or malfunction.

Peritoneum 18

Peritoneal findings generally relate to the presence of free fluid (Table 18.1). Ascites appears "cold" and may cause an attenuation artifact typically affecting the inferior myocardial wall (Chamarthy and Travin 2010; Raza et al. 2005a, b; Shih et al. 2002, 2005; Tallaj et al. 2000; Williams et al. 2003). The volume of ascites in decompensated liver disease may vary significantly (Figs. 18.1, 18.2, and 18.3). Ascites separates the liver dome from the diaphragm on the right side, and the spleen may be displaced inferiorly by ascitic fluid under the left hemidiaphragm. The loops of the small intestine may float more centrally in large volume ascites (Fig. 18.3). Associated findings in cirrhosis include small liver, large spleen, gastric wall uptake (due to gastropathy), and pleural effusion(s) (Joy et al. 2007; Tallaj et al. 2000).

While the presence of ascites will almost always be known, the MPI report should mention it. The report might state:

> The rest and stress raw projection images demonstrate photopenia in the abdominal cavity and under the left hemidiaphragm, consistent with ascites. The liver appears small and the spleen is enlarged. This constellation of imaging findings correlates with the patient's known non-alcoholic steatohepatitis (NASH). There is a fixed inferior and inferior-lateral-basal perfusion defect on non-attenuation-corrected SPECT images that normalizes on the attenuation-corrected SPECT images, consistent with attenuation artifact related to the ascites.

Electronic supplementary material The online version of this chapter (doi:10.1007/978-3-319-25436-4_18) contains supplementary material, which is available to authorized users.

© Springer International Publishing Switzerland 2017
M.E. Oates, V.L. Sorrell, *Myocardial Perfusion Imaging - Beyond the Left Ventricle: Pathology, Artifacts and Pitfalls in the Chest and Abdomen*, DOI 10.1007/978-3-319-25436-4_18

Table 18.1 Differential diagnosis of "hot" and "cold" imaging findings related to the peritoneum

Organ system	"Hot" finding	"Cold" finding	References
Peritoneum	Not reported	Ascites (decompensated cirrhosis, malignancy) Peritoneal dialysate	Chamarthy and Travin (2010) Joy et al. (2007) Raza et al. (2005a, b) Shih et al. (2002, 2005) Tallaj et al. (2000) Williams et al. (2003)

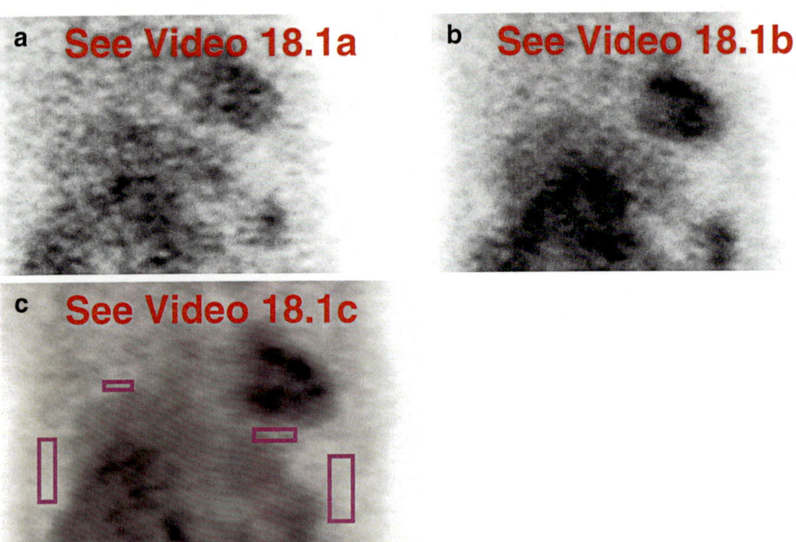

Fig. 18.1 "Cold" ascites. A 34-year-old female has cirrhosis. The abdominal ascites appears photopenic ("cold") (**a–c**). Note how the ascitic fluid outlines the abnormal viscera (small liver, "hot" stomach, enlarged spleen). On processed images (**d**), the ascites produces minimal attenuation artifact on the inferolateral-basal wall (more on the lower dosage rest images compared to the higher dosage stress images), and the examination is essentially normal. On gated images (**e**), all walls move and thicken normally. Even a moderate amount of ascites does not necessarily affect processing nor create a significant artifact, but it can produce striking effects in some patients.

(**a**) Rest raw projection images (Video 18.1a, frame 1), ^{99m}Tc sestamibi. (**b**) Stress raw projection images (Video 18.1b, frame 1), ^{99m}Tc sestamibi. (**c**) Stress raw projection image (Video 18.1c, frame 9), ^{99m}Tc sestamibi, ascites (*pink boxes*). (**d**) Stress/rest processed SPECT images (SA, HLA, VLA) (without and with AC). (**e**) Stress and rest gated SPECT images (Video 18.1d, frame 1) (SA, VLA, HLA)

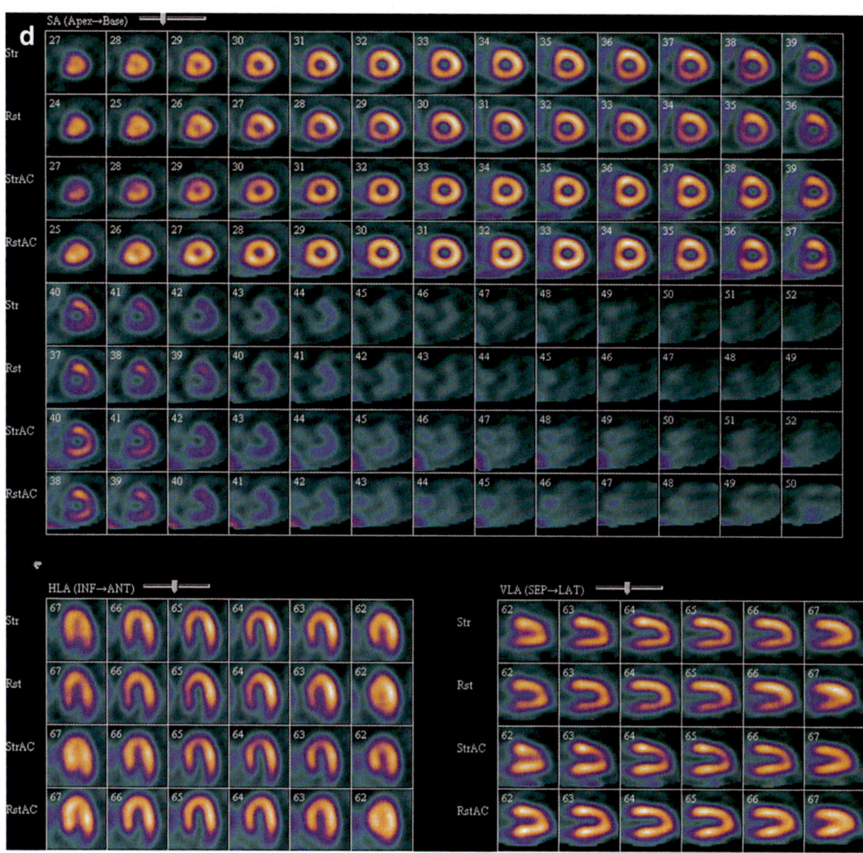

Fig. 18.1 (continued)

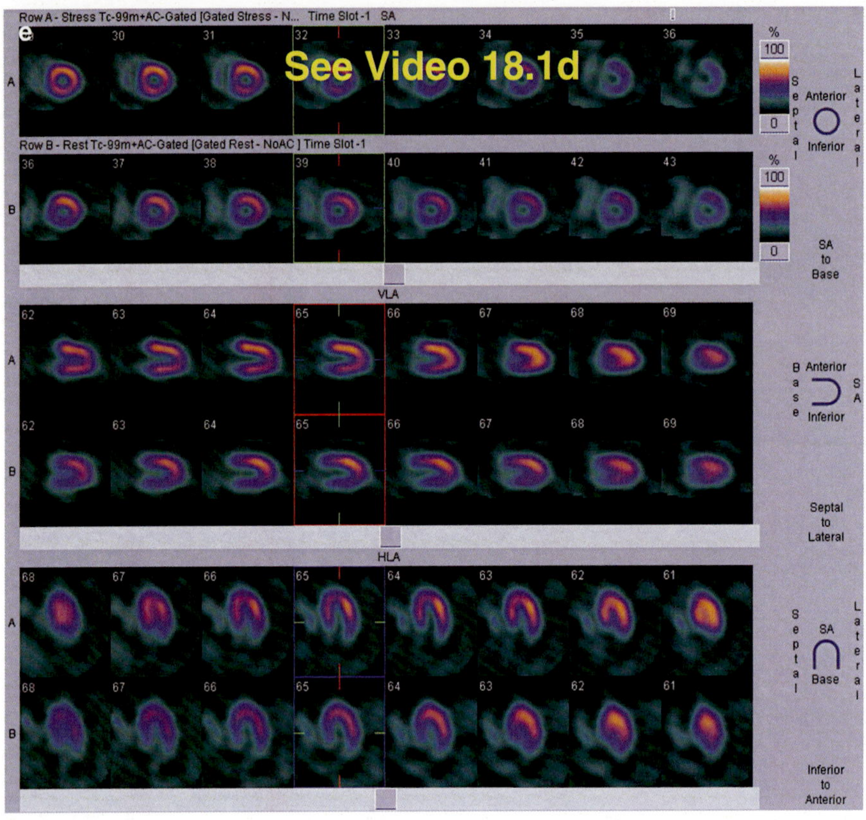

Fig. 18.1 (continued)

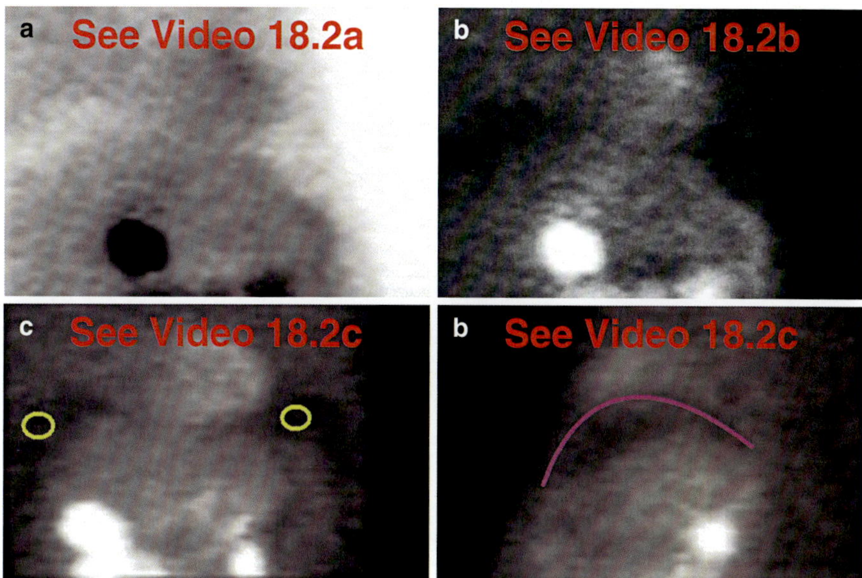

Fig. 18.2 More severe "cold" ascites. A 28-year-old male awaits liver and kidney transplants. Note how the "cold" findings may be easier to discern by adjusting the color display (**a–c**). The inferior and inferobasal wall attenuation artifact is related to a high left hemidiaphragm and the ascites beneath (**d, e**). Gated SPECT images (**f**) are normal.

(**a**) Stress "black-on-white" raw projection images (Video 18.2a, frame 1), ^{99m}Tc sestamibi. (**b**) Stress "white-on-black" raw projection images (Video 18.2b, frame 1), ^{99m}Tc sestamibi. (**c**) Stress "white-on-black" raw projection image (Video 18.2c, frame 20), ^{99m}Tc sestamibi, ascites (*yellow circles*). (**d**) Stress "white-on-black" raw projection image (Video 18.2c, frame 61), ^{99m}Tc sestamibi, left hemidiaphragm (*pink arc*). (**e**) Stress/rest processed SPECT images (SA, HLA, VLA) (without and with AC), fixed inferior and inferobasal defect normalizes on AC (*yellow ovals* and *yellow boxes* on representative SA and VLA images, respectively). (**f**) Stress and rest gated SPECT images (Video 18.2d, frame 1) (SA, VLA, HLA)

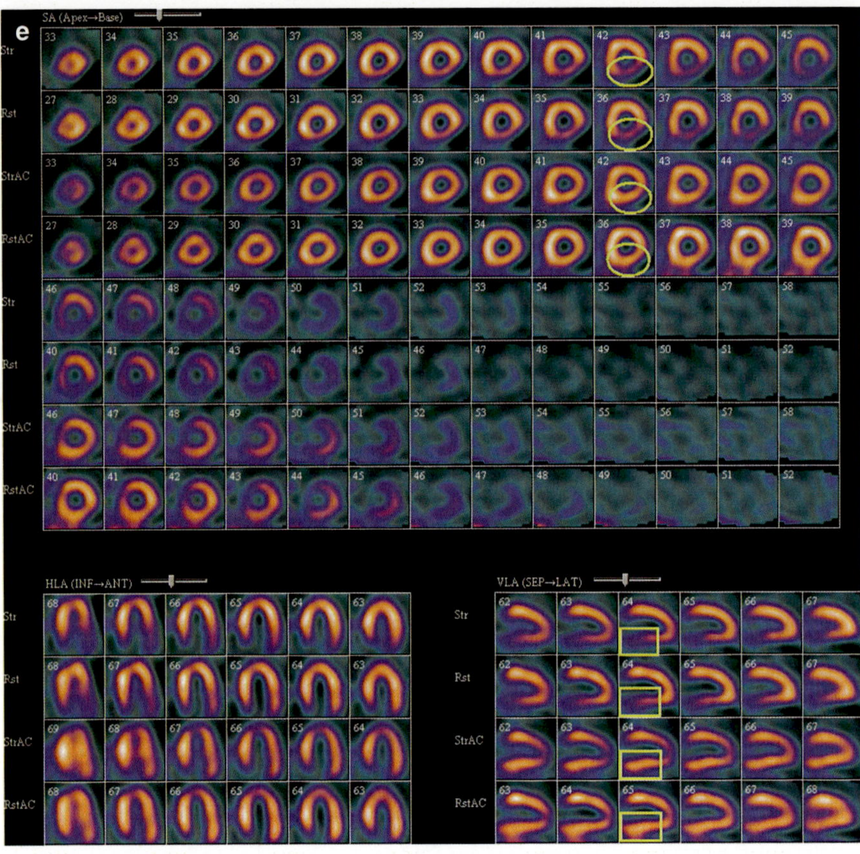

Fig. 18.2 (continued)

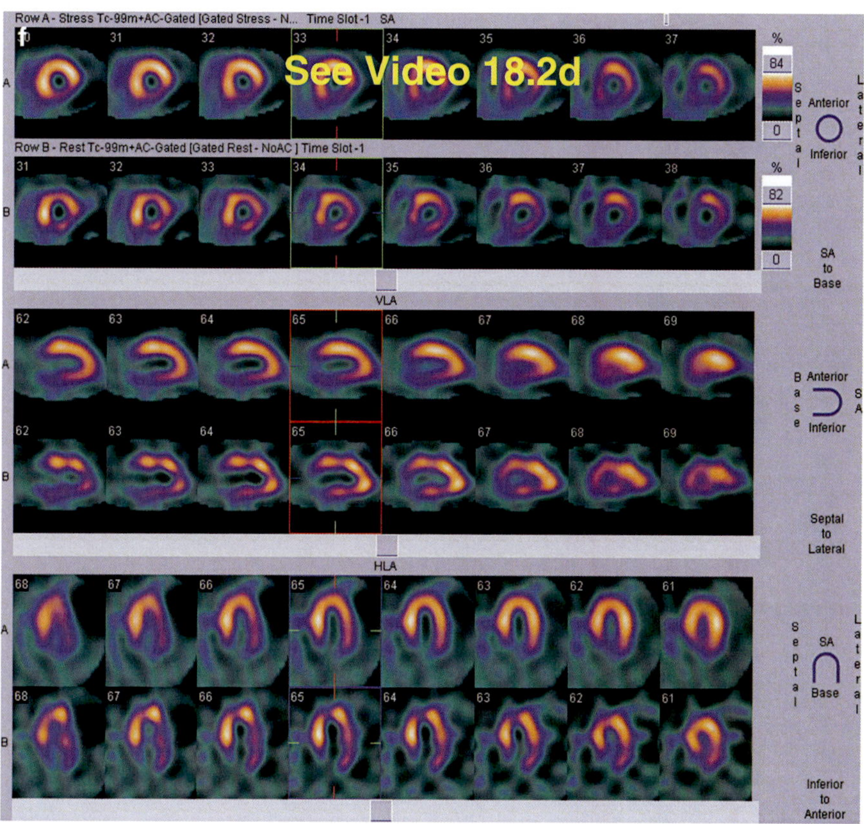

Fig. 18.2 (continued)

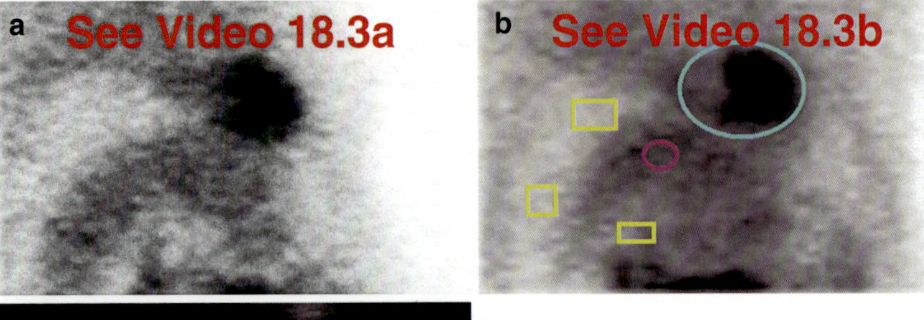

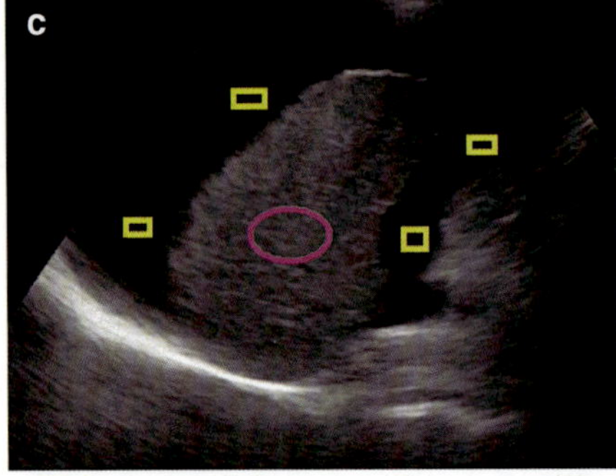

Fig. 18.3 Marked ascites in advanced cirrhosis. Ascites surrounds a shrunken liver (**a–c**). Note splenomegaly (**a**).

(**a**) Stress raw projection images (Video 18.3a, frame 1), ^{99m}Tc sestamibi. (**b**) Stress raw projection image (Video 18.3b, frame 16), ^{99m}Tc sestamibi, perihepatic ascites (*yellow boxes*), liver (*pink oval*), heart for reference (*blue oval*). (**c**) Ultrasonography through liver, ascites (*yellow boxes*), liver (*pink oval*)

> **Key Points**
> - Peritoneal findings generally relate to the presence of free fluid.
> - An understanding of the constellation of findings associated with advanced liver disease is helpful for image interpretation and reporting.

Liver

19

There are many conditions that can be identified in the liver (Table 19.1). The liver is the primary route of clearance of the ^{99m}Tc MPI radiopharmaceuticals and should be visualized to some degree on all SPECT MPI raw data. The degree of visualization depends on liver function, interval between radiopharmaceutical administration and imaging, and type of stress.

Table 19.1 Differential diagnosis of "hot" and "cold" imaging findings related to the liver

Organ system	"Hot" finding	"Cold" finding	References
Liver	Slow physiologic clearance Hepatomegaly Misshapen dome (elevated right hemidiaphragm) Intrahepatic gallbladder Pericholecystic rim sign (acute cholecystitis) *Neoplasm, primary (hepatocellular carcinoma)* *Neoplasm, metastasis (e.g., colon carcinoma)*	Rapid physiologic clearance Cyst/hydatid cyst Post-thermal ablation cyst Polycystic disease *Neoplasm, primary* *Neoplasm, metastasis* Postoperative change	Bhambhvani et al. (2010a, b) Burrell and MacDonald (2006) Chamarthy and Travin (2010) Chatziioannou et al. (1999) Fukushima et al. (1997) Gedik et al. (2007) Ghanbarinia et al. (2008) Hardebeck et al. (2013) Howarth et al. (1996) Joy et al. (2007) Lamont et al. (1996) Raza et al. (2005a, b) Shih et al. (2002, 2005) Tallaj et al. (2000)

Electronic supplementary material The online version of this chapter (doi:10.1007/978-3-319-25436-4_19) contains supplementary material, which is available to authorized users.

© Springer International Publishing Switzerland 2017

M.E. Oates, V.L. Sorrell, *Myocardial Perfusion Imaging - Beyond the Left Ventricle: Pathology, Artifacts and Pitfalls in the Chest and Abdomen,*
DOI 10.1007/978-3-319-25436-4_19

The liver may be diffusely "hot" when there is poor physiologic clearance due to underlying liver disease (Fig. 19.1). An enlarged liver (often accompanied by splenic enlargement) is seen in a variety of liver diseases and may displace other organs (Fig. 19.2) (Ghanbarinia et al. 2008; Raza et al. 2005a, b; Shih et al. 2005). A diffusely "hot" liver, especially when associated with a high right hemidiaphragm, may create processing artifacts, particularly affecting the inferior or inferoseptal myocardial walls, and may require waiting and re-imaging to allow for liver clearance (Fig. 19.3) (Burrell and MacDonald 2006; Howarth et al. 1996). Left ventricular uptake may be falsely increased by "bleeding in" or falsely decreased by normalization of the processed image data (Fig. 19.3) (Burrell and MacDonald 2006).

The shape and size of the liver can be readily evaluated. The right lobe can have an unusual configuration due to elevation of the right hemidiaphragm (Shih et al. 2002). Conversely, a flattened dome (depressed right hemidiaphragm) suggests hyperinflation of the lungs (see Chap. 10, Figs. 10.3, 10.4, and 10.5) (Shih et al. 2002). The left lobe can normally extend into the left upper quadrant (Fig. 19.4); in such cases, it may be misconstrued as gastric activity and it may create processing artifacts.

The degree of uptake within a hepatic neoplasm is variable. Such a lesion may appear relatively "hot" compared to the adjacent normal liver (Fukushima et al. 1997). Focal "hot" lesions may be appreciated on careful review of the raw projection data. Correlation with clinical history and other imaging is paramount as these may represent benign or malignant primary or metastatic lesions (Bhambhvani et al. 2010a, b; Chamarthy and Travin 2010; Chatziioannou et al. 1999; Gedik et al. 2007; Ghanbarinia et al. 2008; Hardebeck et al. 2013). An unusual cause for focal increased uptake in the liver reflects inflammatory changes adjacent to an inflamed gallbladder, the so-called pericholecystic rim sign which is strongly correlated with complicated acute cholecystitis. The gallbladder should not be visualized if this is indeed the underlying pathology (Lamont et al. 1996).

The liver may be faintly visible ("cold") if there is good physiologic clearance (Fig. 19.5). Depending on time intervals, liver clearance may be different between the rest and stress images (Fig. 19.6). Treadmill exercise generally results in less

---

Fig. 19.1 Diffusely "hot" liver. An obese 42-year-old female has hepatitis C and abnormal liver function tests. The liver is diffusely "hot" without focal lesions (**a–c**). Note that the right breast overlying the liver creates a characteristic curvilinear "cold" artifact (**a–c**). The "hot" liver activity can be seen adjacent to the inferoseptal wall on the processed data but does not create a "hot" or "cold" artifact (**d, e**). The left breast overlies the entirety of the heart on both image sets (**a, b**).

(**a**) Day 1: stress raw projection images (Video 19.1a, frame 1), ^{99m}Tc sestamibi. (**b**) Day 2: rest raw projection images (Video 19.1b, frame 1), ^{99m}Tc sestamibi. (**c**) Day 1: stress raw projection image (Video 19.1c, frame 6), ^{99m}Tc sestamibi, right breast (*pink arc*). (**d**) Stress/rest processed SPECT images (SA, HLA, VLA) (without and with AC), selected stress and rest non-AC SA images, liver activity (*white boxes*). (**e**) Gated stress and rest SPECT images (Video 19.1d, frame 1) (SA, VLA, HLA)

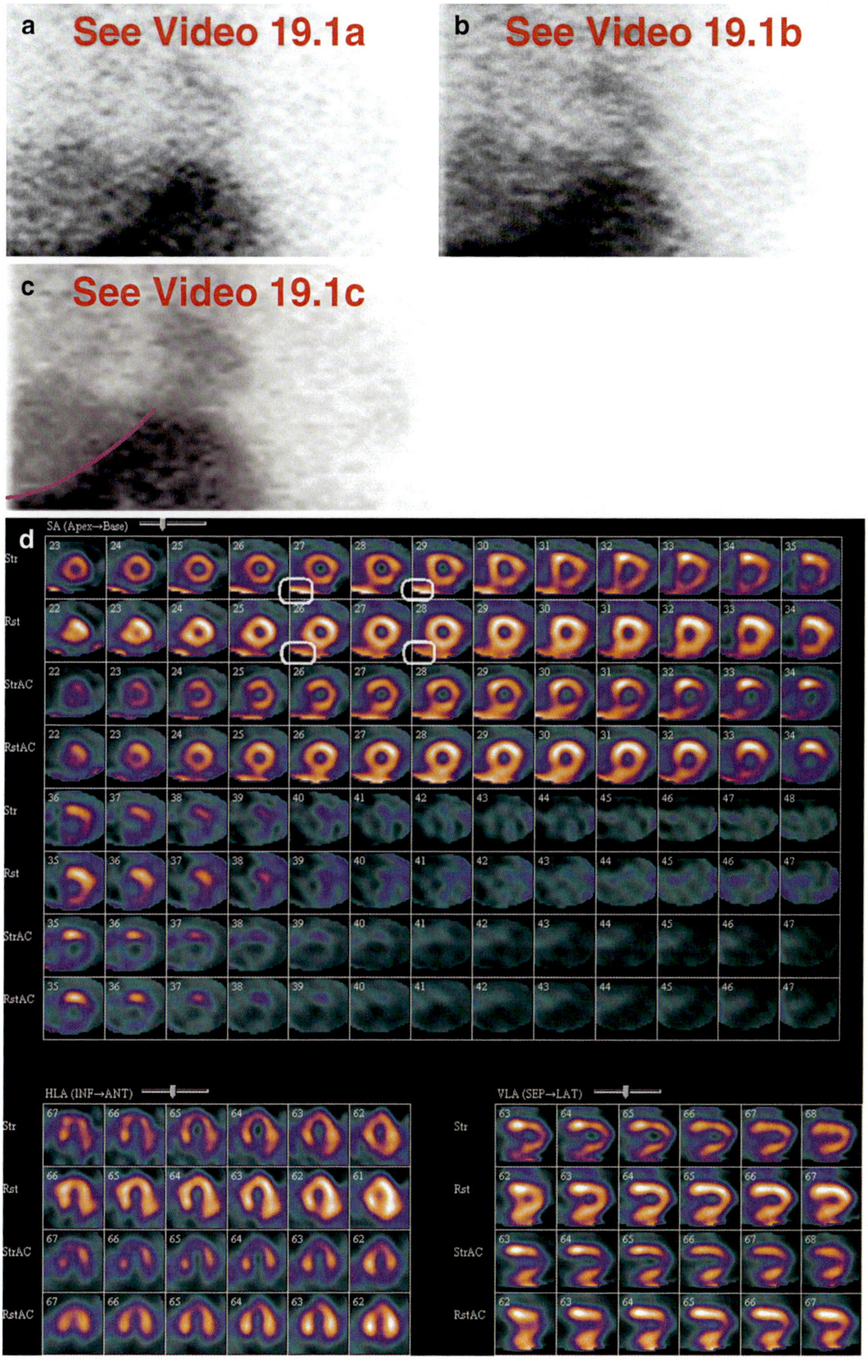

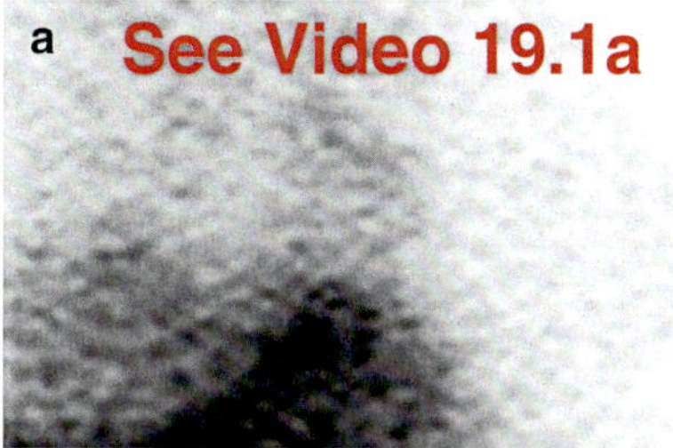
a
See Video 19.1a

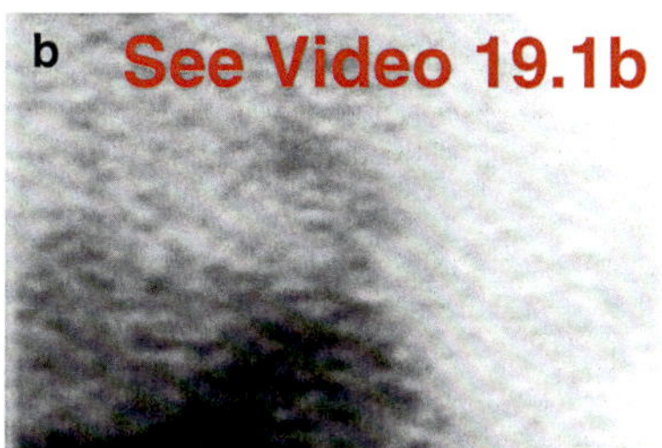
b
See Video 19.1b

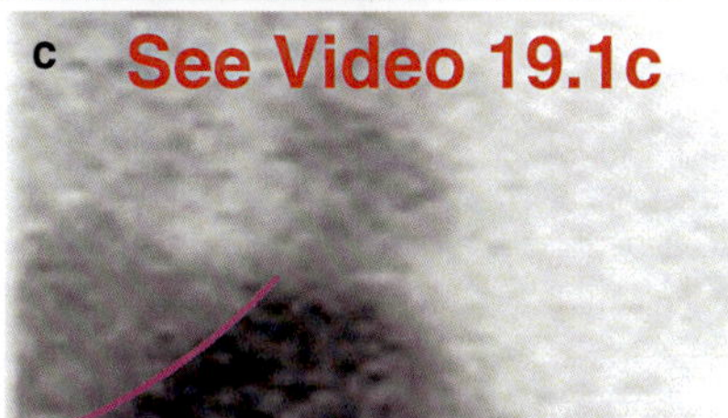
c
See Video 19.1c

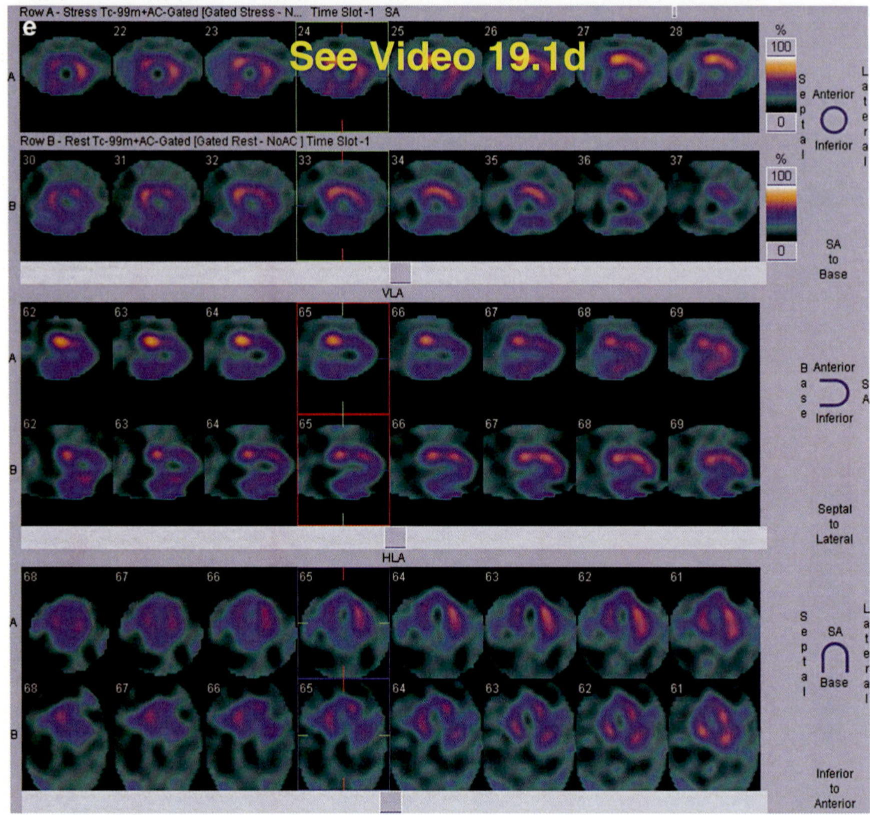

Fig. 19.1 (continued)

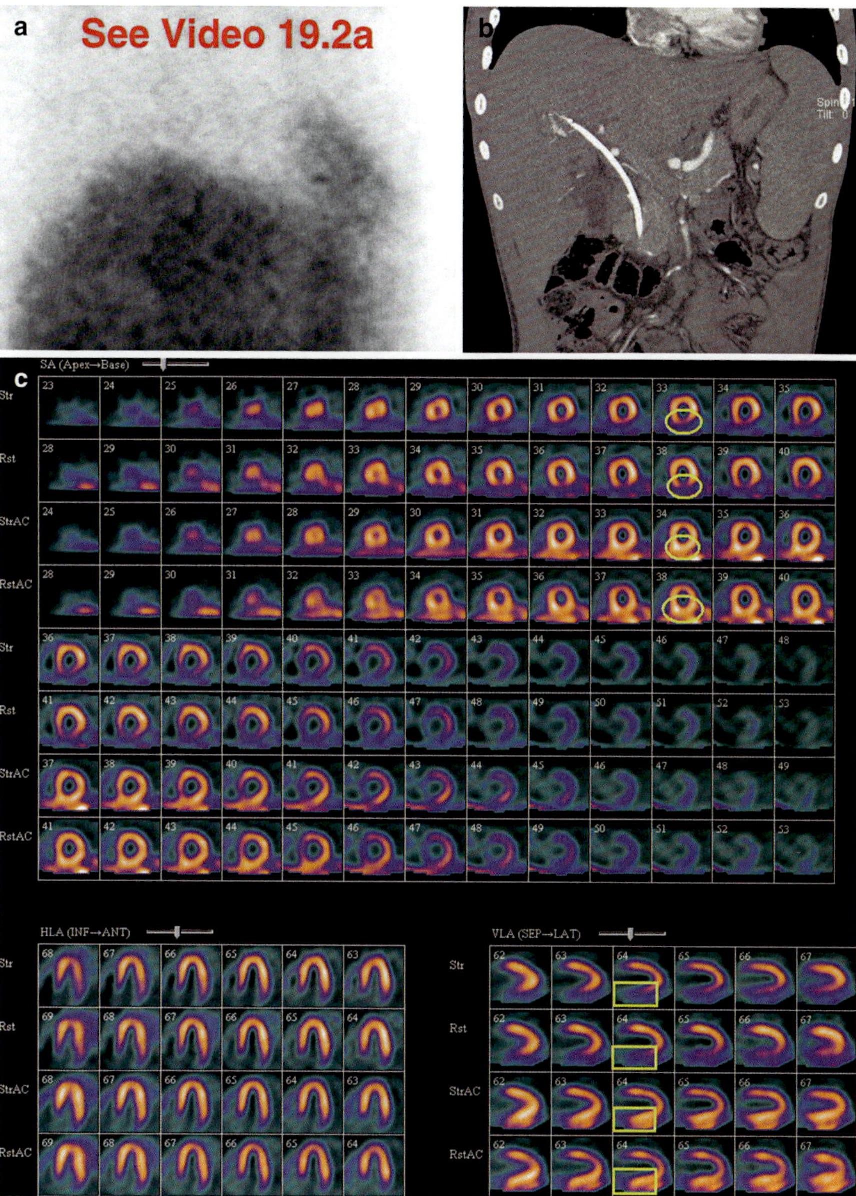

Fig. 19.2 Hepatosplenomegaly due to autoimmune hepatitis and sclerosing cholangitis. A 22-year-old male awaits liver transplant. The enlarged liver and spleen fill the upper abdomen (**a**). Note skeletal activity consistent with chronic anemia. On correlative imaging, there is a biliary stent in place; note splenomegaly (**b**). There is no "cold" pleural effusion or "cold" ascites in this patient. There is a fixed inferior wall defect that normalizes with AC; thus, it is not a scar but rather can be attributed to diaphragmatic attenuation artifact (**c**). The liver activity is only apparent on the AC images (**c**).

(**a**) Stress "black-on-white" raw projection images (Video 19.2a, frame 1), ^{99m}Tc sestamibi. (**b**) Coronal CT of the abdomen through biliary stent and enlarged spleen. (**c**) Stress/rest processed SPECT images (SA, HLA, VLA) (without and with AC), representative SA and VLA images, inferior wall defect (*yellow circles*, SA, and *yellow boxes*, VLA) splanchnic activity due to preferential redistribution of blood flow (and radiopharmaceutical) to the extremities. Conversely, vasodilator stress delivers more radioactivity to the liver.

A shrunken liver or one with poor uptake suggests end-stage chronic disease such as cirrhosis (Fig. 19.7). This finding is often accompanied by easily recognized ascites, splenomegaly, and greater activity in the kidneys, the secondary route of elimination for the ^{99m}Tc MPI radiopharmaceuticals (Chamarthy and Travin 2010; Joy et al. 2007; Shih et al. 2005; Tallaj et al. 2000).

As mentioned above, the degree of uptake within hepatic neoplasms is variable; lesions may appear relatively "cold" compared to the adjacent normal liver (Fukushima et al. 1997). Like focal "hot" lesions, focal "cold" lesions may be appreciated on careful review of the raw projection data because these may represent benign or malignant primary or metastatic lesions (Fig. 19.8) (Bhambhvani et al. 2010a, b; Chamarthy and Travin 2010; Chatziioannou et al. 1999; Gedik et al. 2007; Ghanbarinia et al. 2008; Hardebeck et al. 2013). A deformed or unusual anatomic position of the liver suggests prior surgery, which may be confirmed by history or imaging correlation (Fig. 19.9).

Findings related to the liver may warrant inclusion in the MPI report. For example, a "hot" or "cold" parenchymal lesion should be investigated and its etiology

---

Fig. 19.3 "Hot" liver causing processing artifact. This 75-year-old female underwent uneventful regadenoson stress. On both the rest (**a**) and initial stress (**b**) acquisitions, the liver has pronounced activity. Particularly on both sets of SA and VLA images, there is marked liver activity immediately adjacent to the inferior myocardial wall (**c**). Towards the apex, there is a tiny defect and towards the base, there may be "added" activity. Stress imaging repeated 30 minutes later mitigated the artifactual effect to considerable advantage, and the apical defect is barely perceptible (**d, e**). The case illustrates how it may be strategic to repeat imaging with a longer interval between injection and imaging in some patients; note how the inferior wall can be more confidently interpreted after repeat imaging.

(**a**) Rest raw projection images (75 minutes injection-to-imaging) (Video 19.3a, frame 1), ^{99m}Tc sestamibi. (**b**) Initial stress raw projection images (60 minutes injection-to-imaging) (Video 19.3b, frame 1), ^{99m}Tc sestamibi. (**c**) Initial stress/rest processed SPECT images (SA, HLA, VLA), liver activity adjacent to inferior wall (*yellow boxes* on representative SA images), liver activity and adjacent inferior wall (*yellow boxes* on representative VLA images), tiny apical defect adjacent to "hot" liver (*blue box* on stress SA image). (**d**) Repeat stress raw projection images (90 minutes injection-to-imaging) (Video 19.3c, frame 1), ^{99m}Tc sestamibi. (**e**) Repeat stress/rest processed SPECT images (SA, HLA, VLA), liver activity, and adjacent inferior wall (*yellow boxes* on representative VLA images)

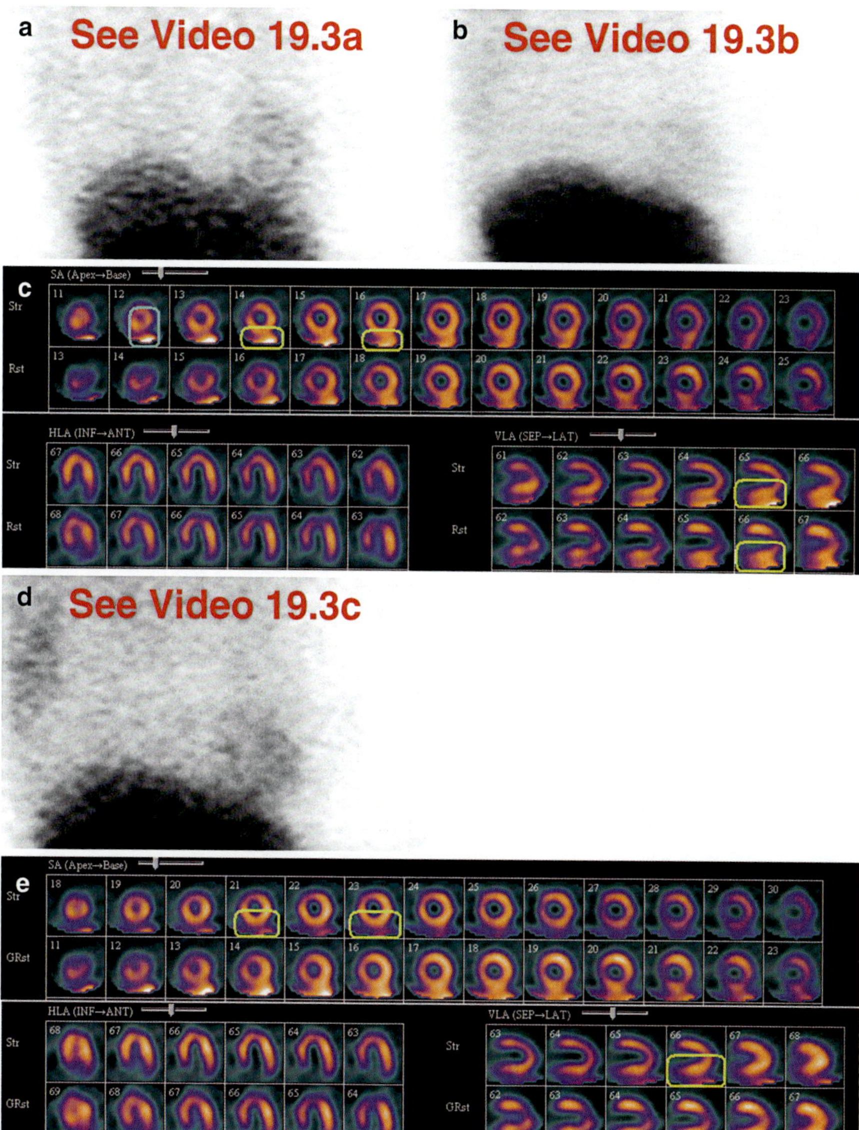
See Video 19.3a
See Video 19.3b
See Video 19.3c

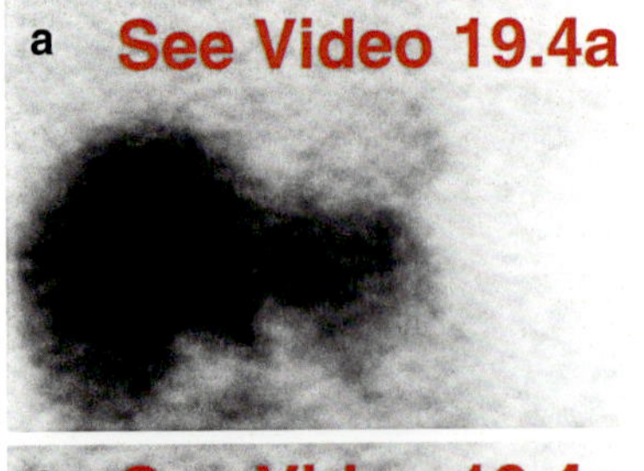
a
See Video 19.4a

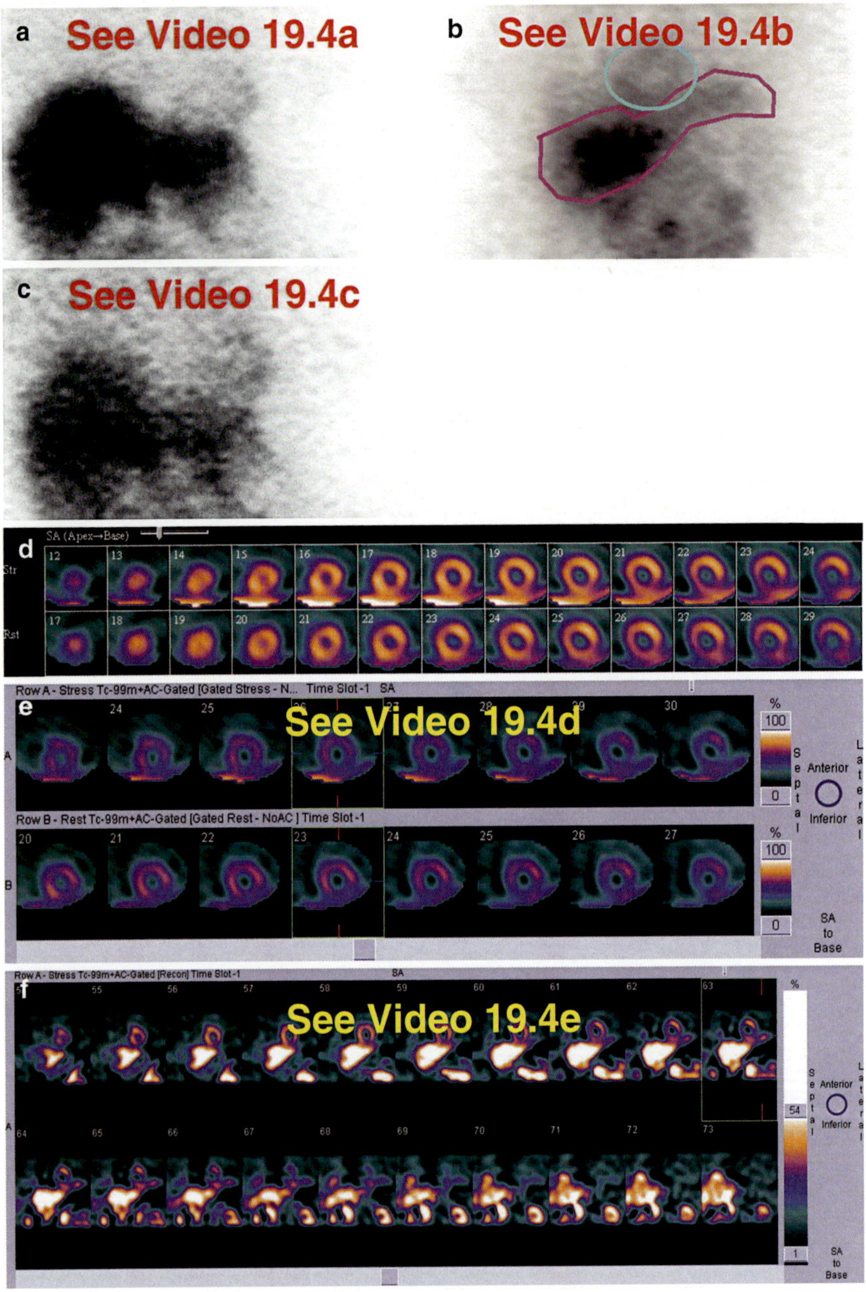

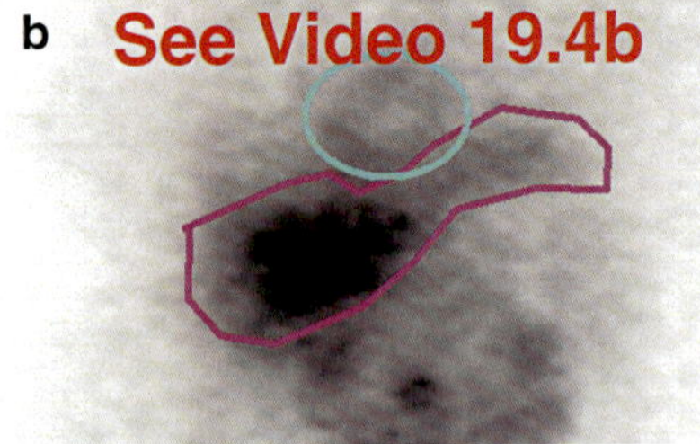
b
See Video 19.4b

c
See Video 19.4c

d
SA (Apex→Base)
Str
Rst
12 13 14 15 16 17 18 19 20 21 22 23 24
17 18 19 20 21 22 23 24 25 26 27 28 29

e
Row A - Stress Tc-99m+AC-Gated [Gated Stress - N...   Time Slot -1   SA
See Video 19.4d
Row B - Rest Tc-99m+AC-Gated [Gated Rest - NoAC] Time Slot -1
%
100
0
Septal   Anterior   Lateral
Inferior
SA to Base

f
Row A - Stress Tc-99m+AC-Gated [Recon] Time Slot -1   SA
54 55 56 57 58 59 60 61 62 63
See Video 19.4e
64 65 66 67 68 69 70 71 72 73
%
54
1
Septal   Anterior   Lateral
Inferior
SA to Base

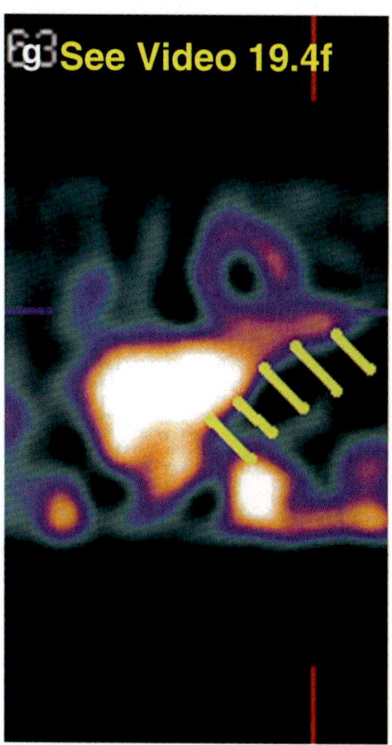

Fig. 19.4 (continued)

Fig. 19.4 Processing artifact related to left lobe of the liver extending into left upper quadrant. This obese 42-year-old female underwent a 2 day protocol. The raw data (**a–c**) show that the liver is positioned immediately subjacent to the left ventricular myocardium and that it extends into the left upper quadrant. Note how it creates an artifactual fixed defect (i.e., processing artifact) involving the inferior and inferolateral walls from apex to base (**d, e**). The "whole-field-of-view reconstruction" (**f, g**) depicts the relationship of the heart to the liver more clearly and demonstrates the continuity of the liver with the tongue of the hepatic tissue extending into the left upper quadrant. The inferior and inferolateral walls move and thicken normally, suggesting artifact rather than scar.

(**a**) Day 1: stress raw projection images (Video 19.4a, frame 1), ^{99m}Tc sestamibi. (**b**) Day 1: stress raw projection image (Video 19.4b, frame 38), ^{99m}Tc sestamibi, outline of the liver (*pink polygon*), left ventricular myocardium outlined in *blue* as reference landmark. (**c**) Day 2: rest raw projection images (Video 19.4c, frame 1), ^{99m}Tc sestamibi. (**d**) Stress/rest processed SPECT images (SA). (**e**) Gated stress and rest SPECT images (Video 19.4d, frame 1) (SA). (**f**) Gated stress SPECT images (Video 19.4e, frame 1), "whole-field-of-view reconstruction", coronal from anterior to posterior. (**g**) Gated stress SPECT image (Video 19.4f, frame 7), "whole-field-of-view reconstruction", coronal, left lobe of the liver (*yellow lines*)

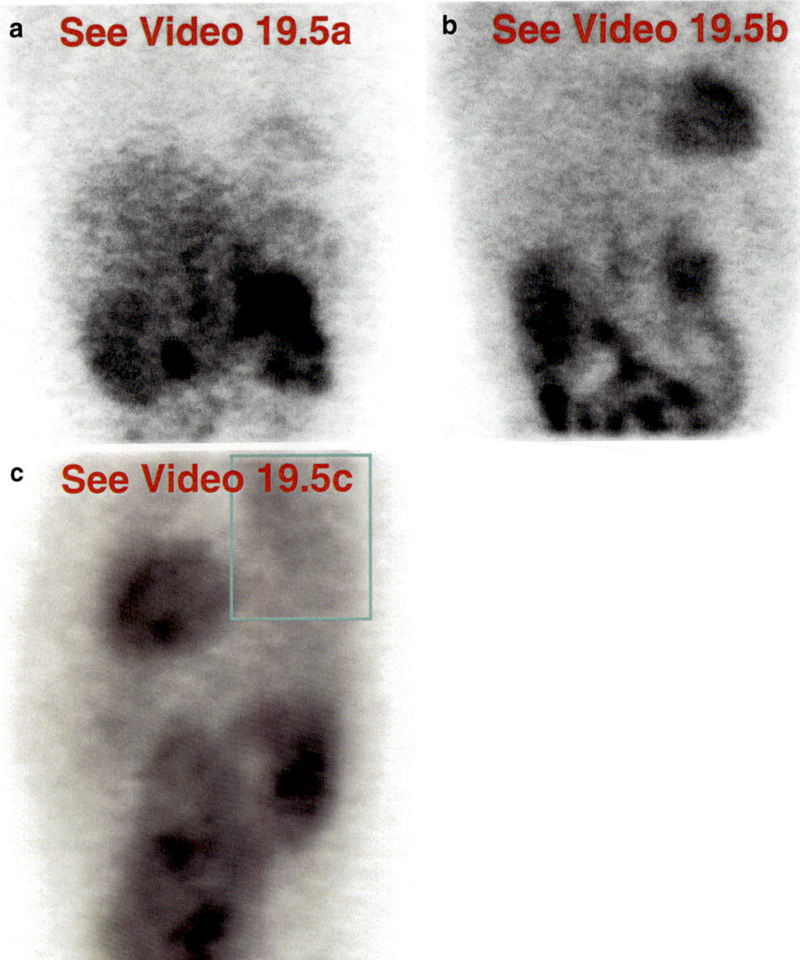

Fig. 19.5 Physiologic faint liver visualization. This 41-year-old male exercised on the treadmill according to the Bruce protocol. During a high workload, there is preferential peripheral distribution of the radiopharmaceutical, thus limiting the delivery to the liver. On both the rest (**a**) and the stress (**b**) images, the liver has cleared nearly completely. Note that the left shoulder musculature is much more apparent on the stress images, a finding often seen after strenuous treadmill exercise (**b**, **c**). Take note of the surgically absent gallbladder (**a**, **b**).

(**a**) Rest raw projection images (Video 19.5a, frame 1), ^{99m}Tc sestamibi. (**b**) Stress raw projection images (Video 19.5b, frame 1), ^{99m}Tc sestamibi. (**c**) Stress raw projection image (Video 19.5c, frame 44), ^{99m}Tc sestamibi, left shoulder (*blue box*)

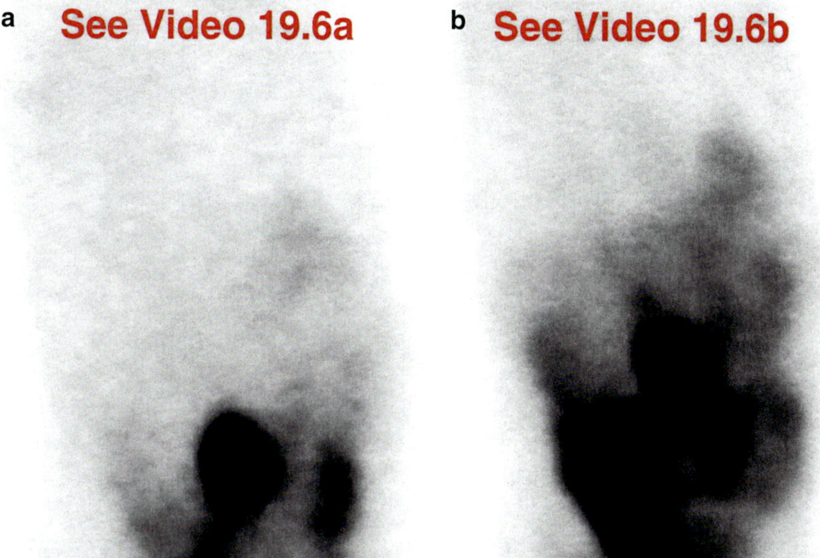

Fig. 19.6 Differential liver clearance between rest and stress. There is much greater liver clearance on the rest raw images (**a**) compared to stress raw images (**b**) because of a 2 hour interval between radiopharmaceutical injection and commencement of the rest acquisition. The liver appears "cold" on the rest images and is faintly visible on the stress images. Note the hyperinflated "cold" emphysematous lungs and flattened diaphragms in a 66-year-old female (see Fig. 10.3).

(**a**) Rest raw projection images (Video 19.6a, frame 1), ^{99m}Tc sestamibi. (**b**) Stress raw projection images (Video 19.6b, frame 1), ^{99m}Tc sestamibi

determined through search of medical and imaging records. Depending on the acuity, personal communication may be appropriate. Such a report could state:

"On the raw projection data, there are multiple "cold" lesions within an enlarged liver. In correlation with the most recent CT scans, these likely correspond to the known multiple hepatic cysts in this patient with polycystic liver disease."

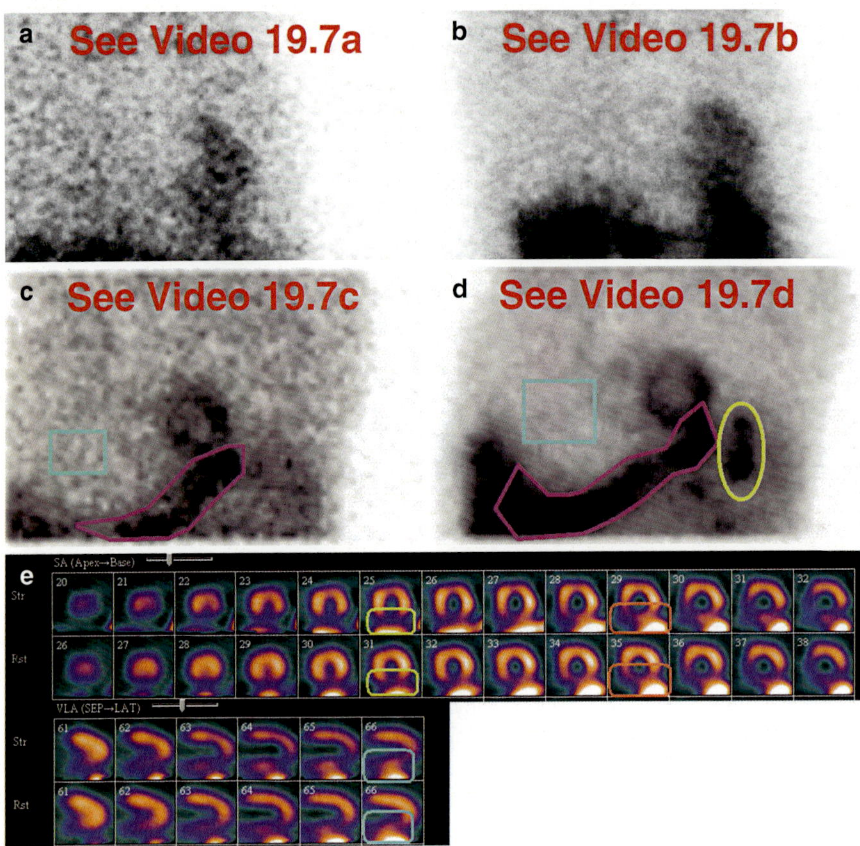

Fig. 19.7 Poor liver visualization due to cirrhosis. A 62-year-old male's MPI shows no discernible hepatic activity on rest and stress raw data (**a–d**). There is, however, marked gastric wall uptake (gastropathy) (**c, d**). The transverse colon and splenic flexure of the large intestine are apparent on the stress raw images (**b, d**). The intensely "hot" stomach next to the heart creates a "cold" and "hot" processing artifact in the adjacent inferior myocardial wall (**e**); preserved wall motion and wall thickening on gated data (**f**) favor artifact rather than scar.

(**a**) Rest raw projection images (Video 19.7a, frame 1), ^{99m}Tc sestamibi. (**b**) Stress raw projection images (Video 19.7b, frame 1), ^{99m}Tc sestamibi. (**c**) Rest raw projection image (Video 19.7c, frame 30), ^{99m}Tc sestamibi, liver (*blue box*) and stomach (*pink outline*). (**d**) Stress raw projection image (Video 19.7d. frame 29), ^{99m}Tc sestamibi, liver (*blue box*) and stomach (*pink outline*), splenic flexure of large intestine (*yellow oval*). (**e**) Stress/rest processed SPECT images (SA, VLA), "cold" effect towards apex (*yellow boxes*, representative SA images), "hot" effect towards lateral basal wall (*blue boxes*, representative VLA images), and mixed "cold" and "hot" towards mid- to basal lateral wall (*orange boxes*, representative SA images). (**f**) Gated stress/rest SPECT images (Video 19.7e, frame 1) (SA, HLA)

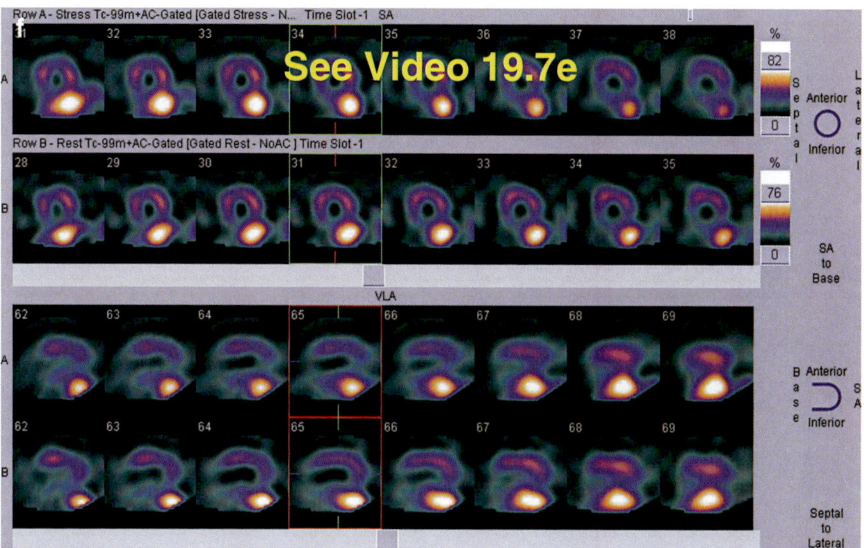

Fig. 19.7 (continued)

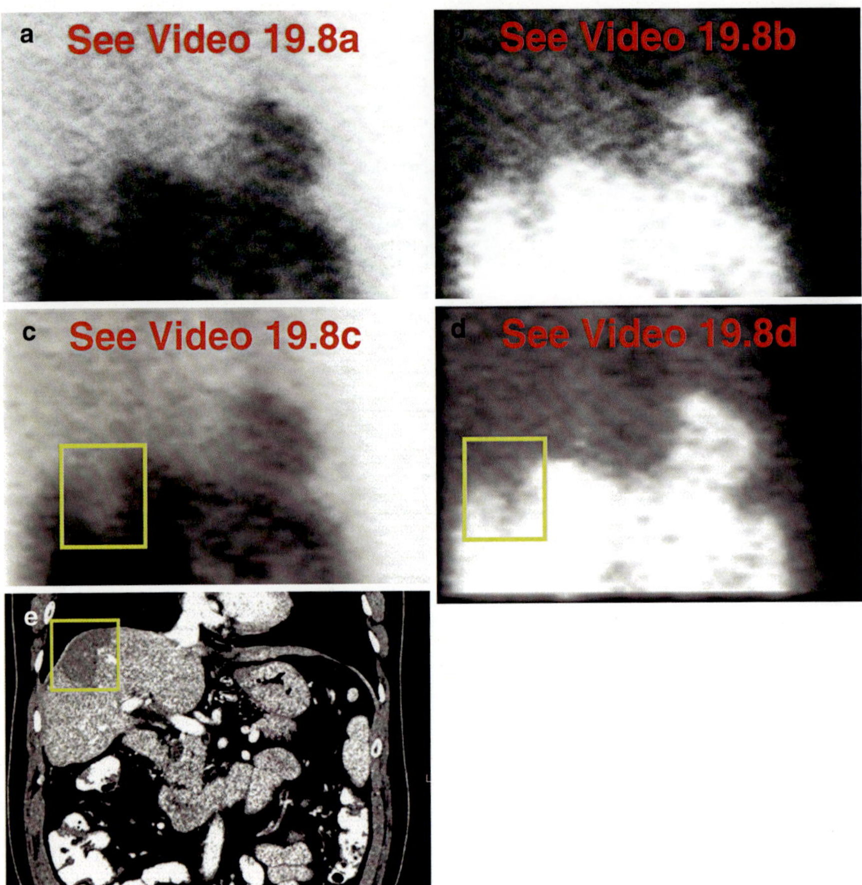

Fig. 19.8 Focal "cold" defect at liver dome due to residual cavity from radiofrequency ablation of hepatocellular cancer 1 year ago. The defect is appreciated on cinematic review (**a**, **b**). Note utility of changing color to better visualize the subtle abnormality (**c**, **d**). Correlation with anatomic imaging is essential (**e**).

(**a**) Stress "black-on-white" raw projection images (Video 19.8a, frame 1), ^{99m}Tc sestamibi. (**b**) Stress "white-on-black" raw projection images (Video 19.8b, frame 1), ^{99m}Tc sestamibi. (**c**) Stress "black-on-white" raw projection image (Video 19.8c, frame 1), ^{99m}Tc sestamibi, lesion (*yellow box*). (**d**) Stress "white-on-black" raw projection image (Video 19.8d, frame 5), ^{99m}Tc sestamibi, lesion (*yellow box*). (**e**) Coronal CT through posterior liver, lesion (*yellow box*)

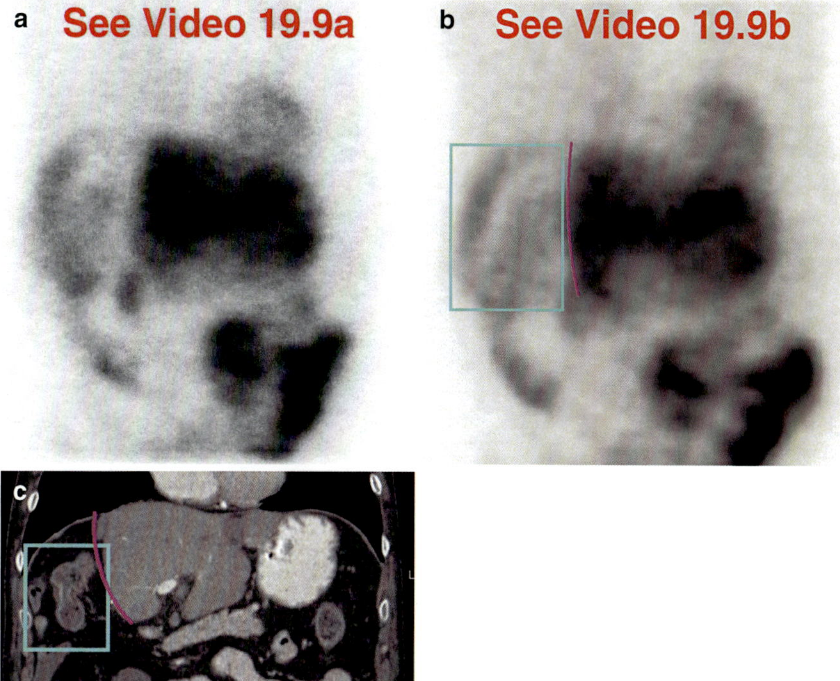

Fig. 19.9 Abnormal liver contour. On the stress raw data (**a**), take note of the distance between the liver edge and the abdominal wall; normally, it abuts it. Large intestinal activity is interposed between the abdominal wall and the liver edge (**a, b**). This 64-year-old male has metastatic colon cancer and underwent resection of the right lobe for metastatic disease. Correlation with anatomic imaging (**c**) greatly aids the interpretation and demonstrates corresponding findings.

(**a**) Stress raw projection images (Video 19.9a, frame 1), ^{99m}Tc sestamibi. (**b**) Stress raw projection image (Video 19.9b, frame 5), ^{99m}Tc sestamibi, hepatic flexure (*blue box*), liver margin (*pink arc*). (**c**) Coronal CT through the liver, hepatic flexure (*blue box*), liver margin (*pink arc*)

Key Points
- The hepatobiliary system is the primary route of clearance of the ^{99m}Tc MPI radiopharmaceuticals.
- The degree of liver visualization depends on liver function, composition (e.g., scarring), interval between radiopharmaceutical administration and imaging, and type of stress performed.
- Liver shape and size can be readily evaluated.
- The degree of uptake within a hepatic neoplasm is variable, and lesions can appear "hot" or "cold."
- Localized hepatic activity adjacent to the (nonfilling) gallbladder fossa may signal complicated acute cholecystitis.

Biliary System and Gallbladder

20

Given that hepatobiliary clearance is the predominant pathway for the ^{99m}Tc MPI radiopharmaceuticals, it is expected that the components of the biliary system (intrahepatic ducts, common hepatic duct, common bile duct) might be visualized and that the gallbladder will be visualized (Figs. 20.1 and 20.2) (Shih et al. 2002). A normal common bile duct is not uncommonly visible and should not be misconstrued as pathologic. While there are relatively few biliary conditions (biliary ectasia, common bile duct obstruction) that can be seen on SPECT MPI, there are multiple physiologic and pathologic conditions of the gallbladder (Table 20.1) (Hesse et al. 2005).

The gallbladder should fill with radioactive bile and appear quite "hot," often the "hottest" finding in the field-of-view. The patient is typically fasting for the stress test, and the gallbladder, as in ^{99m}Tc iminodiacetic acid (IDA) hepatobiliary scintigraphy, should fill. Diaphragmatic motion may produce a moving ("beating") gallbladder (Fig. 20.3). The gallbladder generally has a characteristic round to ovoid shape and is tucked under the inferior right lobe; however, it may be intrahepatic in location (Howarth et al. 1996). Figure 20.4 shows an unusually elongated and superiorly displaced gallbladder; it is adjacent to the right hemidiaphragm by anatomic CT correlation. A very "hot" and "high" gallbladder may create a processing artifact on the reconstructed MPI (Fig. 20.5). The degree of gallbladder visualization can vary from rest to stress imaging on both 1-day and 2-day protocols (Figs. 20.6 and 20.7). The gallbladder is usually well-distended and a contracted gallbladder is considered abnormal (Fig. 20.8).

Electronic supplementary material The online version of this chapter (doi:10.1007/978-3-319-25436-4_20) contains supplementary material, which is available to authorized users.

© Springer International Publishing Switzerland 2017

M.E. Oates, V.L. Sorrell, *Myocardial Perfusion Imaging - Beyond the Left Ventricle: Pathology, Artifacts and Pitfalls in the Chest and Abdomen,*
DOI 10.1007/978-3-319-25436-4_20

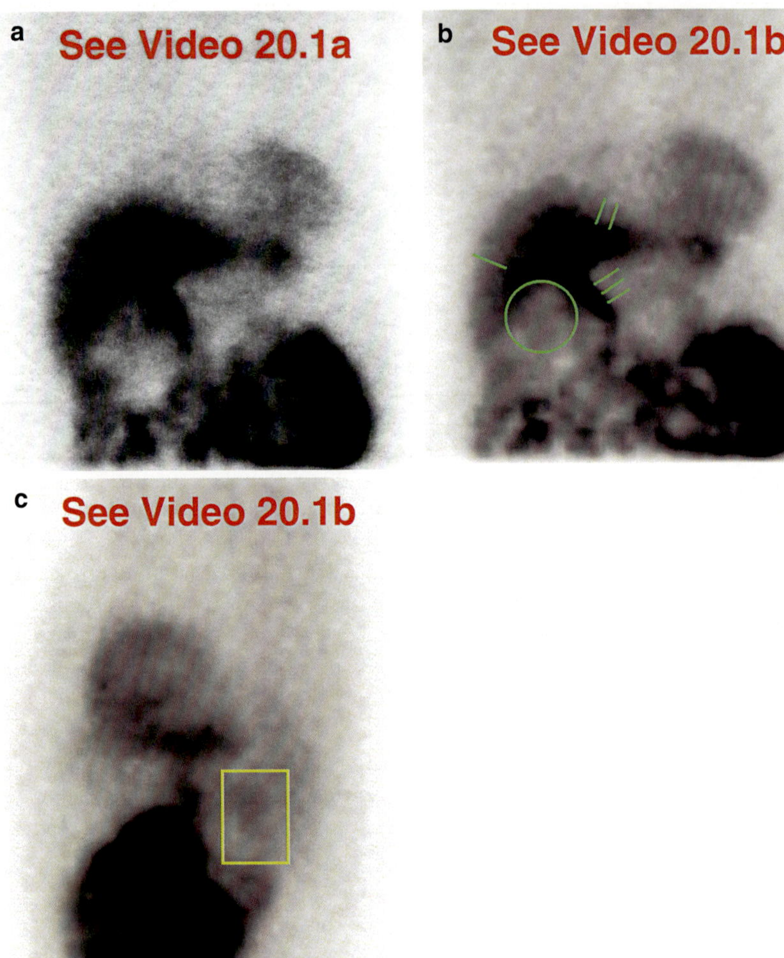

Fig. 20.1 Normal intrahepatic bile ducts and common bile duct. The non-dilated bile ducts are prominent (**a**, **b**). Note absence of a gallbladder (cholecystectomy) (**b**). The left kidney is atrophic (**a**, **c**) in this patient on dialysis for end-stage kidney disease.

(**a**) Stress raw projection images (Video 20.1a, frame 1), ^{99m}Tc sestamibi. (**b**) Stress raw projection image (Video 20.1b, frame 6), ^{99m}Tc sestamibi, right hepatic duct (*one green line*), left hepatic duct (*two green lines*), common bile duct (*three green lines*), gallbladder fossa (*green circle*). (**c**) Stress raw projection images (Video 20.1b, frame 47), ^{99m}Tc sestamibi, left kidney (*yellow box*)

If not surgically absent, non-visualization of the gallbladder signals acute cholecystitis or chronic cholecystitis, and clinical correlation is warranted (Fig. 20.9) (Chamarthy and Travin 2010; Gedik et al. 2007). In a series of 697 consecutive patients undergoing ^{99m}Tc sestamibi SPECT MPI, the gallbladder failed to visualize in 16 %. Of those, a significant minority (27 %) had not had a cholecystectomy, and acute cholecystitis, chronic cholecystitis, or cholelithiasis was diagnosed as the underlying condition (Toran et al. 1997). In another series of 566 patients who

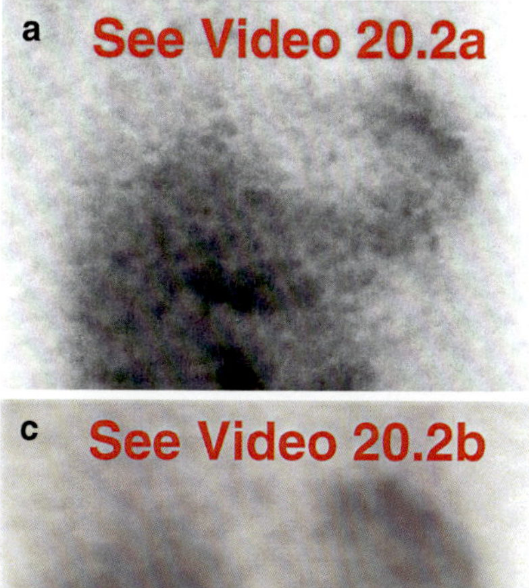

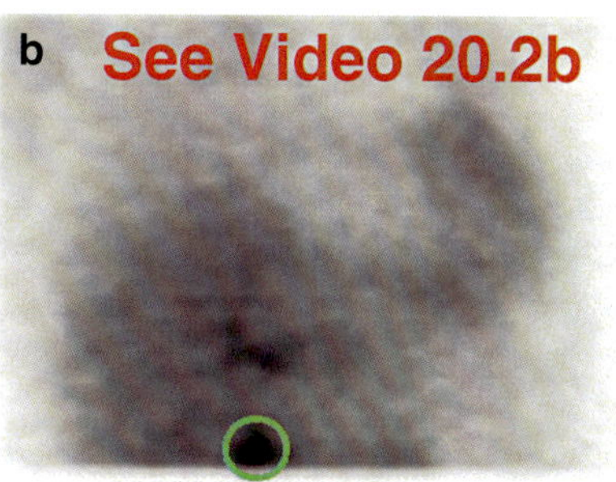

Fig. 20.2 Contracted gallbladder in patient with dilated cardiomyopathy. The gallbladder is small and just seen "at the edge of the field-of-view" (**a**, **b**). Note the confluence of biliary ducts at the porta hepatis (**a**, **c**). The heart is enlarged with a dilated left ventricular cavity (**a**).

(**a**) Stress raw projection images (Video 20.2a, frame 1), ^{99m}Tc sestamibi. (**b**) Stress raw projection image (Video 20.2b, frame 2), ^{99m}Tc sestamibi, gallbladder (*green circle*). (**c**) Stress raw projection image (Video 20.2b, frame 7), ^{99m}Tc sestamibi, porta hepatis bile ducts (*green box*)

Table 20.1 Differential diagnosis of "hot" and "cold" imaging findings related to the biliary system and gallbladder

Organ system	"Hot" finding	"Cold" finding	References
Biliary system and gallbladder	Biliary ectasia with stasis Common bile duct obstruction	Inadequate or prolonged fasting *Cholecystitis* (*acute*, chronic) Biliary stricture/stone at ampulla of Vater	Chamarthy and Travin (2010) Gedik et al. (2007) Hesse et al. (2005) Howarth et al. (1996) Meesala et al. (2006) Panjrath et al. (2004) Shih et al. (2002, 2005) Toran et al. (1997)

underwent ^{99m}Tc tetrofosmin SPECT MPI, 47 (8.3 %) had non-visualization of the gallbladder associated with acute or chronic cholecystitis or cholecystectomy (Shih et al. 2005).

A distended "cold" gallbladder is distinctly abnormal and indicates underlying gallbladder disease (Fig. 20.10). Focal increased uptake in the liver adjacent to a "cold" or non-visualized gallbladder is termed the "pericholecystic rim sign" and

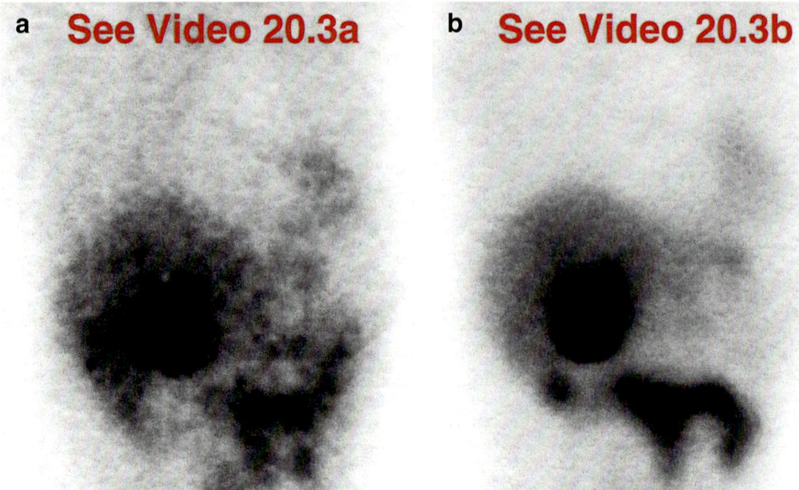

Fig. 20.3 "Beating gallbladder." Note how the gallbladder appears to be fluttering throughout both acquisitions (**a**, **b**); this is a clue to right hemidiaphragmatic breathing motion which could lead to motion artifact on processed SPECT MPI. The gallbladder should be stationary; however, the small intestinal activity should change with normal peristalsis as seen here (**a**, **b**).

(**a**) Rest raw projection images (Video 20.3a, frame 1), ^{99m}Tc sestamibi. (**b**) Stress raw projection images (Video 20.3b, frame 1), ^{99m}Tc sestamibi

signals acute cholecystitis. This imaging finding raises the likelihood of more complicated or advanced gallbladder disease (Lamont et al. 1996). There may be an associated incomplete common bile duct stricture or a common bile duct stone in chronic calculous cholecystitis; radioactivity in the small intestine excludes complete or high-grade common bile duct obstruction (Meesala et al. 2006; Panjrath et al. 2004).

As for the MPI report, it should document the absence of gallbladder visualization when there is confidence in this finding (e.g., the gallbladder fossa is included in the field-of-view). Two sample reports follow:

The gallbladder is not visualized, consistent with history of cholecystectomy.

The gallbladder is not visualized; this is an unexpected, abnormal finding. Recent ultrasonography demonstrated gallstones. Differential diagnosis includes acute or chronic calculous cholecystitis. The finding and differential diagnosis were discussed personally with the referring physician at the time of interpretation.

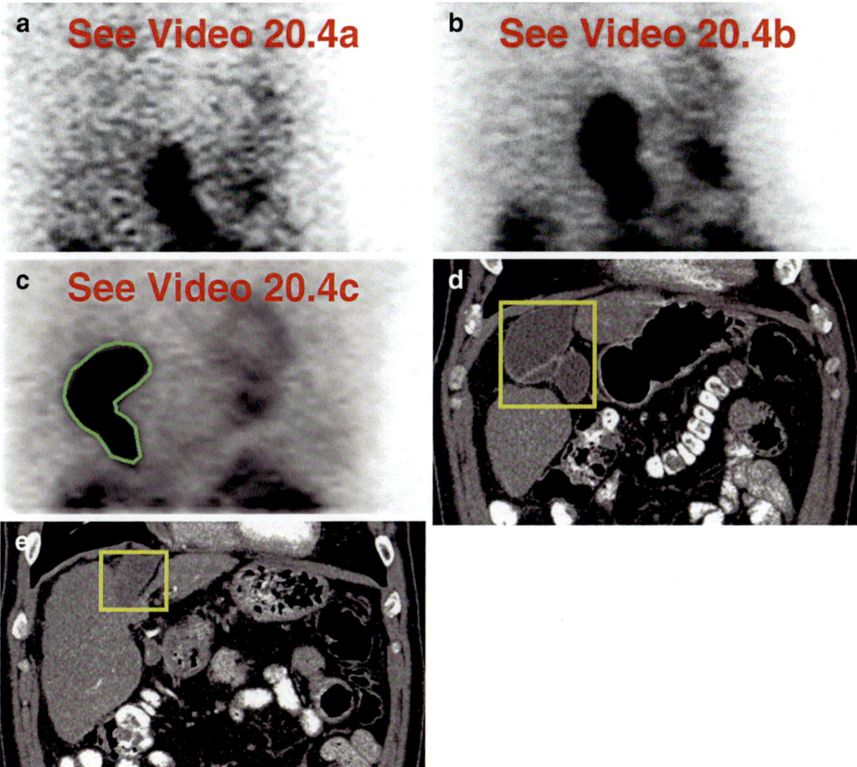

Fig. 20.4 Elongated, elevated gallbladder. Note the unusual shape and position of the gallbladder (**a–c**). The CT images define its anatomic position and morphology (**d, e**).

(**a**) Rest raw projection images (Video 20.4a, frame 1), ^{99m}Tc sestamibi. (**b**) Stress raw projection images (Video 20.4b, frame 1), ^{99m}Tc sestamibi. (**c**) Stress raw projection image (Video 20.4c, frame 18), ^{99m}Tc sestamibi, gallbladder (*green outline*). (**d**) Coronal CT through more anterior liver and gallbladder, septate gallbladder abuts right hemidiaphragm (*yellow box*). (**e**) Coronal CT through more posterior liver and gallbladder, posteriormost tail of gallbladder (*yellow box*) abuts right hemidiaphragm

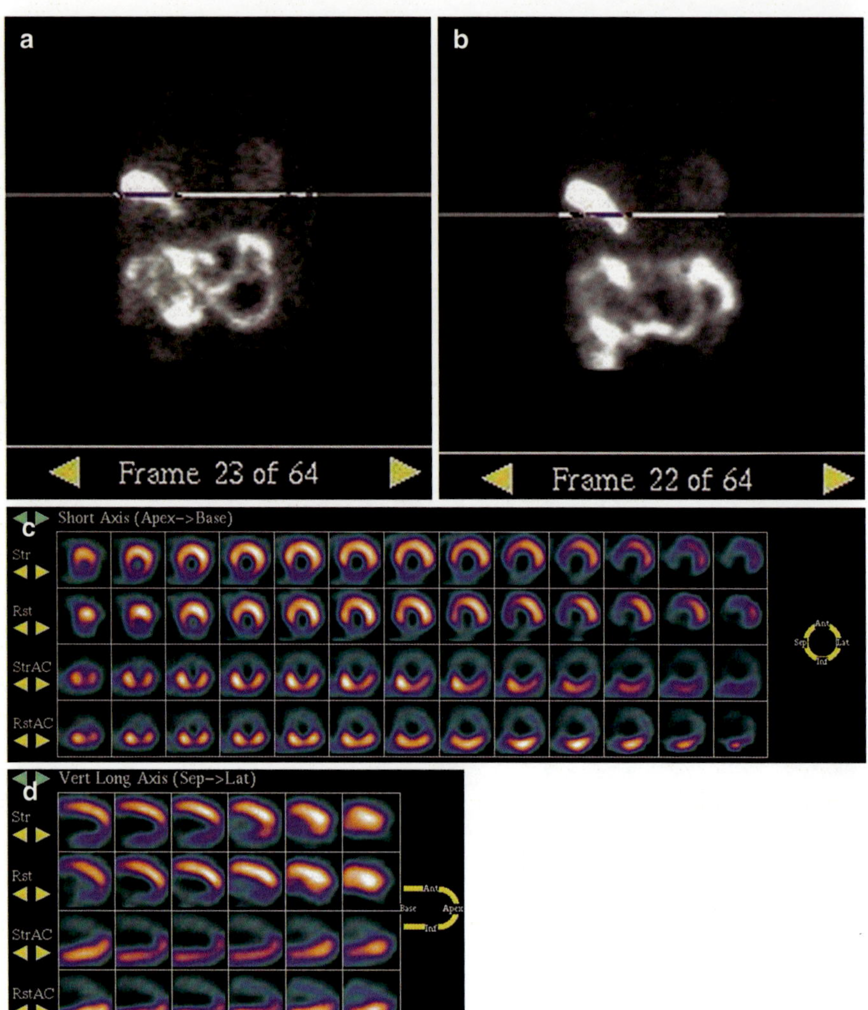

Fig. 20.5 "Sunrise/sunset" processing/reconstruction artifact. The gallbladder is "hot" and "high" (most of it lies above the line defining the lower aspect of the heart) (**a, b**). The anterior wall is "hot" and the inferior wall is "cold" on non-AC images (**c–e**), but the opposite is apparent on the AC images (**c–e**), giving rise to an unusual "sunrise/sunset" pattern. The AC algorithm overcorrects the inferior wall and undercorrects the anterior wall. Although the gallbladder is distant from the heart, its intensity leads to this unusual artifact.

(**a**) Rest raw projection images, ^{99m}Tc tetrofosmin, white line defines lower aspect of heart. (**b**) Stress raw projection images, ^{99m}Tc tetrofosmin, white line defines lower aspect of heart. (**c**) Stress/rest processed SPECT images (SA) (without and with AC). (**d**) Stress/rest processed SPECT images (VLA) (without and with AC). (**e**) Polar maps without and with AC (from *top* to *bottom*: stress, rest, stress AC, rest AC)

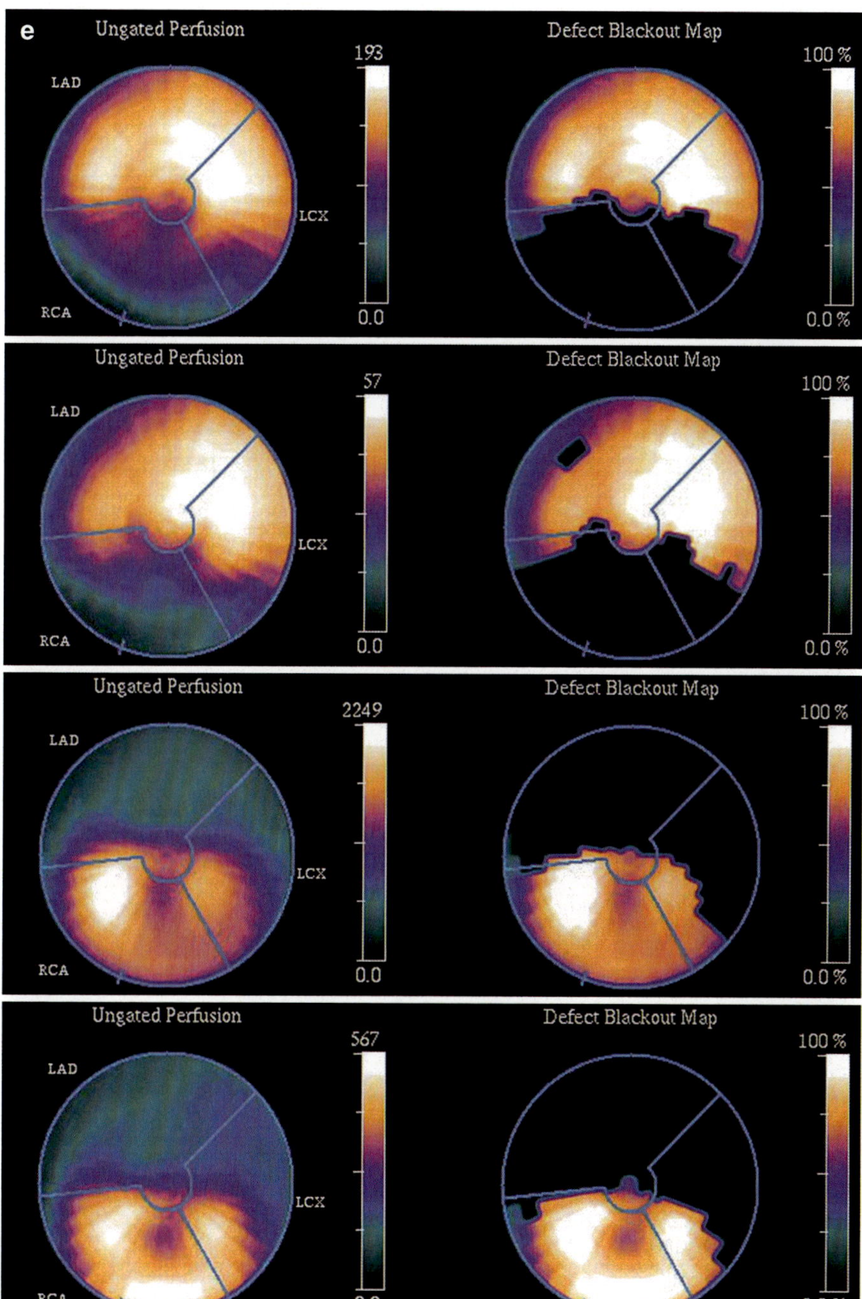

Fig. 20.5 (continued)

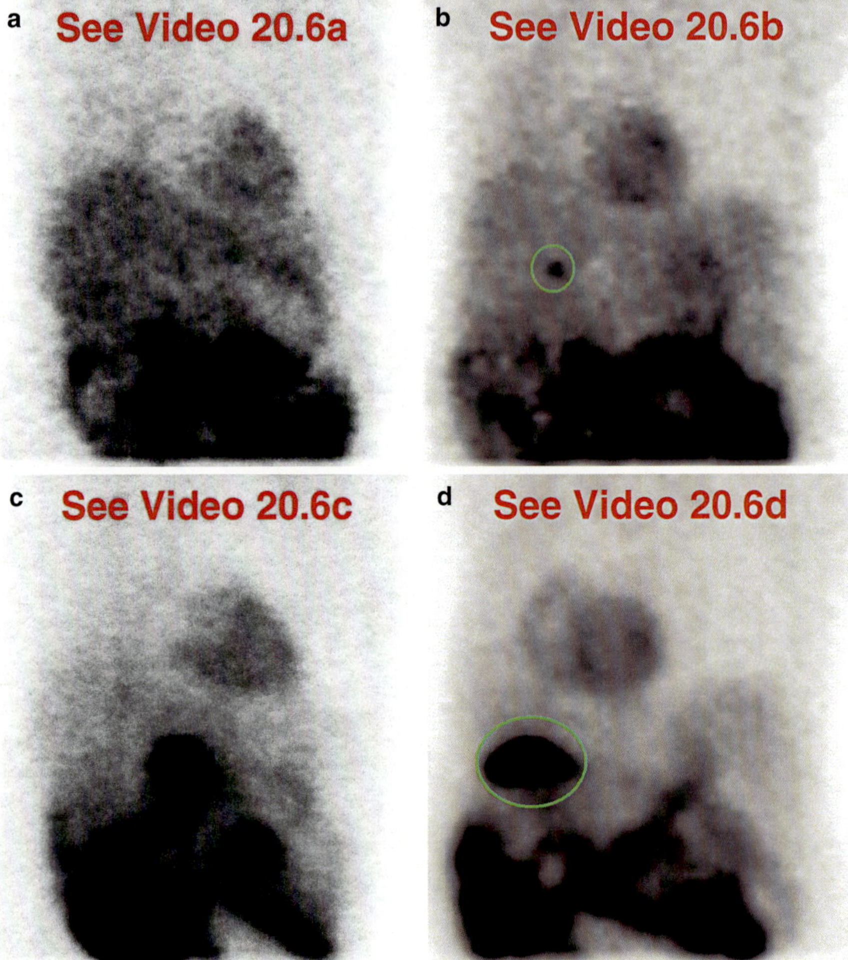

Fig. 20.6 Differential gallbladder visualization, 1-day rest/stress protocol. There is incomplete filling of the gallbladder at rest (**a**, **b**), but it appears complete at stress (**b**, **d**) in a 1-day protocol. This may represent chronic cholecystitis vs. incomplete fasting before the rest imaging. This patient had undergone right lung transplant. Did you observe the asymmetry in the lungs? Did you recognize these images from Fig. 10.7?

(**a**) Rest raw projection images (Video 20.6a, frame 1), ^{99m}Tc sestamibi. (**b**) Rest raw projection image (Video 20.6b, frame 17), ^{99m}Tc sestamibi, gallbladder (*green oval*). (**c**) Stress raw projection images (Video 20.6c, frame 1), ^{99m}Tc sestamibi. (**d**) Stress raw projection image (Video 20.6d frame 26), ^{99m}Tc sestamibi, gallbladder (*green oval*)

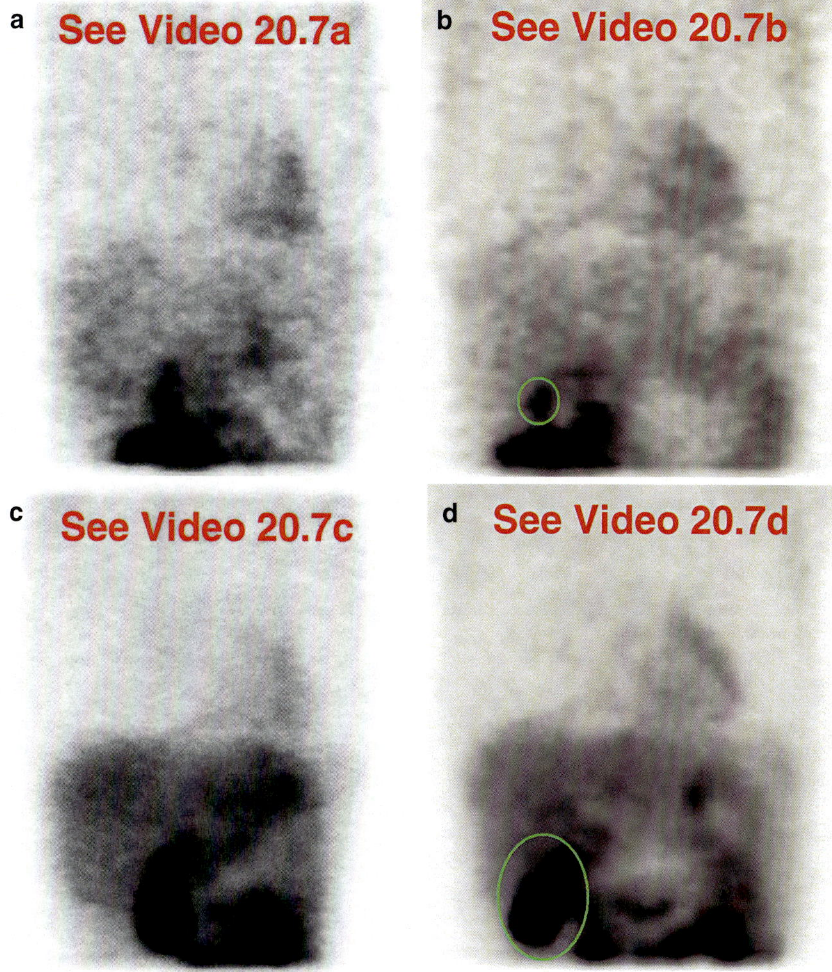

Fig. 20.7 Differential gallbladder visualization, 2-day rest/stress protocol. For rest imaging on the first day of a 2-day rest/stress protocol, the patient was not fasting; therefore, there is minimal visualization of the gallbladder (**a, b**). For the stress test on the second day, the patient was fasting and there is the expected degree of gallbladder visualization (**c, d**). The hospitalized patient underwent the rest component the afternoon before ("a late add-on") and the stress early the following day to facilitate management.

(**a**) Day 1: rest raw projection images (Video 20.7a, frame 1), ^{99m}Tc sestamibi (non-fasting). (**b**) Day 1: rest raw projection image (Video 20.7b, frame 12), ^{99m}Tc sestamibi (non-fasting), gallbladder (*green circle*). (**c**) Day 2: stress raw projection images (Video 20.7c, frame 1), ^{99m}Tc sestamibi (fasting). (**d**) Day 2: stress raw projection image (Video 20.7d, frame 16), ^{99m}Tc sestamibi (fasting), gallbladder (*green oval*)

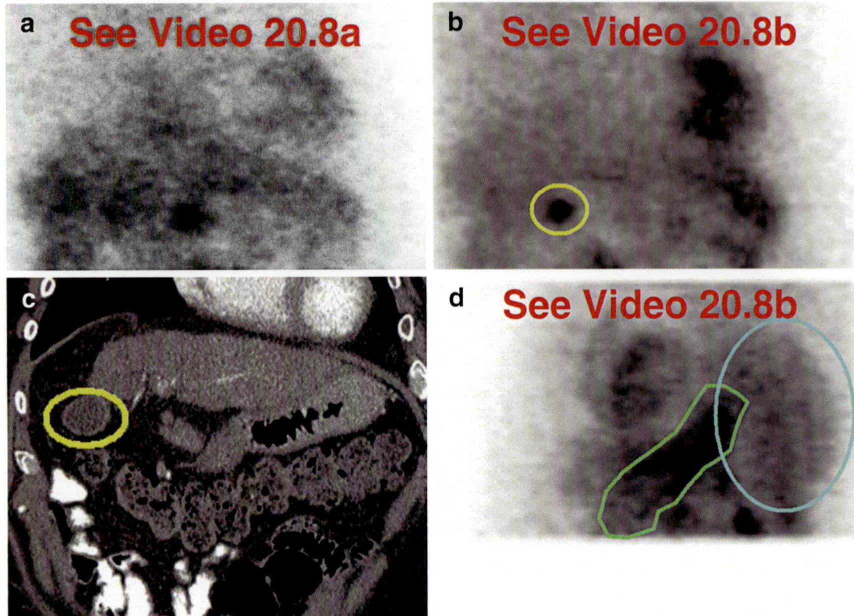

Fig. 20.8 Contracted gallbladder. The gallbladder appears contracted (**a, b**) on MPI and on correlative CT (**c**). This patient had undergone TIPS; note small liver (**a, c**), splenomegaly (**a, d**) and a "hot" stomach (gastropathy) (**a, d**), characteristic signs of cirrhosis.

(**a**) Stress raw projection images (Video 20.8a, frame 1), ^{99m}Tc sestamibi. (**b**) Stress raw projection image (Video 20.8b, frame 9), ^{99m}Tc sestamibi, gallbladder (*yellow oval*). (**c**) Coronal CT through gallbladder (*yellow oval*). (**d**) Stress raw projection image (Video 20.8b, frame 43), ^{99m}Tc sestamibi, stomach (*green outline*), spleen (*blue oval*)

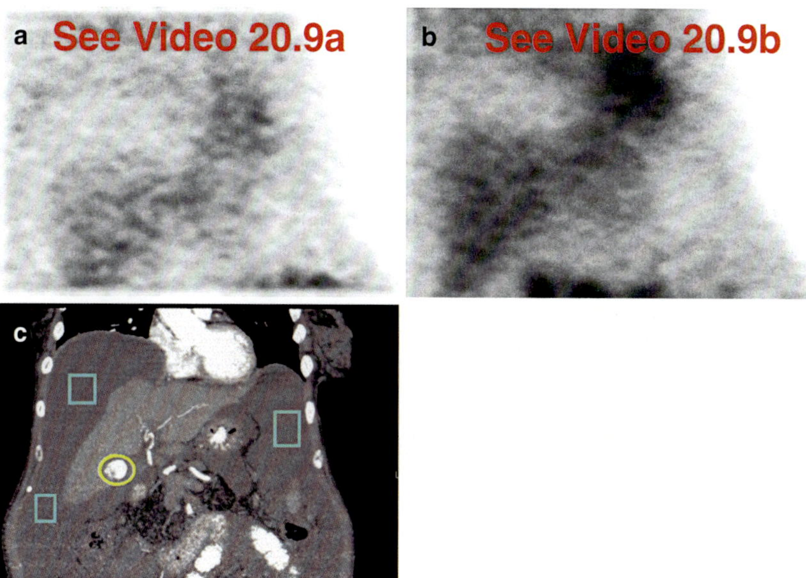

Fig. 20.9 Non-visualized gallbladder due to chronic calculous cholecystitis. The gallbladder fails to fill (**a, b**). The activity at the lower edge of the field-of-view represents small intestine with peristaltic movements; when there is large volume ascites, the small intestine loops float centrally. There is a large gallstone in a contracted gallbladder on CT (**c**). Note marked "cold" ascites surrounding the liver (**a–c**), splenomegaly (**a, b**), and a medially displaced, shrunken liver (**a–c**).

(**a**) Rest raw projection images (Video 20.9a, frame 1), ^{99m}Tc sestamibi. (**b**) Stress raw projection images (Video 20.9b, frame 1), ^{99m}Tc sestamibi. (**c**) Coronal CT through gallbladder, gallstone (*yellow oval*), ascites (*green boxes*)

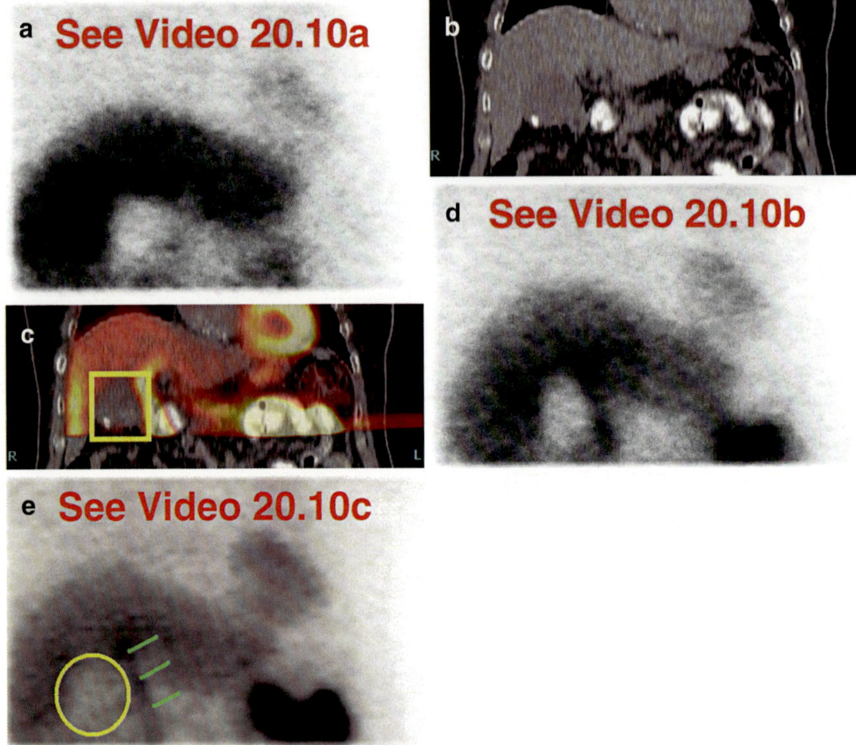

Fig. 20.10 "Cold" gallbladder due to chronic calculous cholecystitis. The gallbladder is not simply non-visualized; it actually appears round, distended, and frankly "cold." It is located in the usual position at the inferior aspect of the right hepatic lobe (**a**). Note the small gallstone in a distended gallbladder by CT (**b**). The "whole-field-of-view" fusion images confirm the relationship between the "cold" scintigraphic finding and the bile-filled, stone-containing gallbladder (**c**). Interestingly, comparison with previous MPI (**d**, **e**) shows a similar pattern in this chronic condition.

(**a**) Stress raw projection images (Video 20.10a, frame 1), ^{99m}Tc sestamibi. (**b**) Coronal CT at level of gallbladder and gallstone. (**c**) Coronal SPECT/CT fusion, whole-field-of-view reconstruction, gallbladder with gallstone (*yellow box*). (**d**) Two years previously: stress raw projection images (Video 20.10b, frame 1), ^{99m}Tc sestamibi. (**e**) Two years previously: stress raw projection image (Video 20.10c, frame 6), ^{99m}Tc sestamibi, gallbladder fossa (*yellow circle*), common bile duct (*green lines*)

Key Points
- The gallbladder should fill with radioactive bile and appear "hot"; it is often the "hottest" finding in the field-of-view.
- When superiorly displaced, the "hot" gallbladder can create a processing artifact on the reconstructed SPECT MPI.
- The degree of gallbladder visualization can vary between rest and stress imaging on both 1-day and 2-day protocols and is dependent on the fasting state of the patient.
- The gallbladder is usually well-distended in the fasting state; a contracted gallbladder is considered abnormal.
- Non-visualization of the gallbladder, if not surgically absent, or a distended "cold" gallbladder signifies underlying gallbladder disease; such findings warrant clinical correlation and communication with the referring physician.
- Radioactivity in the small intestine excludes high-grade or complete common bile duct obstruction.

The differential diagnosis of conditions affecting the spleen is limited (Table 21.1). The spleen is typically faintly visualized (Shih et al. 2002). The most common diffuse finding is splenomegaly, usually in association with hepatomegaly or cirrhosis (Chamarthy and Travin 2010; Joy et al. 2007; Shih et al. 2005; Tallaj et al. 2000). Splenomegaly can displace the left kidney (Shih et al. 2002). The incidence of patients with splenomegaly varies considerably with the patient population evaluated. For example, liver transplantation programs have a much higher likelihood of splenomegaly than community practices. Focal splenic lesions can be seen if sufficiently large. Figures 21.1, 21.2, and 21.3 show three different patients with splenomegaly in association with underlying liver disease.

The written report could include wording along the lines of:

Incidentally noted is an enlarged spleen. This finding is expected in the context of the patient's underlying cirrhosis and portal hypertension.

Personal communication with the referring physician is optional in such cases and usually not necessary if the cirrhosis is known.

Electronic supplementary material The online version of this chapter (doi:10.1007/978-3-319-25436-4_21) contains supplementary material, which is available to authorized users.

© Springer International Publishing Switzerland 2017
M.E. Oates, V.L. Sorrell, *Myocardial Perfusion Imaging - Beyond the Left Ventricle: Pathology, Artifacts and Pitfalls in the Chest and Abdomen,*
DOI 10.1007/978-3-319-25436-4_21

Table 21.1 Differential diagnosis of "hot" and "cold" imaging findings related to the spleen

Organ system	"Hot" finding	"Cold" finding	References
Spleen	Splenomegaly	Cyst Infarct	Chamarthy and Travin (2010) Joy et al. (2007) Shih et al. (2002) Shih et al. (2005) Tallaj et al. (2000)

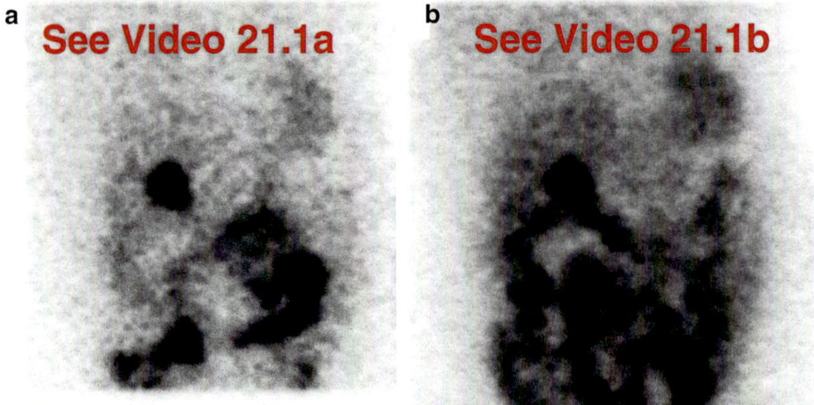

Fig. 21.1 Splenomegaly. This 48-year-old male has NASH (nonalcoholic steatohepatitis) and marked splenomegaly (**a–d**). Although photopenic regions appear to surround the small intestine mimicking ascites, there is not significant ascites by contemporaneous CT scan; there is only minimal perihepatic ascites (**d**). This point underscores the value of correlation during MPI interpretation. Note how an enlarged spleen, which lies immediately below the left hemidiaphragm, can overlie the inferior wall during MPI (**e**); this can potentially create a processing artifact. The left kidney is well seen and displaced by the large spleen (**f**). The gallbladder is visualized (**a–c**).

(**a**) Rest raw projection images (Video 21.1a, frame 1), ^{99m}Tc sestamibi. (**b**) Stress raw projection images (Video 21.1b, frame 1), ^{99m}Tc sestamibi. (**c**) Stress raw projection image (Video 21.1c, frame 30, LAO), ^{99m}Tc sestamibi, long-axis of spleen (*yellow line*), gallbladder (*pink circle*). (**d**) Coronal CT scan through spleen, long-axis of spleen (*yellow line*), perihepatic fluid (*green lines*), gallbladder (*pink circle*). (**e**) Stress raw projection image (Video 21.1c, frame 41), ^{99m}Tc sestamibi, top of spleen (*yellow arc*), level of inferior myocardial wall (*red line*). (**f**) Stress raw projection image (Video 21.1c, frame 58, left lateral projection), ^{99m}Tc sestamibi, left kidney length and width (*blue lines*), center of enlarged spleen for reference (*yellow circle*)

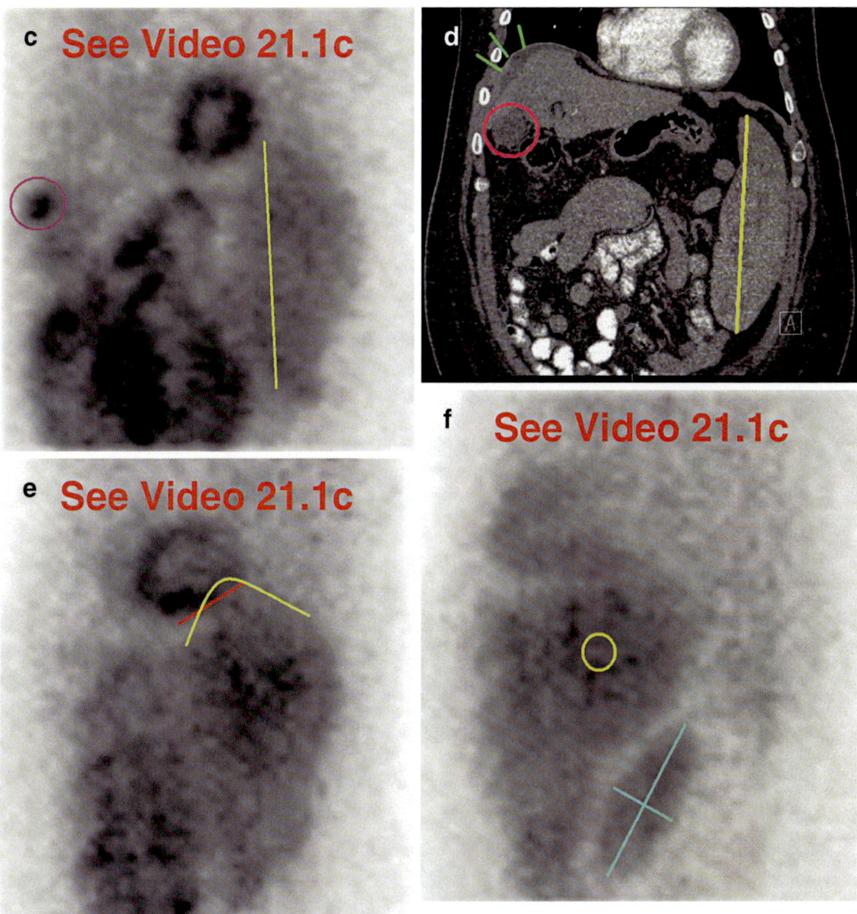

Fig. 21.1 (continued)

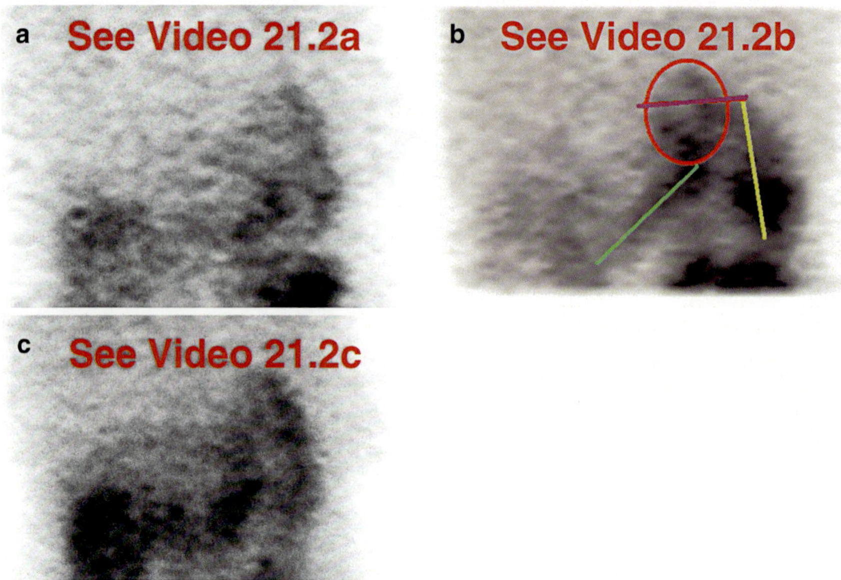

Fig. 21.2 Splenomegaly with similarly intense "hot stomach" (associated gastropathy). The cirrhotic patient has an enlarged "hot" spleen; the stomach is also "hot" and neighbors the spleen (**a–f**). Note the effect of the "hot" stomach on the adjacent inferior myocardial wall on the reconstructed SPECT data; it creates an artifactual fixed defect (**d, f**). Although the top of the "hot" spleen under the left hemidiaphragm is near the heart, it is more laterally positioned and has less of an effect on the stress reconstructed images. It does, however, contribute to an artifactual lateral wall defect on the rest processed images (**d, f**). Wall motion and wall thickening are preserved, favoring artifact and not scar (**e**).

(**a**) Rest raw projection images (Video 21.2a, frame 1), ^{99m}Tc sestamibi. (**b**) Rest raw projection image (Video 21.2b, frame 19), ^{99m}Tc sestamibi, spleen (*yellow line*), stomach (*green line*), heart (*red oval*), top of spleen/left hemidiaphragm through the mid left ventricle (*pink line*). (**c**) Stress raw projection images (Video 21.2c, frame 1), ^{99m}Tc sestamibi. (**d**) Stress/rest processed SPECT images (SA, HLA, VLA) (without and with AC), spleen (*yellow ovals*), stomach (*green boxes*) on selected images. (**e**) Stress and rest gated SPECT (Video 21.2d, frame 1) (SA, VLA, HLA). (**f**) Stress and rest gated SPECT image (Video 21.2e, frame 7) (SA, VLA, HLA), spleen (*yellow ovals*), stomach (*green boxes*) on selected images

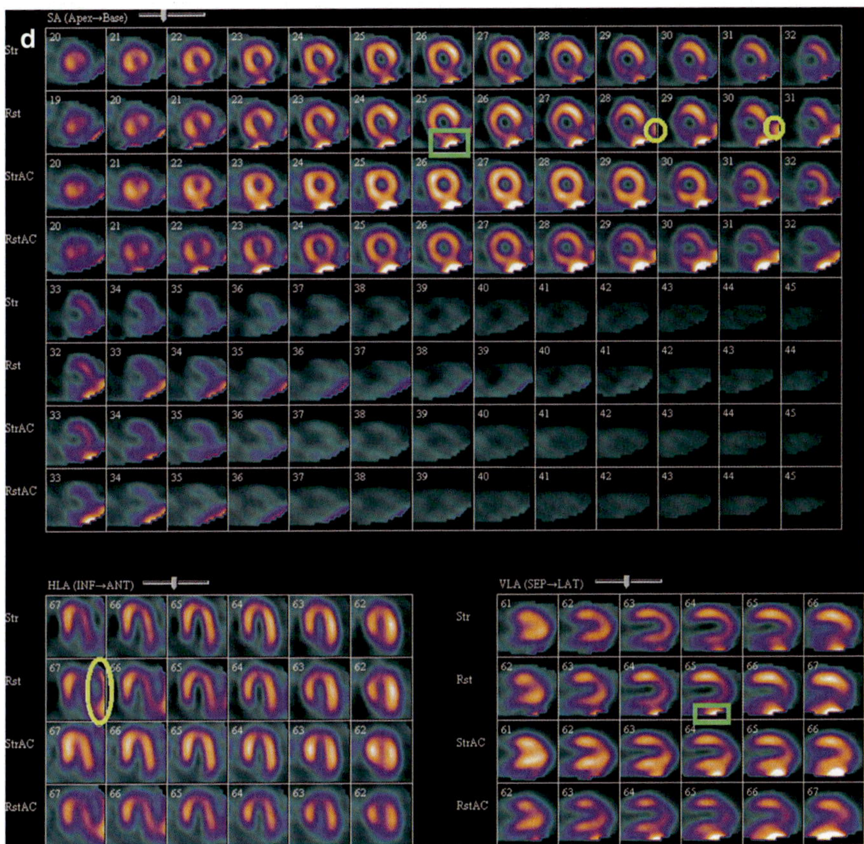

Fig. 21.2 (continued)

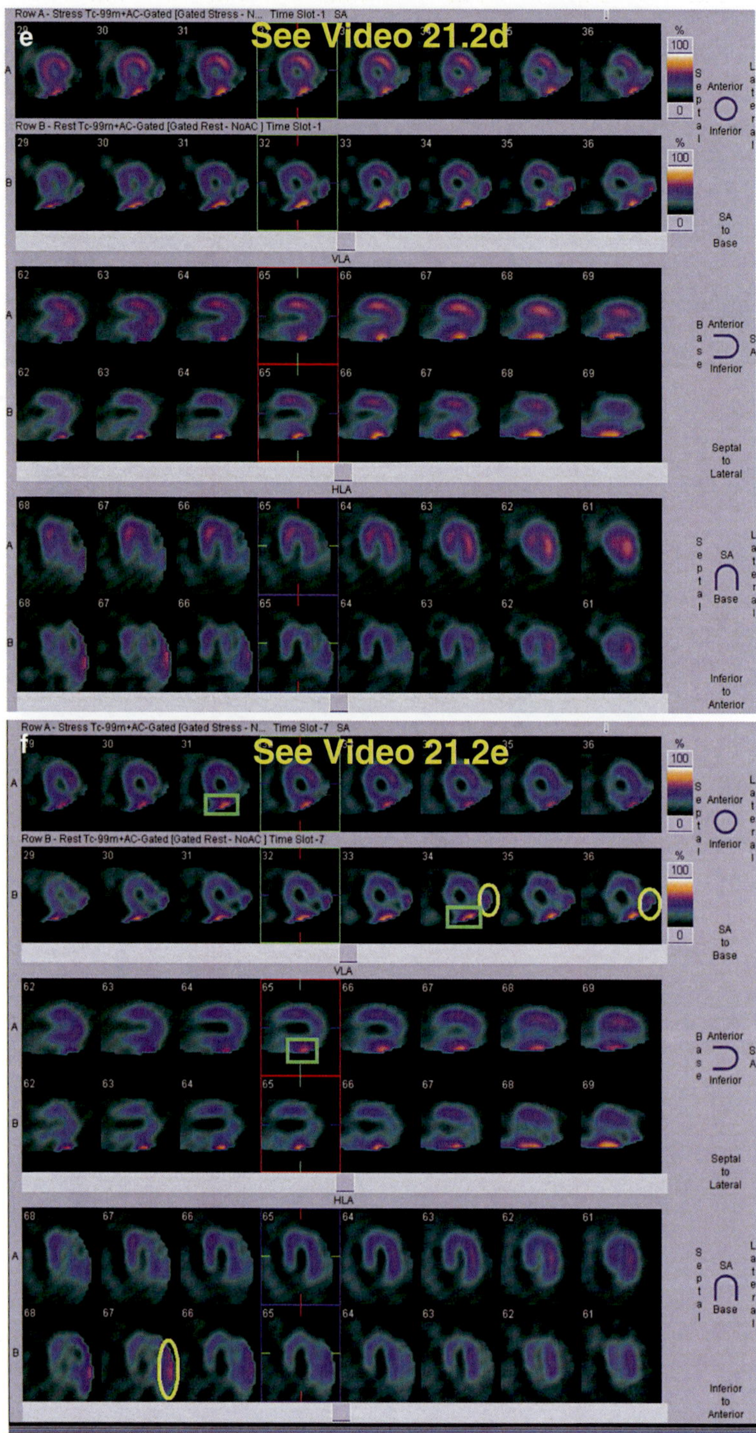

Fig. 21.2 (continued)

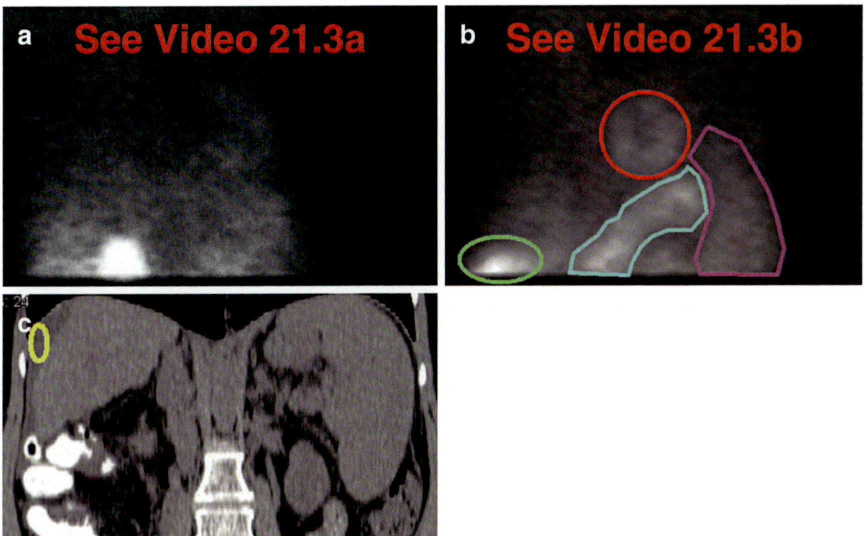

Fig. 21.3 Splenomegaly with much more intense "hot" stomach (associated gastropathy). The spleen is enlarged but not nearly as "hot" as the nearby "hot" stomach (**a, b**). The gallbladder visualizes normally (**a, b**). Note minimal ascites and splenomegaly by CT (**c**).

(**a**) Stress raw projection images (Video 21.3a, frame 1), ^{99m}Tc sestamibi. (**b**) Stress raw projection image (Video 21.3b, frame 32), ^{99m}Tc sestamibi, spleen (*pink outline*), stomach (*blue outline*), gallbladder (*green oval*), heart for reference (*red circle*). (**c**) Coronal CT scan through posterior liver and spleen, perihepatic fluid (*yellow oval*)

Key Points
- The most common finding regarding the spleen in SPECT MPI is splenomegaly, often associated with underlying liver pathology.
- Splenomegaly can result in displacement of the left kidney.
- Focal splenic lesions can be seen if sufficiently large.

Stomach

22

Table 22.1 lists various causes for a "hot" or "cold" stomach on MPI. Gastric activity can be quite confounding with respect to reconstruction processing artifacts affecting the inferior myocardial wall. Most often, gastric activity is related to intraluminal duodenogastric bile reflux that may occur to different degrees of severity between patients and between rest and stress imaging in the same patient (Fig. 22.1). Gastric activity obscures the inferior myocardial wall and frequently creates processing artifacts. Ideally, subdiaphragmatic gastric activity is avoided altogether (Burrell and MacDonald 2006; Middleton and Williams 1994).

Drinking, eating, changing to a prone position, waiting, and repeating MPI are often the most practical maneuvers to lessen this common artifact (Fig. 22.2) (Burrell and MacDonald 2006). Refluxed duodenogastric activity may persist within the gastric lumen for a long time in patients with gastroparesis; sometimes ingestion of water or food helps clear it (Fig. 22.3), but at other times, there is no significant benefit (Gedik et al. 2007). Patients with repeat examinations may show the same pattern (Fig. 22.4); knowing this at the time of the follow-up MPI may prompt modifications to the imaging protocol such as a longer fasting state if possible, particularly in diabetics who are at risk to develop gastroparesis. In one series, three patients out of 76 had uninterpretable examinations (Middleton and Williams 1996). Because the fundus is dependent, laying the patient with right side down for 20 minutes facilitated clearance of the stomach, resulting in all examinations being interpretable; the frequency and degree of duodenogastric reflux were considerably lower with the maneuver (Middleton and Williams 1996). This maneuver might be an option for facilities with semi-upright/recumbent dedicated cardiac gamma camera systems that cannot be easily configured for prone image acquisition.

Electronic supplementary material The online version of this chapter (doi:10.1007/978-3-319-25436-4_22) contains supplementary material, which is available to authorized users.

© Springer International Publishing Switzerland 2017
M.E. Oates, V.L. Sorrell, *Myocardial Perfusion Imaging - Beyond the Left Ventricle: Pathology, Artifacts and Pitfalls in the Chest and Abdomen,*
DOI 10.1007/978-3-319-25436-4_22

Table 22.1 Differential diagnosis of "hot" and "cold" imaging findings related to the stomach

Organ system	"Hot" finding	"Cold" finding	References

Stomach	Duodenogastric reflux
	Gastroparesis
	Gastropathy (dyspepsia/
	  gastritis, cirrhosis)
	Free ^{99m}Tc pertechnetate
		Ingestion of fluids
		Distension, acute
		  or chronic
			Burrell and
			  MacDonald (2006)
			Cote and Dumont (2004)
			Gedik et al. (2007)
			Gholamrezanezhad
			  et al. (2006)
			Gupta et al. (2015)
			Khary et al. (1995)
			Middleton
			  and Williams (1994)
			Middleton
			  and Williams (1996)

The stomach may be positioned adjacent to the heart in patients with eventration of the left hemidiaphragm. A "hot" stomach in this location can cause significant processing artifacts (Fig. 22.5). A "hot" stomach can also interfere with gated SPECT processing because the computer program may consistently flag the region of interest incorrectly including the "hot" stomach as part of the left ventricular myocardium despite efforts to manually correct this miscontouring (Burrell and MacDonald 2006). The stomach may be separated from the heart by an interposed left lobe of the liver (Fig. 22.6).

The gastric wall itself may accumulate the radiopharmaceutical in patients with a gastropathy as seen in cirrhosis (Figs. 22.7 and 22.8). A "hot" gastric wall tends to have a uniform biodistribution from antrum to fundus and it can be quite intense. It can resemble railroad tracks (Fig. 22.9) (Gupta et al. 2015). Unlike duodenogastric reflux, it cannot be cleared by water or food ingestion. The stomach may have a more horizontal position; a "hot" gastric wall can cause processing artifact in the inferior myocardial wall (Fig. 22.10). In a study of 819 patients imaged with ^{99m}Tc sestamibi, 1.6 % had significant gastric wall uptake, and they tended to have gastric-related symptoms (Cote and Dumont 2004). In another study of 1056 patients, 1.9 % had gastric wall activity, and they were more likely to have gastric symptoms as well (Gholamrezanezhad et al. 2006). Gastric localization of ^{201}Tl chloride has been strongly associated with symptomatology, suggesting hyperemia as a potential mechanism (Khary et al. 1995). The lumen of the "hot" stomach may appear to be collapsed ("hot") or distended ("cold") (Figs. 22.11 and 22.12).

Although gastric activity is commonplace, it should be described as to whether it represents intramural gastric wall uptake as in gastropathy or intraluminal activity as in bile reflux. Any maneuvers employed to mitigate it should be mentioned, and the impact on the processed data should be acknowledged. The report could state:

On both rest and stress images, there is marked gastric activity, which appears to be intraluminal, suggesting duodenogastric bile reflux. The patient was fluid-restricted and could not drink water to try to clear it. There is a medium-size, moderately severe, fixed defect in the adjacent inferior myocardial wall; this defect demonstrates normal wall motion and wall thickening on gated SPECT imaging. It is likely due to Ramp filter artifact and not scar.

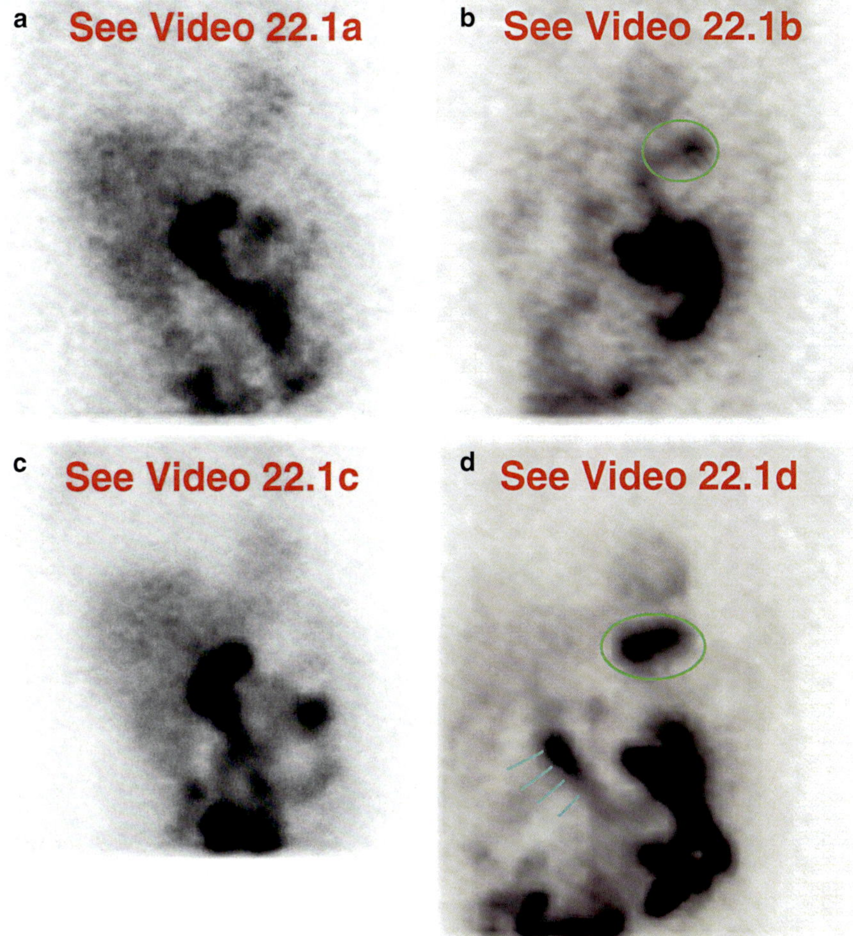

Fig. 22.1 Variable degrees of intermittent duodenogastric reflux. On rest (**a**, **b**) and stress (**c**, **d**) imaging, there are different degrees (intensities) of gastric activity: on rest, there is much less with only a few episodes of duodenogastric reflux, while on stress, there is much more refluxed activity that persists longer. The variable appearance indicates intraluminal activity; gastric wall uptake will not change between rest and stress. Note that gastric activity is clearly apparent only on stress processed SPECT and gated SPECT images (**e**, **f**); there is no significant artifactual effect on the adjacent inferior myocardial wall. A previous cholecystectomy is the reason for non-visualization of the gallbladder (**a**, **c**).

(**a**) Rest raw projection images (Video 22.1a, frame 1), ^{99m}Tc sestamibi. (**b**) Rest raw projection image (Video 22.1b, frame 31), ^{99m}Tc sestamibi, gastric activity (*green oval*). (**c**) Stress raw projection images (Video 22.1c, frame 1), ^{99m}Tc sestamibi. (**d**) Stress raw projection image (Video 22.1d, frame 24), ^{99m}Tc sestamibi, gastric activity (*green oval*), duodenal activity (*blue lines*). (**e**) Stress/rest processed SPECT images (SA, VLA, HLA), gastric activity (*green box*) on selected SA and VLA images. (**f**) Stress gated SPECT images (Video 22.1e, frame 1) (SA, VLA, HLA)

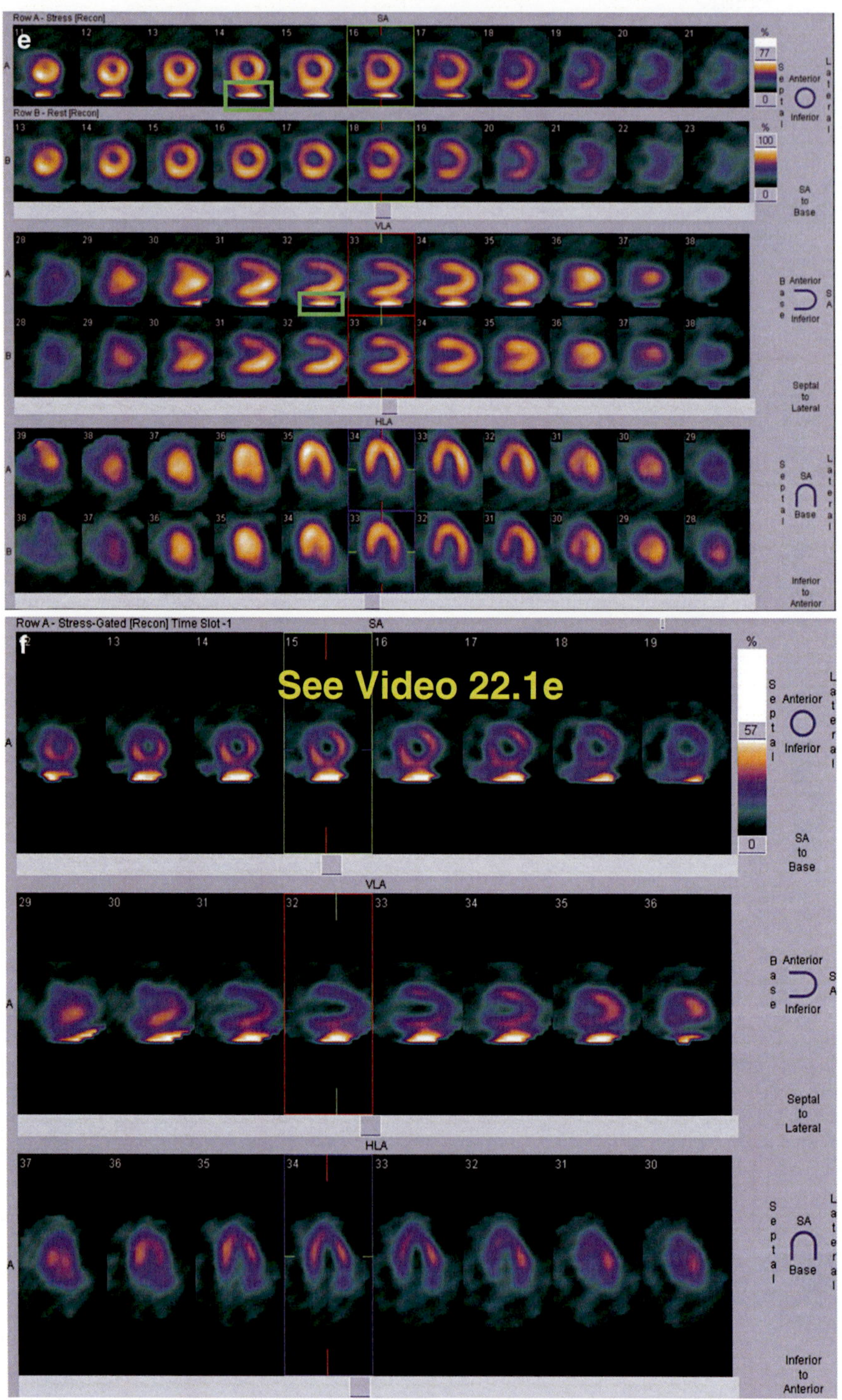

Fig. 22.1 (continued)

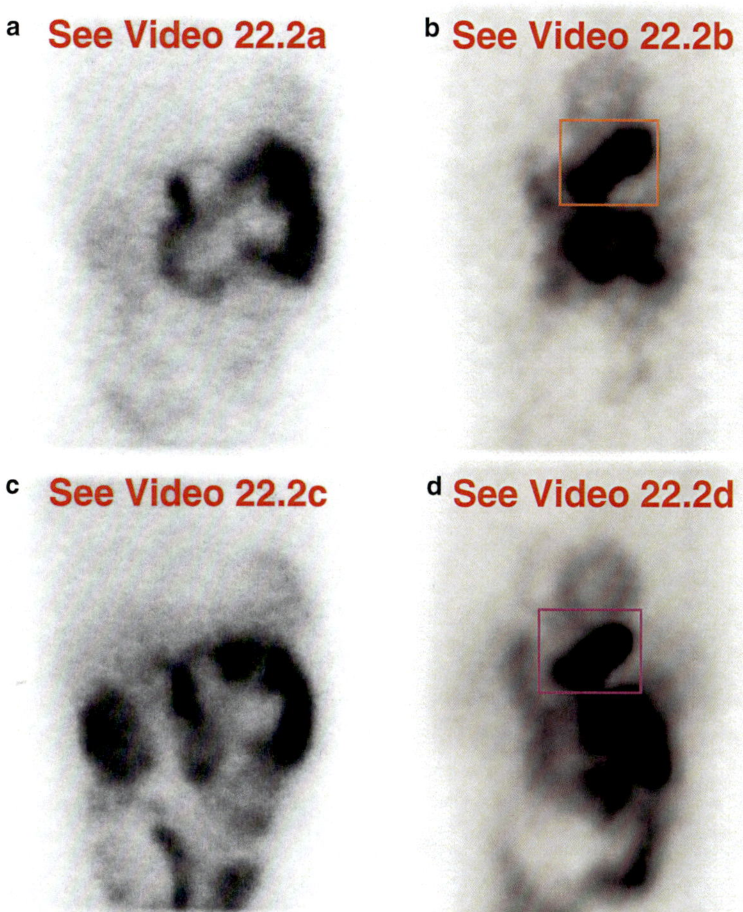

Fig. 22.2 Problematic gastric activity, clearing after water and waiting. This 60-year-old male has a history of previous myocardial infarction and hypertension; he underwent a regadenoson stress test. The "hot" stomach on the initial rest (**a**, **b**) and stress (**c**, **d**) images creates a significant defect in the inferior myocardium (**e**–**g**). The gastric activity clears on the repeat stress images (**h**, **i**) after water and waiting, and there is improvement in the artifact (**j**, **k**). There is an apparent small, mild perfusion defect in the inferior wall, but its characterization is compromised by the adjacent gastric activity; it was interpreted as a possible scar or processing artifact. On the gated SPECT images (**g**, **k**), the inferior wall shows mild hypokinesis, but its evaluation is limited by the gastric activity. Visually, left ventricular function was low normal.

(**a**) Rest raw projection images (Video 22.2a, frame 1), ^{99m}Tc sestamibi. (**b**) Rest raw projection image (Video 22.2b, frame 36), ^{99m}Tc sestamibi, gastric activity (*orange box*). (**c**) Initial stress raw projection images (Video 22.2c, frame 1), ^{99m}Tc sestamibi. (**d**) Initial stress raw projection image (Video 22.2d, frame 38), ^{99m}Tc sestamibi, gastric activity (*pink box*). (**e**) Initial stress/rest processed SPECT images optimized for stress images (SA, HLA, VLA). (**f**) Initial stress/rest processed SPECT images optimized for rest images (SA, HLA, VLA). (**g**) Initial stress gated SPECT images (Video 22.2e, frame 1) (SA, VLA, HLA). (**h**) Repeat stress raw projection images after water and 20 minute wait (Video 22.2f, frame 1), ^{99m}Tc sestamibi. (**i**) Repeat stress raw projection image after water and 20 minute wait (Video 22.2g, frame 39), ^{99m}Tc sestamibi, gastric activity (*blue box*). (**j**) Repeat stress/rest processed SPECT images optimized for stress images (SA), gastric activity (*blue oval*), inferior wall defect (*vertical yellow line*). (**k**) Repeat stress gated SPECT images (Video 22.2h, frame 1) (SA, VLA, HLA)

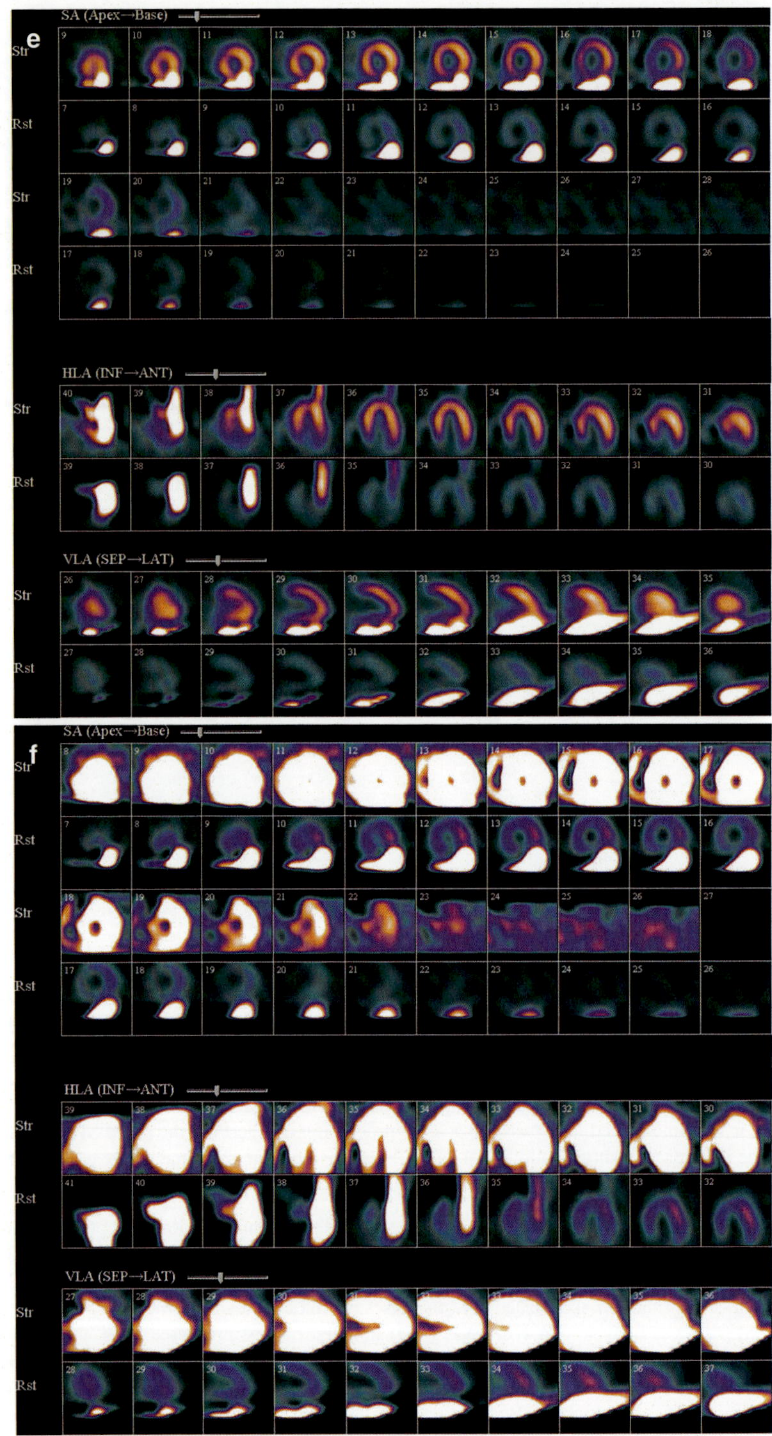

Fig. 22.2 (continued)

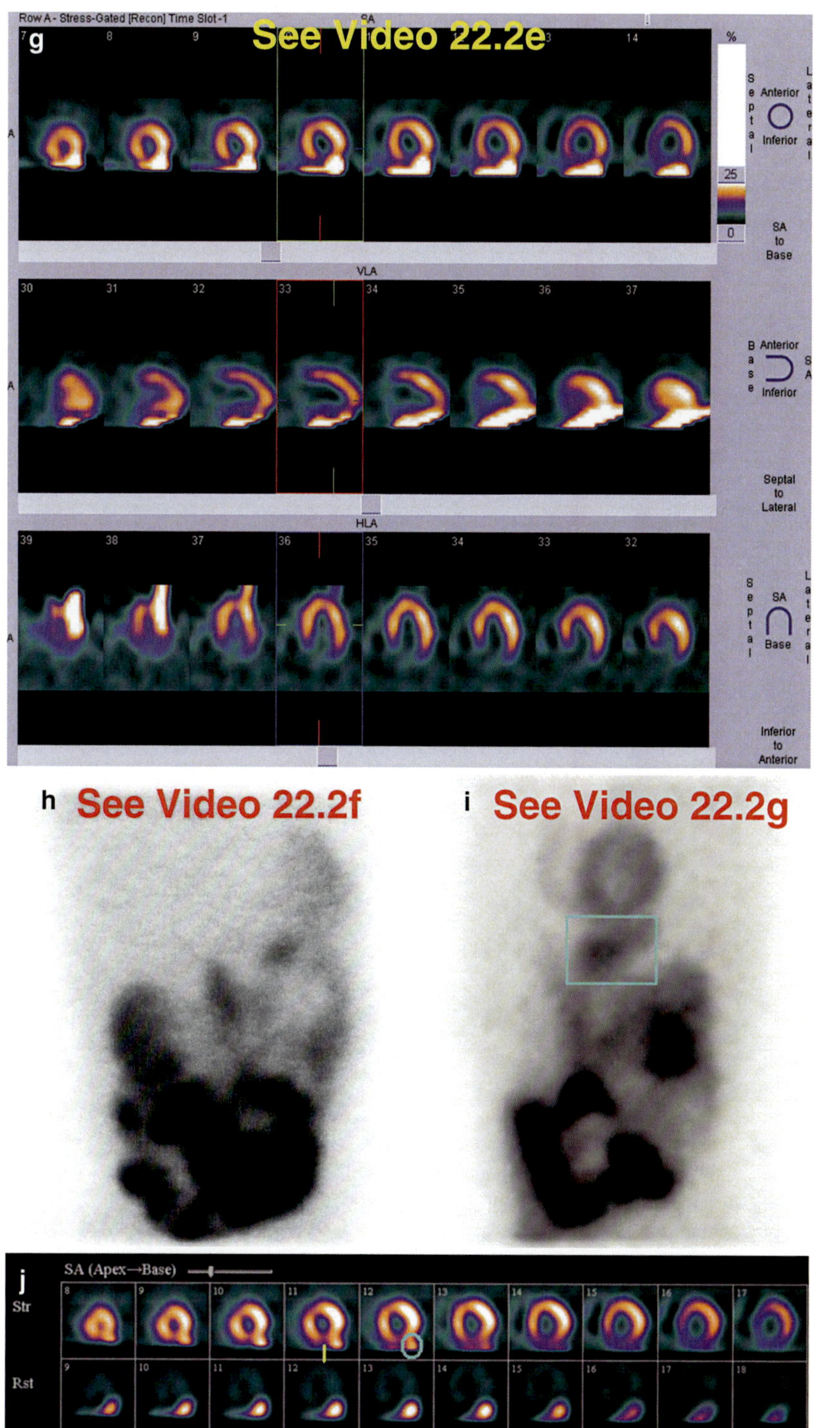

Fig. 22.2 (continued)

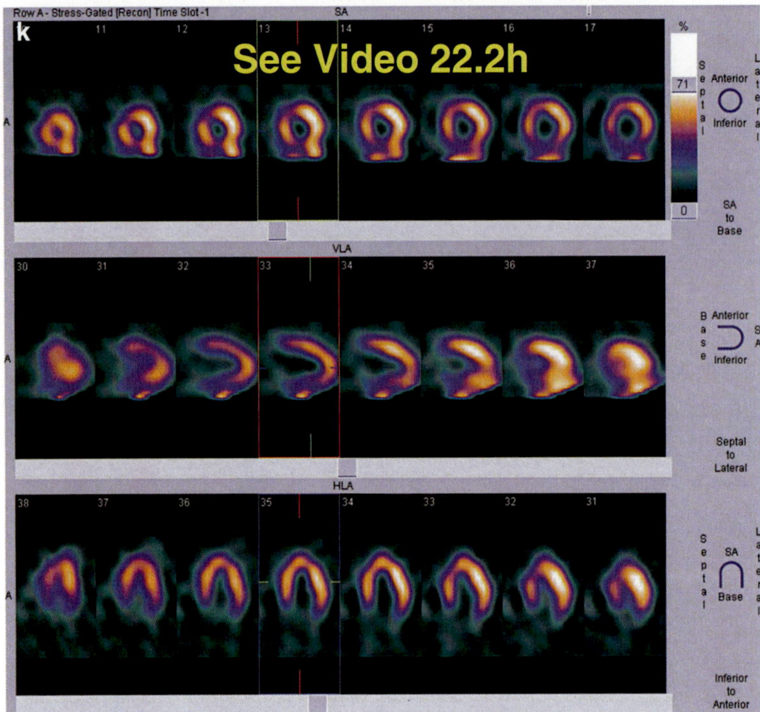

Fig. 22.2 (continued)

Fig. 22.3 Diabetic gastroparesis, minimal clearing of problematic gastric activity with water. There is a "hot" stomach on the initial stress images (**a–c**). It is partially mitigated by re-imaging after water (**d, e**); the stomach may empty slowly in functional motility disorders. There is a small inferior wall defect on rest images; the inferior and inferolateral walls from apex to base are almost impossible to evaluate on initial stress images (**c**), and only somewhat evaluable on repeat stress images (**e**).

(**a**) Selected rest raw projection image, ^{99m}Tc tetrofosmin, level of inferior wall (*white line*). (**b**) Selected stress raw projection image, ^{99m}Tc tetrofosmin, level of inferior wall (*white line*). (**c**) Stress/rest processed SPECT images (SA) (without and with AC). (**d**) Selected repeat stress raw projection image 90 minutes after water ingestion, level of inferior wall (*white line*). (**e**) Repeat stress/original rest processed SPECT images (SA) (without and with AC)

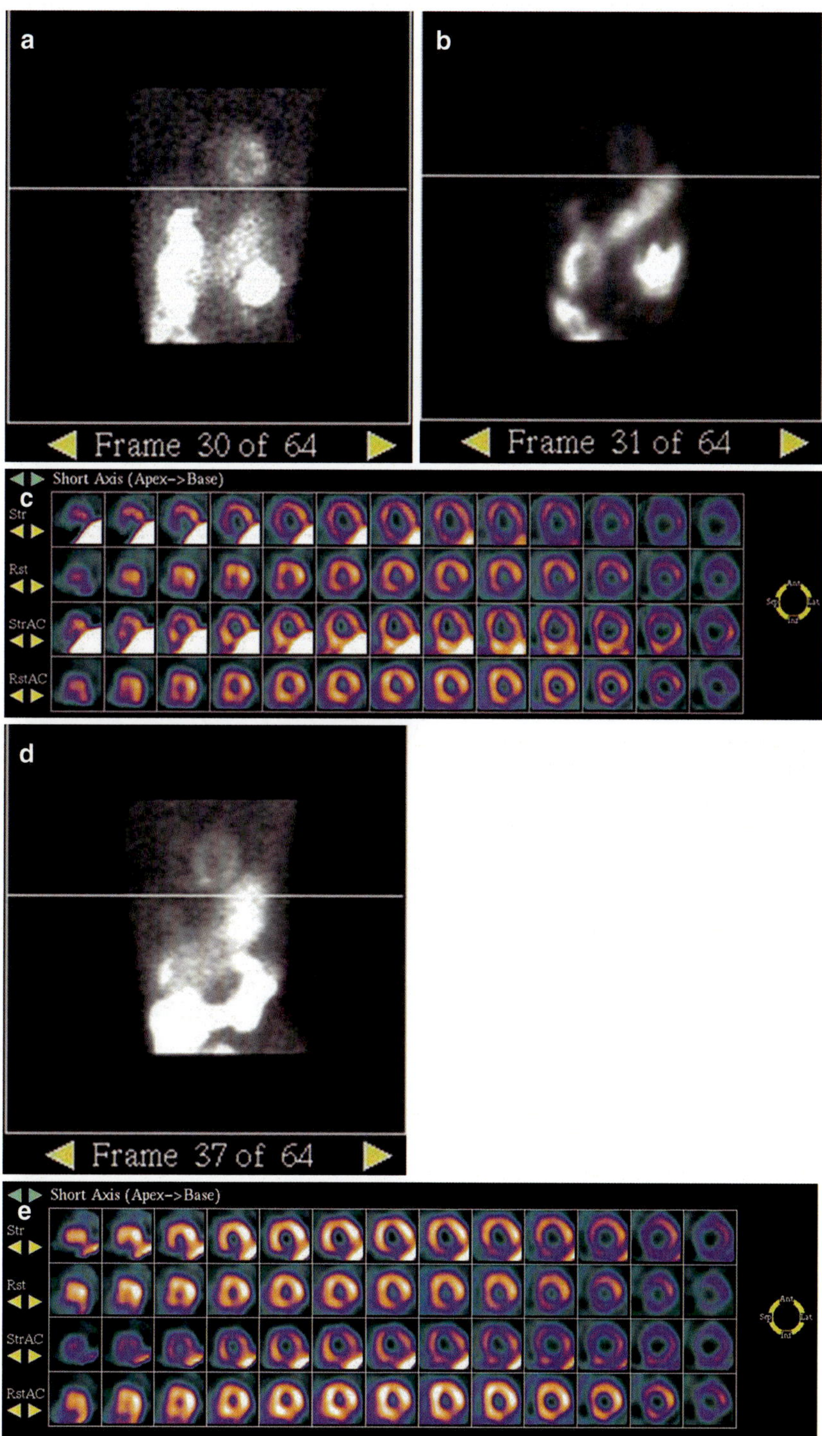

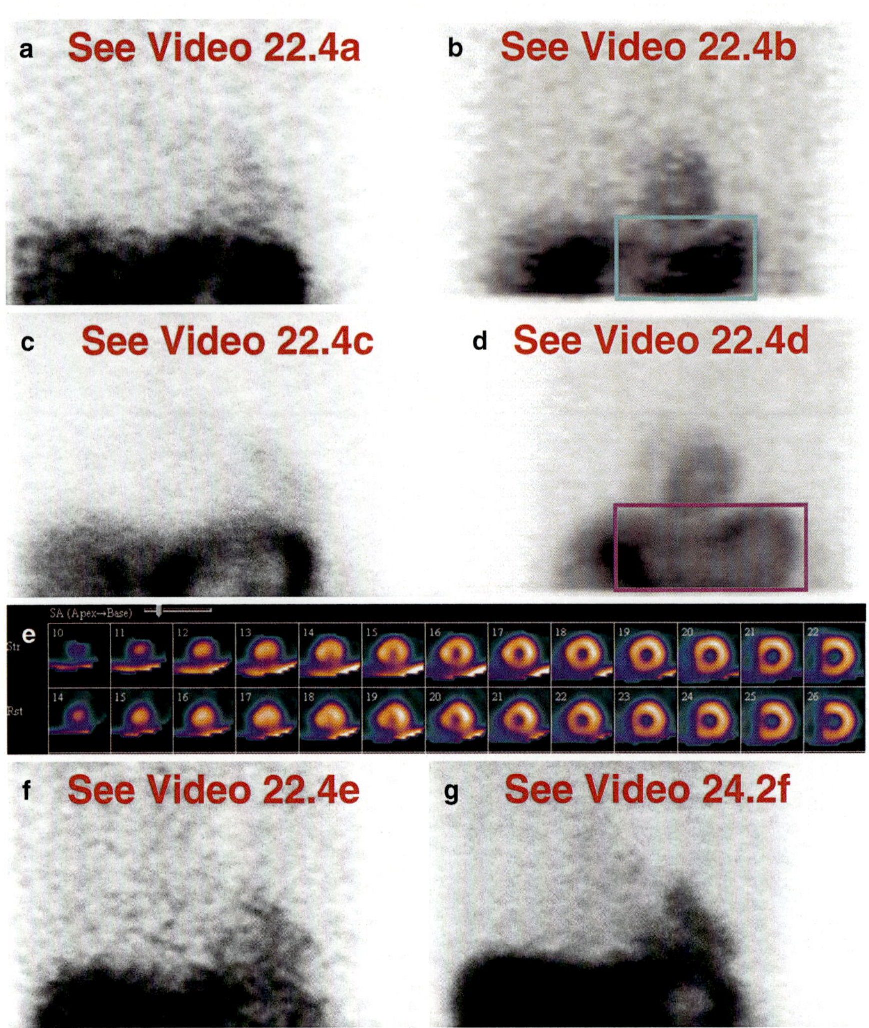

Fig. 22.4 Nondiabetic gastroparesis with "hot" and "cold" stomach. The current MPI demonstrates a distended "cold" stomach with a "hot" wall on both rest (**a**, **b**) and stress (**c**, **d**) raw projection images. Although the gastric activity is clearly apparent on the processed images (**e**), there is only a small, mild, fixed inferoapical defect. Interestingly, the raw data patterns are similar to those seen four years earlier (**f**, **g**); at that time, the processed data did not demonstrate significant artifact from the gastric activity (**h**). Although stomach-related artifactual effects are not always predictable, as shown here, comparison with previous images and reports can guide follow-up imaging techniques. Note the stomach morphology; it extends from anterior to posterior and lies immediately inferior to the heart (**i**).

(**a**) Rest raw projection images (Video 22.4a, frame 1), ^{99m}Tc sestamibi. (**b**) Rest raw projection image (Video 22.4b, frame 31), ^{99m}Tc sestamibi, stomach (*blue box*). (**c**) Stress raw projection images (Video 22.4c, frame 1), ^{99m}Tc sestamibi. (**d**) Stress raw projection image (Video 22.4d, frame 38), ^{99m}Tc sestamibi, stomach (*pink box*). (**e**) Stress/rest processed SPECT images (SA). (**f**) Four years earlier: rest raw projection images (Video 22.4e, frame 1), ^{99m}Tc sestamibi. (**g**) Four years earlier: stress raw projection images (Video 22.4f, frame 1), ^{99m}Tc sestamibi. (**h**) Four years earlier: stress/rest processed SPECT images (SA). (**i**) Sagittal CT image of the upper abdomen and stomach (outlined in *green*, within *yellow box*)

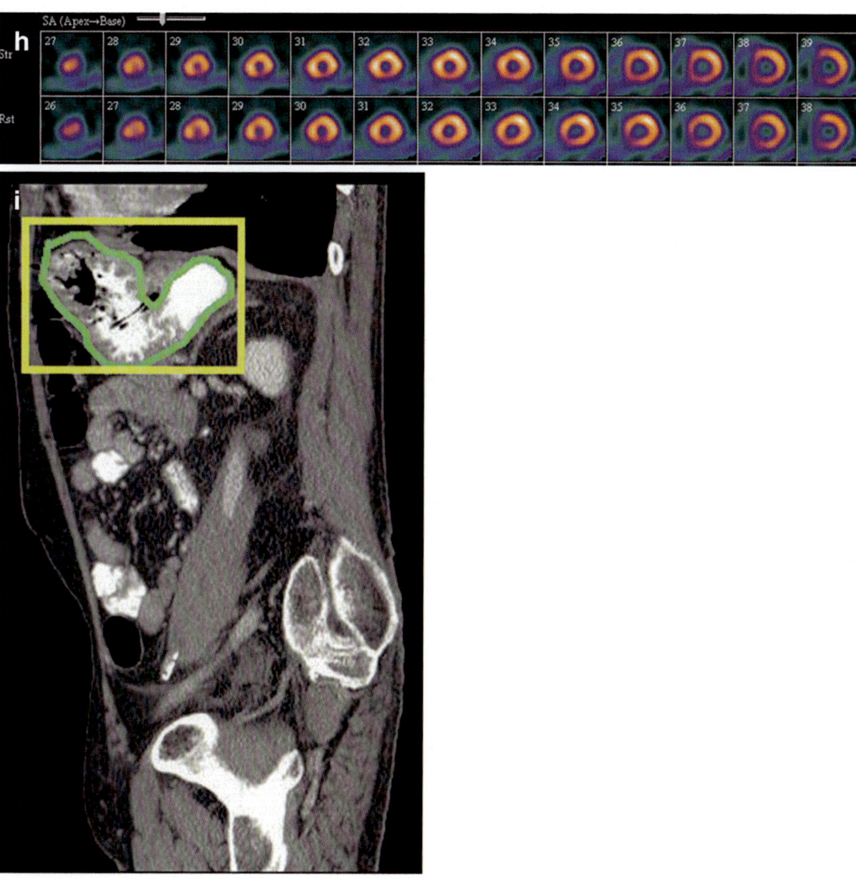

Fig. 22.4 (continued)

Alternatively,

On both rest and stress images, there is marked gastric activity, which appears to be intramural and involves the entire stomach; this pattern is consistent with gastropathy in association with known cirrhosis and portal hypertension. There is a small, severe, fixed defect in the adjacent inferior myocardial wall; this defect demonstrates normal wall motion and wall thickening on gated SPECT imaging. Same-day echocardiography shows a normal inferior wall. Thus, the perfusion defect is most likely artifactual and is much less likely to represent scar.

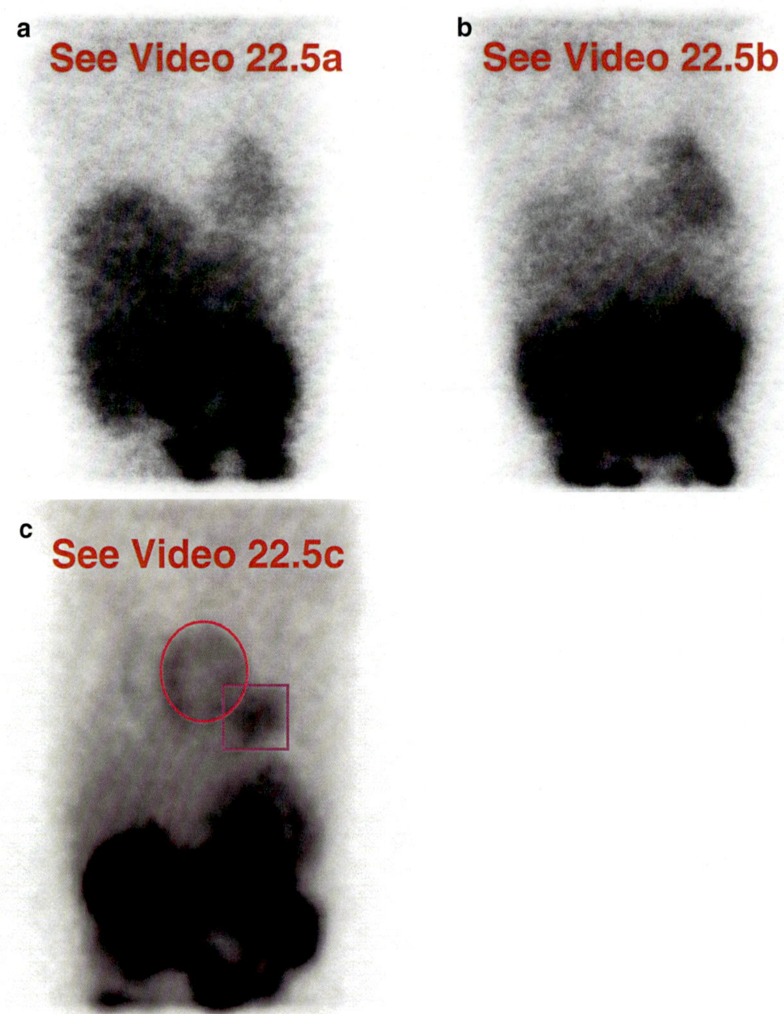

Fig. 22.5 "High" stomach due to eventration of the left hemidiaphragm. On a 1-day protocol in a 61-year-old female, there is minimal gastric activity on rest (**a**) and considerably more on stress (**b, c**) images. On processed images (**d**), there is no adjacent "hot" or "cold" artifact even though the "hot" stomach clearly abuts the inferolateral myocardium. The contour region of interest (ROI) aids appreciation of the slight tethering of the lateral wall by the "hot" stomach on the gated images (**e**). The stomach is positioned more superiorly than usual and is adjacent to the left ventricle on correlative CT images (**f**). The effects of an adjacent "hot" stomach on MPI interpretation are variable and unpredictable.

(**a**) Rest raw projection images (Video 22.5a, frame 1), ^{99m}Tc sestamibi. (**b**) Stress raw projection images (Video 22.5b, frame 1), ^{99m}Tc sestamibi. (**c**) Stress raw projection image (Video 22.5c, frame 35), ^{99m}Tc sestamibi, stomach activity (*pink box*), heart (*red oval*). (**d**) Stress/rest processed SPECT images (SA, HLA), stomach activity (stress, *pink boxes*; rest, *yellow boxes*) on selected images. (**e**) Stress gated SPECT images (Video 22.5d, frame 1) (SA), with left ventricular contour region-of-interest (ROI) (*white outline*). (**f**) Coronal CT image of the abdomen including lower chest and the stomach (*yellow box*) adjacent to left ventricle

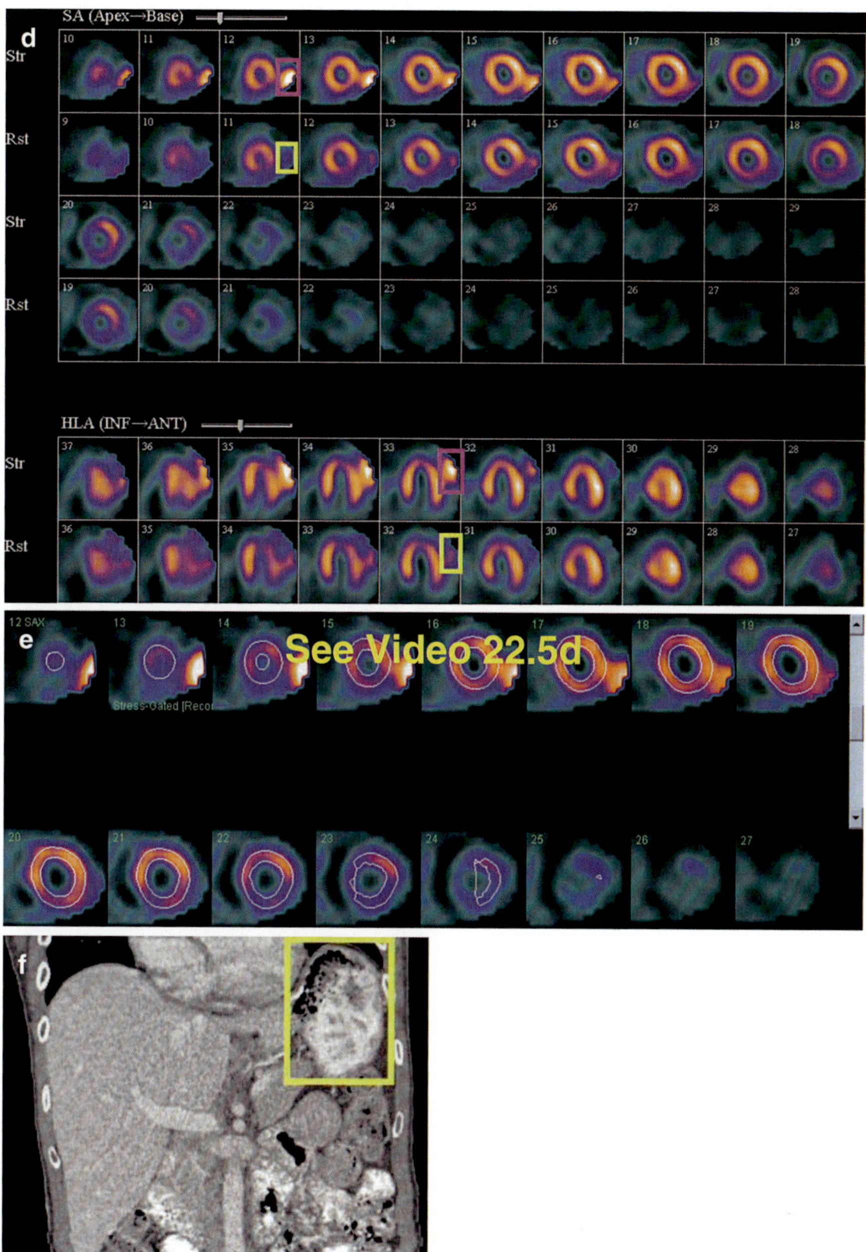

Fig. 22.5 (continued)

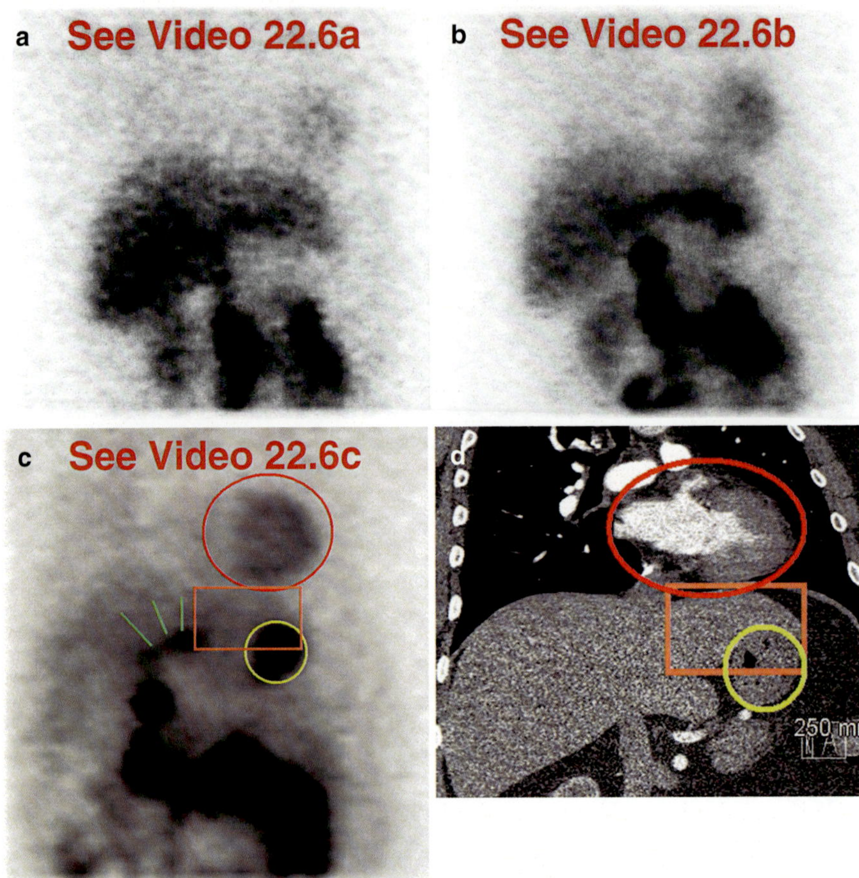

Fig. 22.6 Interposition of left hepatic lobe separating the heart from the stomach. The left lobe of the liver is positioned beneath the heart on the rest images (**a**). There is pronounced gastric reflux on the stress images (**b**), providing an opportunity to discern that the left hepatic lobe buffers this source of potential artifact from the inferior myocardial wall (**c**). Note biliary prominence (**c**) and absent gallbladder (known cholecystectomy) (**a, b**).

(**a**) Rest raw projection images (Video 22.6a, frame 1), ^{99m}Tc sestamibi. (**b**) Stress raw projection images (Video 22.6b, frame 1), ^{99m}Tc sestamibi. (**c**) Stress raw projection image (Video 22.6c, frame 21), ^{99m}Tc sestamibi, left lobe of the liver (*orange box*), left bile duct (*green lines*), stomach (*yellow circle*), and heart for reference (*red oval*). (**d**) Coronal CT image through left lobe of the liver (*orange box*), stomach (*yellow circle*), and heart (*red oval*)

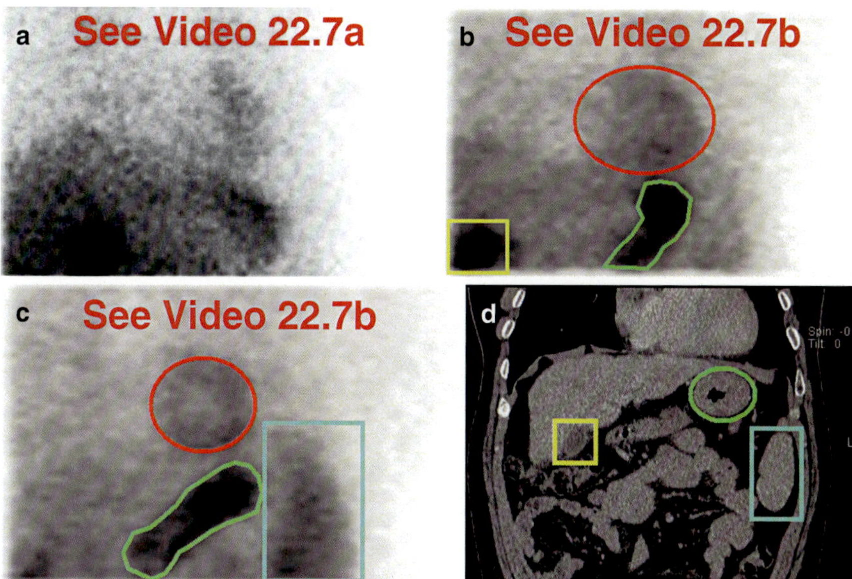

Fig. 22.7 Diffusely "hot" stomach wall characteristic of cirrhotic gastropathy. A 48-year-old male presents with shortness of breath during pre-transplant evaluation. Note the "hot" gastric wall with a relatively "cold" center; the gallbladder fills and there is splenomegaly (**a–c**). By CT, the liver is shrunken but there is no ascites (**d**). The heart is normal.

(**a**) Stress raw projection images (Video 22.7a, frame 1), ^{99m}Tc sestamibi. (**b**) Stress raw projection image (Video 22.7b, frame 15), ^{99m}Tc sestamibi, stomach (*green outline*), gallbladder (*yellow box*), heart for reference (*red oval*). (**c**) Stress raw projection image (Video 22.7b, frame 29), ^{99m}Tc sestamibi, stomach (*green outline*), spleen (*blue box*), heart for reference (*red oval*). (**d**) Coronal CT image through the liver and stomach (*green oval*), gallbladder (*yellow box*), and inferior tip of the spleen (*blue box*)

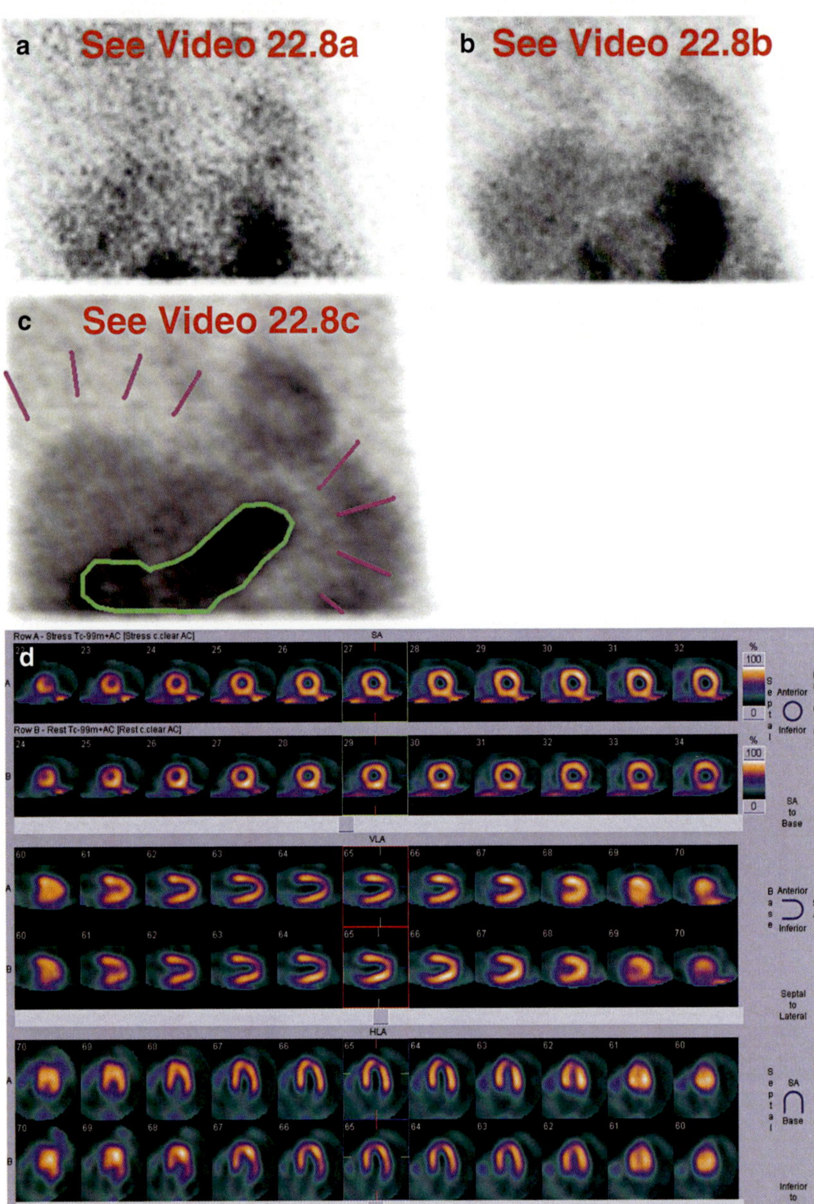

Fig. 22.8 Diffusely "hot" stomach wall in cirrhotic gastropathy. Note how the intensity of gastric activity exceeds that of the myocardium on both the rest (**a**) and the stress (**b, c**) raw data. Interestingly, there is no significant processing artifact on the adjacent myocardium; the heart is normal (**d–f**). The 67-year-old male has a small liver, splenomegaly, and "cold" ascites (**a–c**).

(**a**) Rest raw projection images (Video 22.8a, frame 1), ^{99m}Tc sestamibi. (**b**) Stress raw projection images (Video 22.8b, frame 1), ^{99m}Tc sestamibi. (**c**) Stress raw projection image (Video 22.8c, frame 18), ^{99m}Tc sestamibi, stomach (*green outline*), ascites (*pink lines*). (**d**) Stress/rest processed SPECT images (SA, VLA, HLA). (**e**) Stress/rest processed SPECT images (SA), gastric activity (*green boxes*) on selected stress and rest images. (**f**) Stress and rest gated SPECT images (Video 22.8d, frame 1) (SA, VLA, HLA)

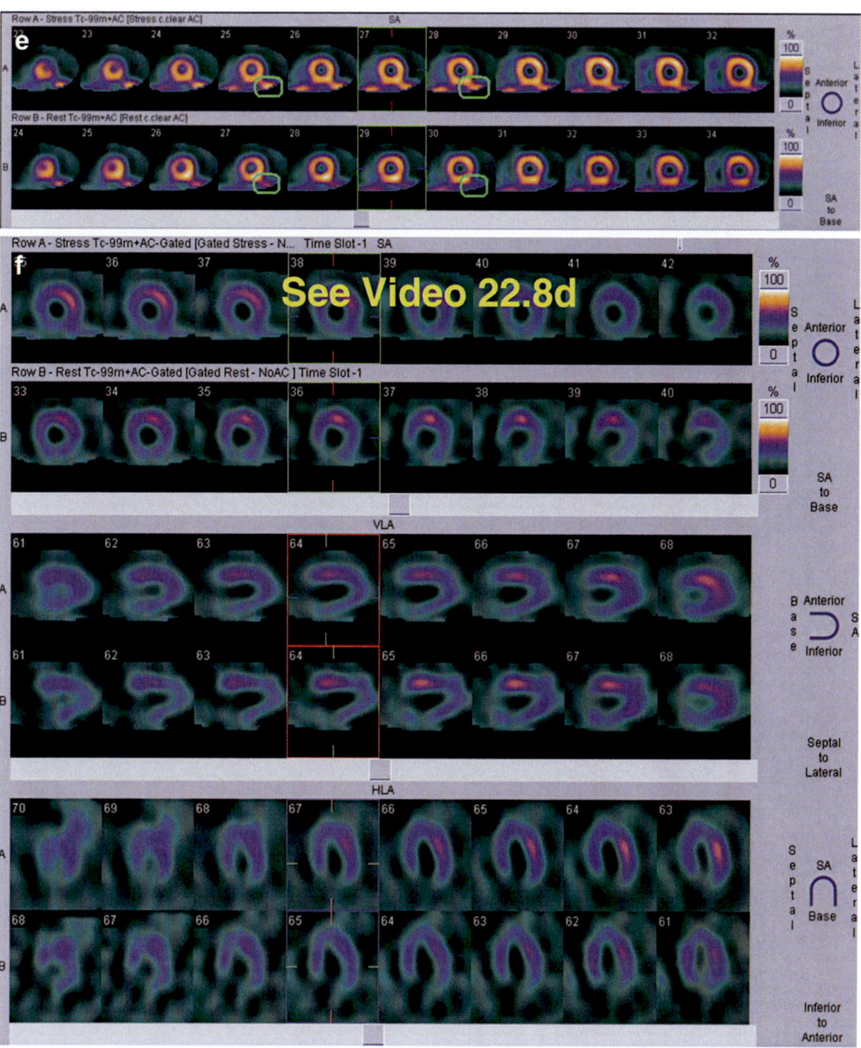

Fig. 22.8 (continued)

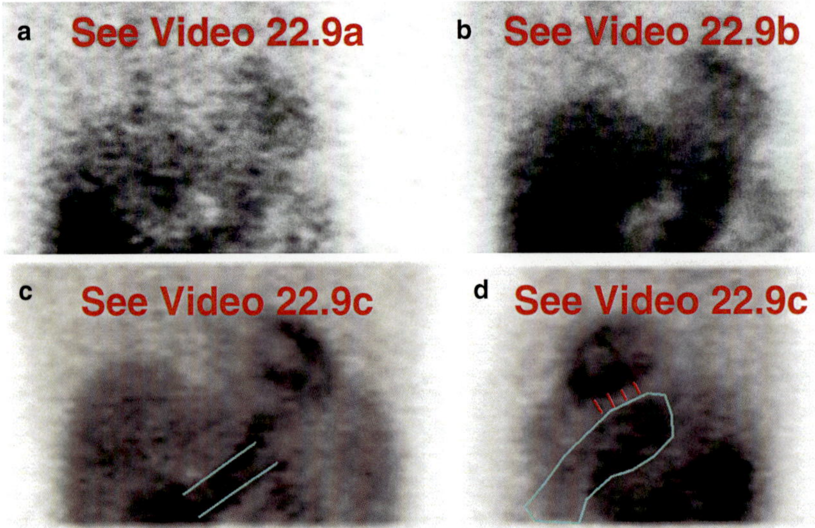

Fig. 22.9 "Railroad track" pattern of gastric wall uptake in cirrhosis. A 52-year-old male's raw data (**a**, **b**) show gastric wall uptake. There is separation of the "hot" gastric walls with a "cold" central lumen (**a**, **b**); this pattern resembles railroad tracks (**c**). In contradistinction, intraluminal duodenogastric reflux would have a "hot" lumen. Note the distance between the heart and the "hot" stomach; despite the markedly abnormal stomach, there is no artifactual effect on the normal processed and gated images (**e**, **f**). Note splenomegaly and a prominent left kidney (**a**, **b**); renal activity may be prominent in the setting of liver disease (refer to Chap. 25).

(**a**) Rest raw projection images (Video 22.9a, frame 1), ^{99m}Tc sestamibi. (**b**) Stress raw projection images (Video 22.9b, frame 1), ^{99m}Tc sestamibi. (**c**) Stress raw projection image (Video 22.9c, frame 16), ^{99m}Tc sestamibi, gastric walls (*blue lines*). (**d**) Stress raw projection image (Video 22.9c, frame 42), ^{99m}Tc sestamibi, stomach (*blue outline*), distance between the heart and stomach (*red lines*). (**e**) Stress/rest processed SPECT images (SA, HLA, VLA) (without and with AC). (**f**) Stress and rest gated SPECT images (Video 22.9d, frame 1) (SA, VLA, HLA)

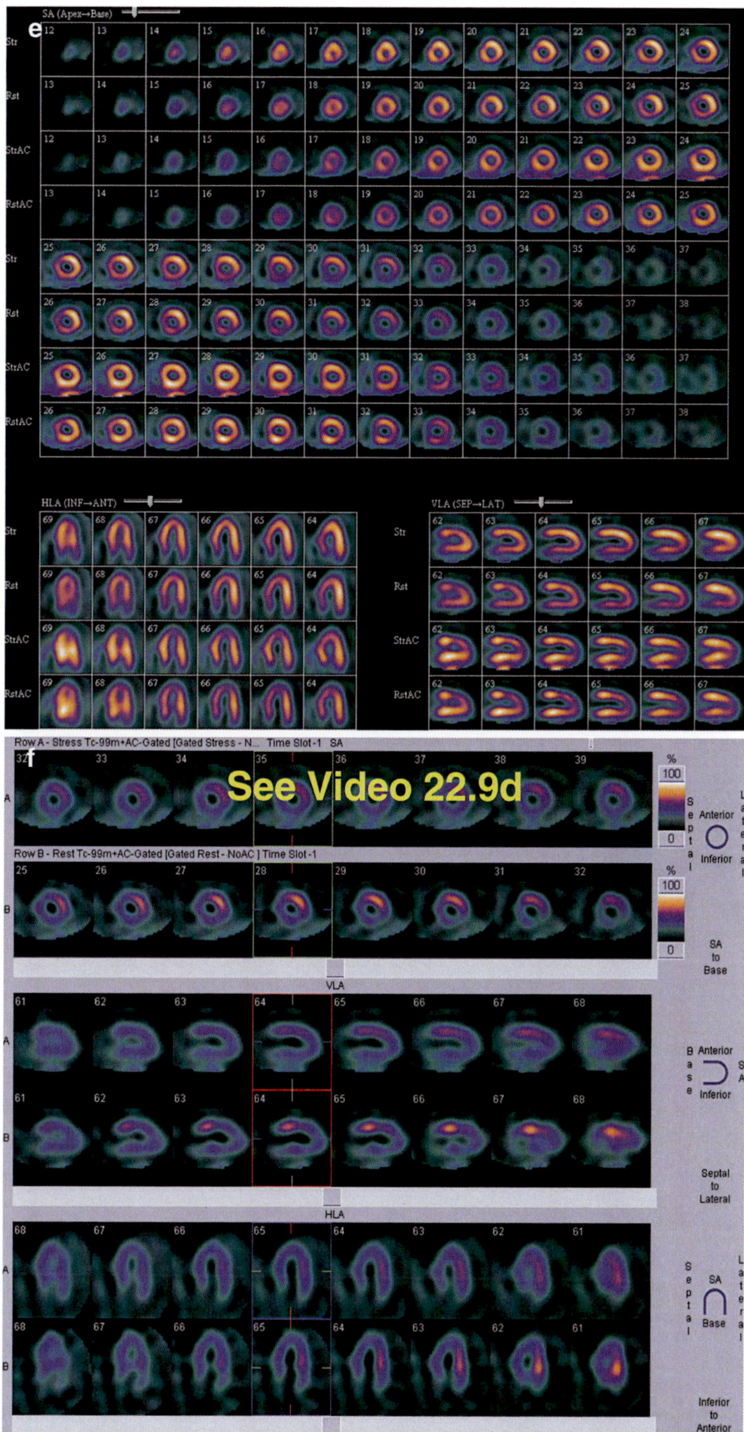

Fig. 22.9 (continued)

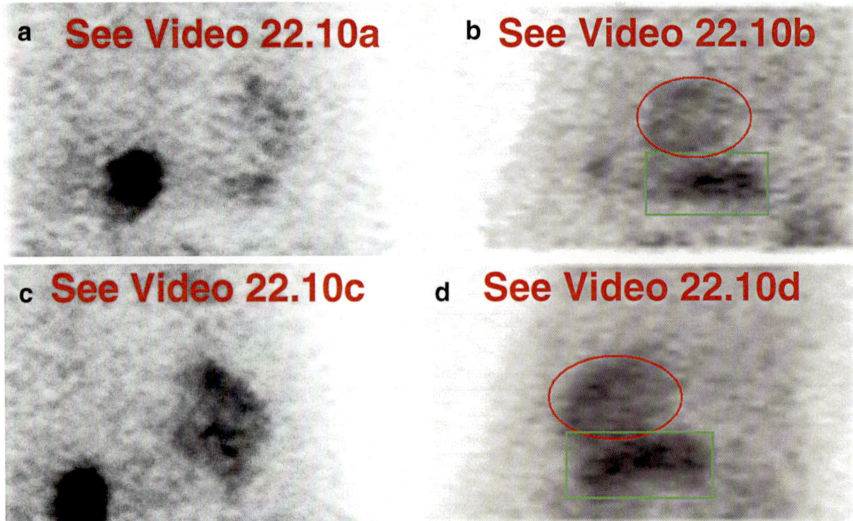

Fig. 22.10 Horizontal "hot" stomach. This patient has cirrhotic gastropathy. The "hot" stomach has a horizontal lie (**a–d**). On careful inspection, the stomach activity is more related to the inferior wall on the rest processed images but more closely related to the inferolateral wall on stress processed images (**e, f**). Thus, slight differences in patient position during image acquisition can result in interpretative challenges. The gastric activity creates a fixed defect in the adjacent inferior myocardial wall (**e, f**). Note that the liver is faintly perceptible, yet the gallbladder is well visualized (**a, c**).

(**a**) Rest raw projection images (Video 22.10a, frame 1), ^{99m}Tc sestamibi. (**b**) Rest raw projection image (Video 22.10b, frame 40), ^{99m}Tc sestamibi, stomach (*green box*), heart for reference (*red oval*). (**c**) Stress raw projection images (Video 22.10c, frame 1), ^{99m}Tc sestamibi. (**d**) Stress raw projection image (Video 22.10d, frame 45), ^{99m}Tc sestamibi, stomach (*green box*), heart for reference (*red oval*). (**e**) Stress/rest processed SPECT images (SA, HLA, VLA) (without and with AC), gastric activity with adjacent inferior wall defect (*blue boxes* on representative SA and VLA images). (**f**) Stress and rest gated SPECT images (Video 22.10e, frame 1) (SA, VLA, HLA)

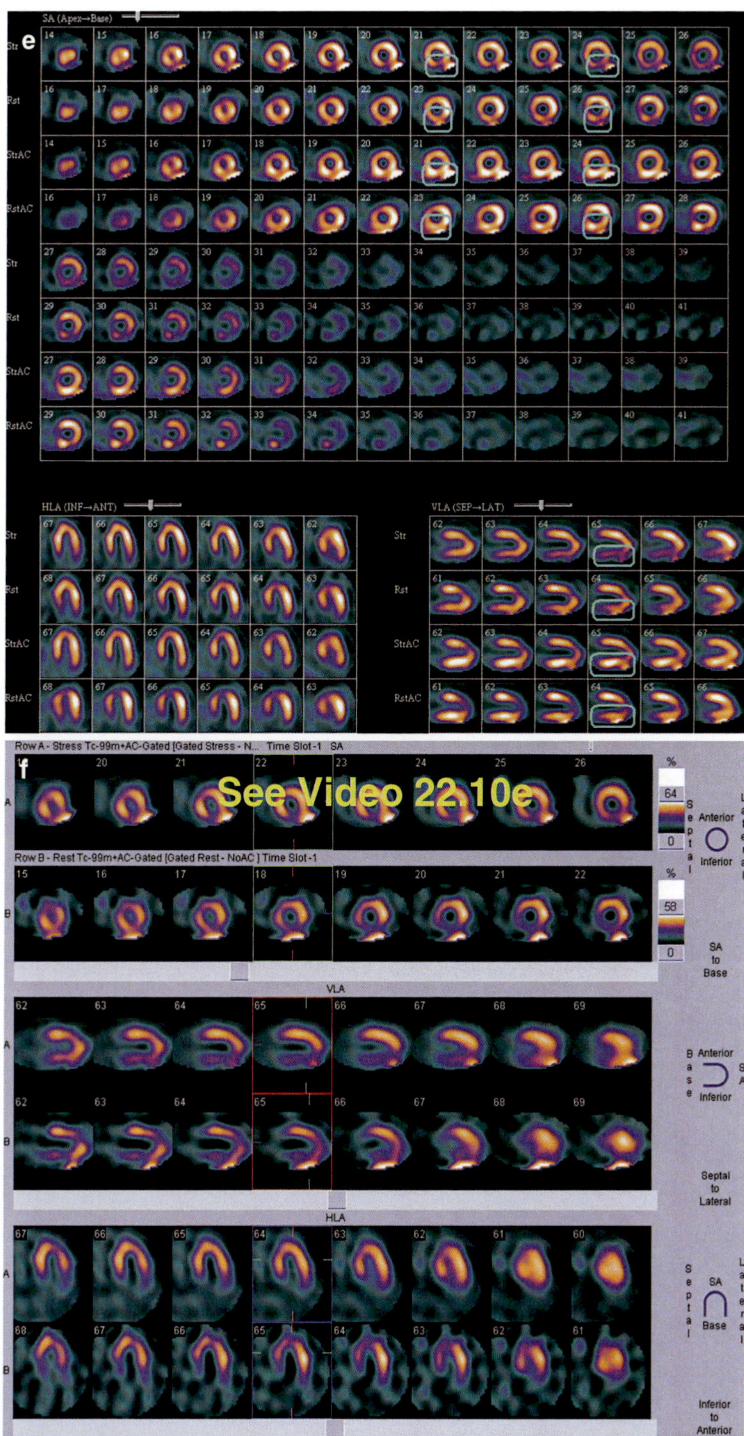

Fig. 22.10 (continued)

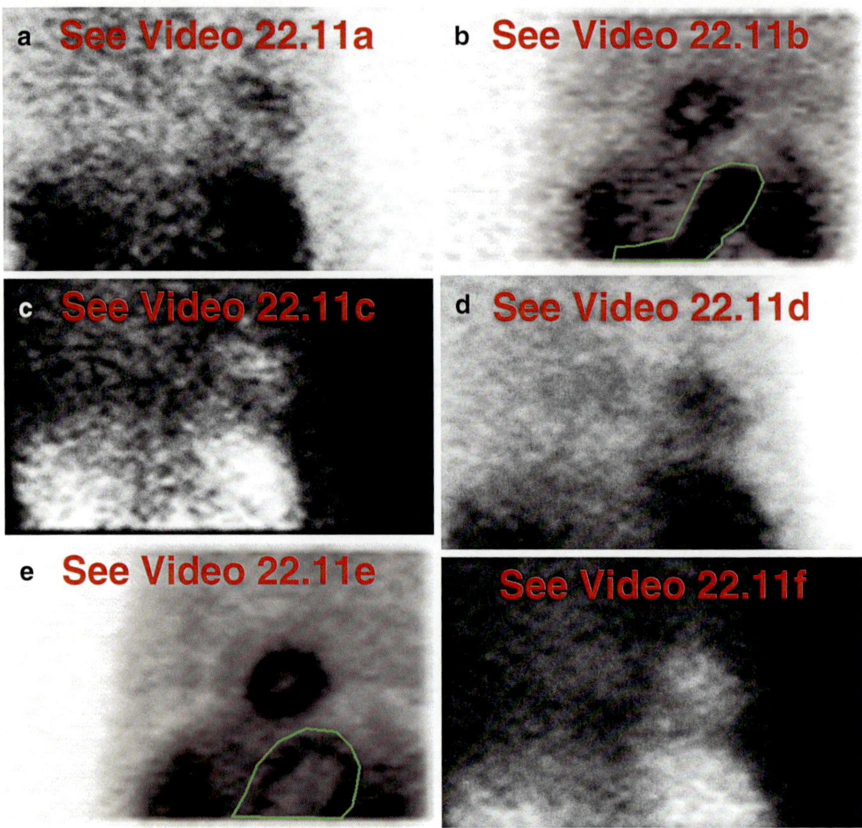

Fig. 22.11 Cirrhotic gastropathy with variable stomach distension. The "hot" stomach is collapsed on rest images (closely approximated "hot" walls with no discernible lumen) (**a–c**) yet quite distended on stress images ("hot" walls widely separated by a "cold" center) (**d–g**). Note how the ascites causes a well-demarcated "cold" region overlying the liver; this is better appreciated on the "white-on-black" raw data (**c, f**). MRI (**h**) demonstrates ascites.

(**a**) Rest "black-on-white" raw projection images (Video 22.11a, frame 1), ^{99m}Tc sestamibi. (**b**) Rest "black-on-white" raw projection image (Video 22.11b, frame 37), ^{99m}Tc sestamibi, stomach (*green outline*). (**c**) Rest "white-on-black" raw projection images (Video 22.11c, frame 1), ^{99m}Tc sestamibi. (**d**) Stress "black-on-white" raw projection images (Video 22.11d, frame 1), ^{99m}Tc sestamibi. (**e**) Stress "black-on-white" raw projection image (Video 22.11e, frame 36), ^{99m}Tc sestamibi, stomach (*green outline*). (**f**) Stress "white-on-black" raw projection images (Video 22.11f, frame 1), ^{99m}Tc sestamibi. (**g**) Stress "white-on-black" raw projection image (Video 22.11g, frame 27), ^{99m}Tc sestamibi, stomach (*green outline*), ascites (*pink outlines*). (**h**) Coronal MRI through the liver, ascites (*yellow ovals*)

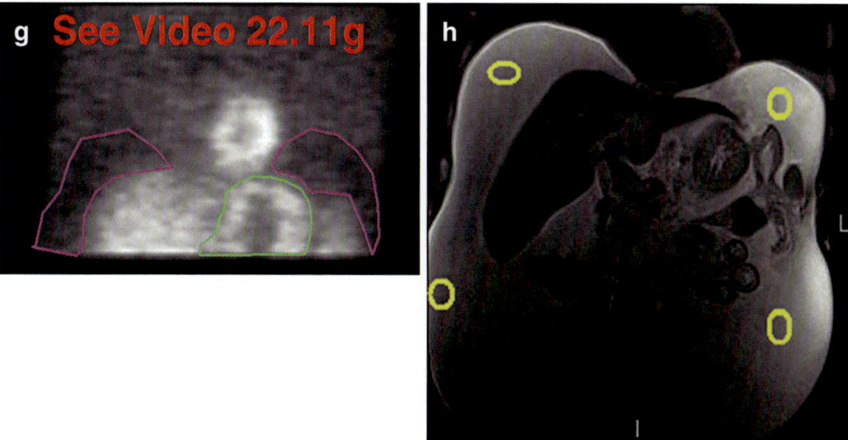

Fig. 22.11 (continued)

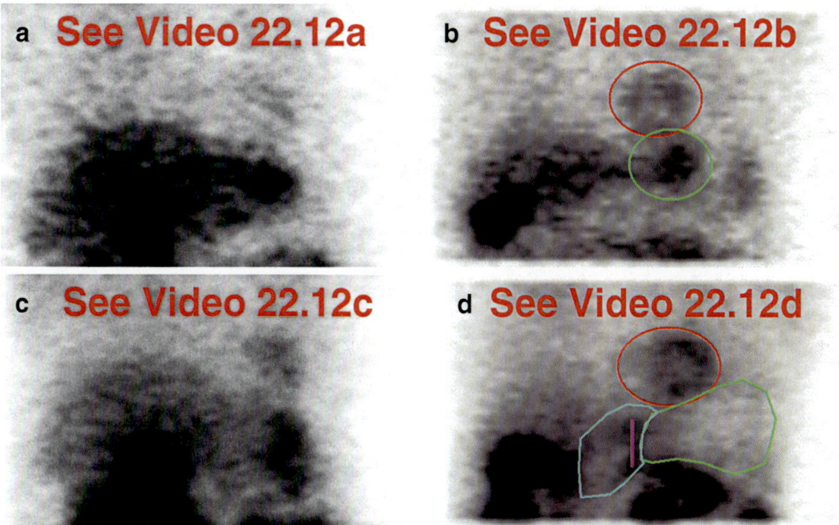

Fig. 22.12 Collapsed "hot" stomach on rest, distended "cold" stomach on stress. In this fasting patient, the "hot" stomach is collapsed at rest (**a, b**); the activity is more fundal in location, suggesting duodenogastric reflux as the etiology. On stress images (**c, d**), the stomach – from antrum to fundus – appears quite distended and "cold" due to water ingestion; the "hot" activity at rest has cleared with minimal residual gastric wall uptake evident. Note that the stomach appears "folded on itself" in the distended state (**c, d**). On the processed images (**e**), gastric activity is problematic only on rest images; there is an associated small inferior wall defect; since this region is normal on the stress images, it is of no clinical consequence.

(**a**) Rest raw projection images (Video 22.12a, frame 1), ^{99m}Tc sestamibi. (**b**) Rest raw projection image (Video 22.12b, frame 31), ^{99m}Tc sestamibi, stomach activity (*green oval*), heart for reference (*red oval*). (**c**) Stress raw projection images (Video 22.12c, frame 1), ^{99m}Tc sestamibi. (**d**) Stress raw projection image (Video 22.12d, frame 30), ^{99m}Tc sestamibi, stomach antrum (*blue outline*), stomach fundus (*green outline*), overlapping stomach wall due to fold (*pink line*), heart for reference (*red oval*). (**e**) Stress/rest processed SPECT images (SA, HLA, VLA) (without and with AC)

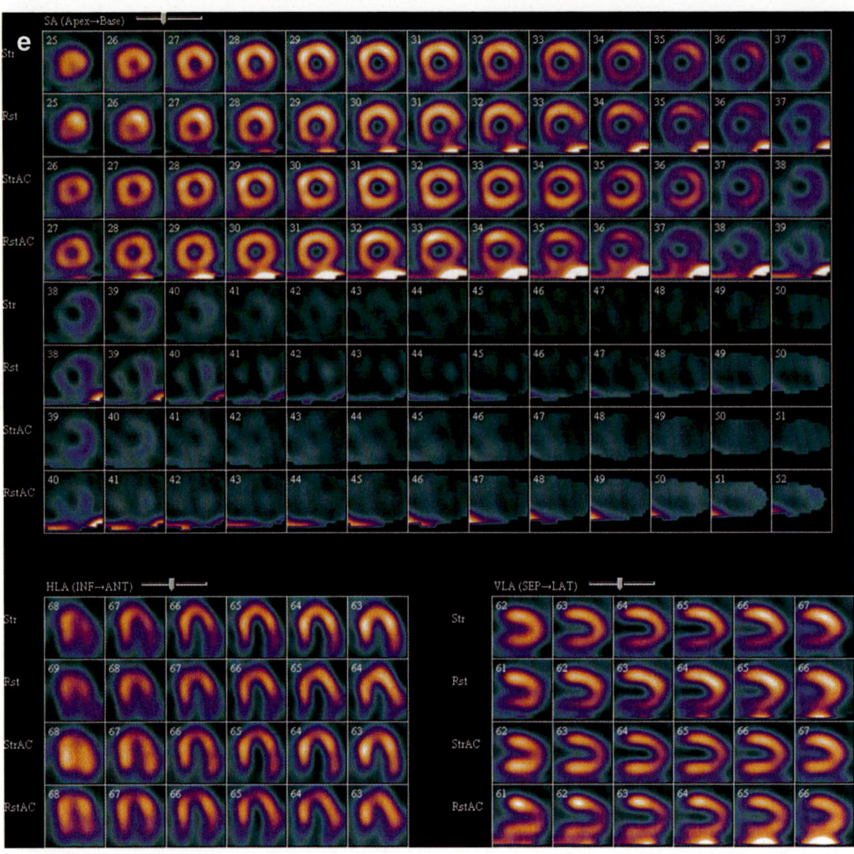

Fig. 22.12 (continued)

Key Points
- Radiopharmaceutical activity within the stomach is commonly encountered in SPECT MPI.
- It can be intraluminal due to duodenogastric bile reflux or can be intramural due to underlying gastropathy; in either case, gastric activity can be a vexing source of artifact.
- Modification of the imaging protocol and other strategies may be necessary to prevent or limit intraluminal gastric activity.

Small Intestine and Large Intestine

23

There are many conditions that impact the appearance of the small intestine and large intestine on SPECT MPI (Table 23.1). The small intestine is always visualized due to clearance through the hepatobiliary system (Chamarthy and Travin 2010; Gedik et al. 2007). Normal peristalsis may be apparent during the course of imaging (Fig. 23.1). Duodenogastric bile reflux (Fig. 23.2) and intense jejunal activity may create reconstruction processing artifacts. The jejunum may herniate through the diaphragm and appear in the chest (Gedik et al. 2007; Hendel et al. 1999). Waiting and re-imaging usually allows for peristalsis to clear the problematic jejunal activity. An unusual case of focal "hot" activity due to a duodenal leiomyosarcoma has been reported; this case used ^{201}Tl chloride, but the ^{99m}Tc radiopharmaceuticals could show this pattern after the physiologic intraluminal activity clears (Shuke et al. 1995).

The large intestine may be seen if gastrointestinal motility is relatively rapid or there is a long interval between injection and imaging. Figure 23.3 shows that activity has reached the transverse colon and splenic flexure. Figure 23.4 illustrates visualization of the entire colon. Radioactivity in the large intestine may be related to a previous radionuclide examination, and it should be evident on the first SPECT MPI performed (e.g., rest imaging in a 1-day rest/stress protocol) (Gedik et al. 2007; Hendel et al. 1999). A "cold" large intestine may be related to retained barium, which is a dense metal (Hendel et al. 1999).

Generally speaking, small intestinal activity is dealt with routinely and does not require special mention in the MPI report. It rarely interferes with interpretation. It is less common to visualize the large intestine, but, again, it generally is not

---

Electronic supplementary material The online version of this chapter (doi:10.1007/978-3-319-25436-4_23) contains supplementary material, which is available to authorized users.

© Springer International Publishing Switzerland 2017
M.E. Oates, V.L. Sorrell, *Myocardial Perfusion Imaging - Beyond the Left Ventricle: Pathology, Artifacts and Pitfalls in the Chest and Abdomen*, DOI 10.1007/978-3-319-25436-4_23

Table 23.1 Differential diagnosis of "hot" and "cold" imaging findings related to the small intestine and large intestine

Organ system	"Hot" finding	"Cold" finding	References
Small intestine and large intestine	Herniation Stasis/slow peristalsis Neoplasm, primary (e.g., duodenal leiomyosarcoma) Previous radiopharmaceutical	Barium	Chamarthy and Travin (2010) Gedik et al. (2007) Hendel et al. (1999) Shuke et al. (1995)

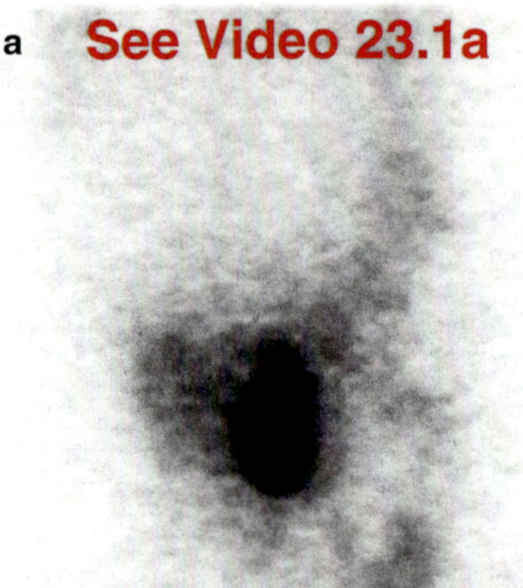

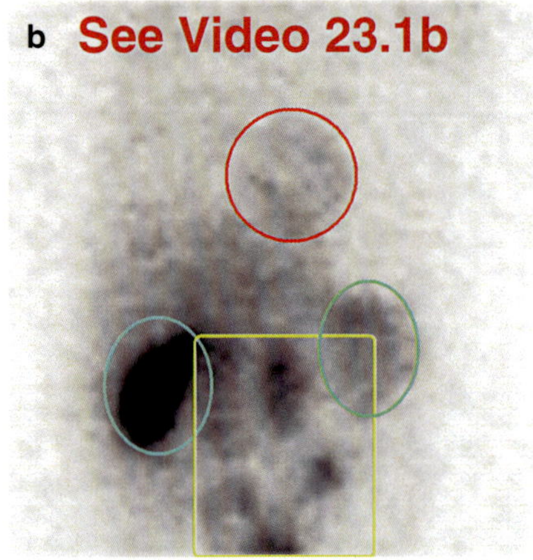

Fig 23.1 Normal small bowel peristalsis. A obese 39-year-old female underwent a normal pharmacologic stress test. As expected on a 1-day rest/stress protocol, there is more small intestinal activity on the stress images compared to the rest images (**a–d**). The normal gallbladder and the normal left kidney are visualized (**a–d**). There is duodenogastric reflux and retained liver activity, more evident on stress images, requiring tight limits for the reconstruction (**e**). A small, partially reversible inferolateral-apical perfusion defect is likely related to a "hot" stomach and/or a "hot" liver processing artifact (**e**). On gated SPECT images, the liver and stomach activity is much more apparent (**f**). There is preserved wall motion and wall thickening, and normal global left ventricular function with a LVEF of 57 %. Note that the large pendulous "cold" breasts seen on the raw data (**a, c**) do not create an anterior wall attenuation artifact.

(**a**) Rest raw projection images (Video 23.1a, frame 1), ^{99m}Tc sestamibi. (**b**) Rest raw projection image (Video 23.1b, frame 30), ^{99m}Tc sestamibi, small intestine (*yellow box*), gallbladder (*blue oval*), left kidney (*green oval*), heart for reference (*red oval*). (**c**) Stress raw projection images (Video 23.1c, frame 1), ^{99m}Tc sestamibi. (**d**) Stress raw projection image (Video 23.1d, frame 25), ^{99m}Tc sestamibi, small intestine (*yellow box*), gallbladder (*blue oval*), gastric activity (*green oval*), heart for reference (*red oval*). (**e**) Stress/rest processed SPECT images (SA, VLA, HLA), small defect adjacent to "hot" extracardiac activity (*yellow boxes* on representative images). (**f**) Stress gated SPECT (Video 23.1e, frame 1) (SA, VLA, HLA). (**g**) Stress gated SPECT (Video 23.1f, frame 3) (SA), liver (*blue box*), stomach (*green box*) on selected images

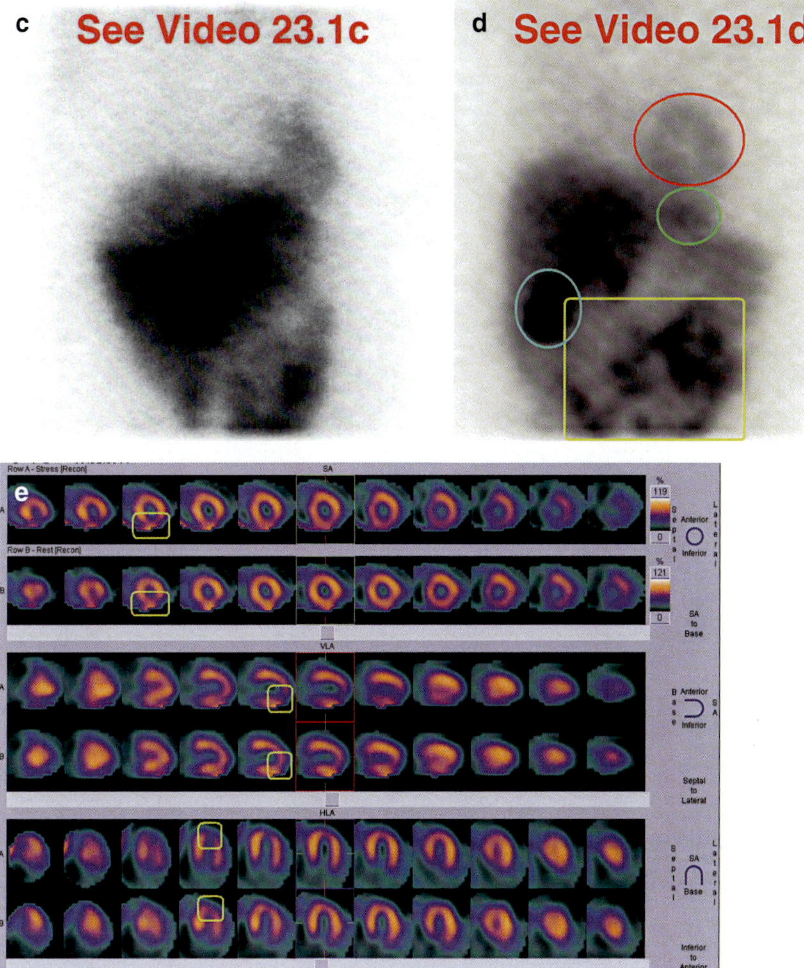

Fig 23.1 (continued)

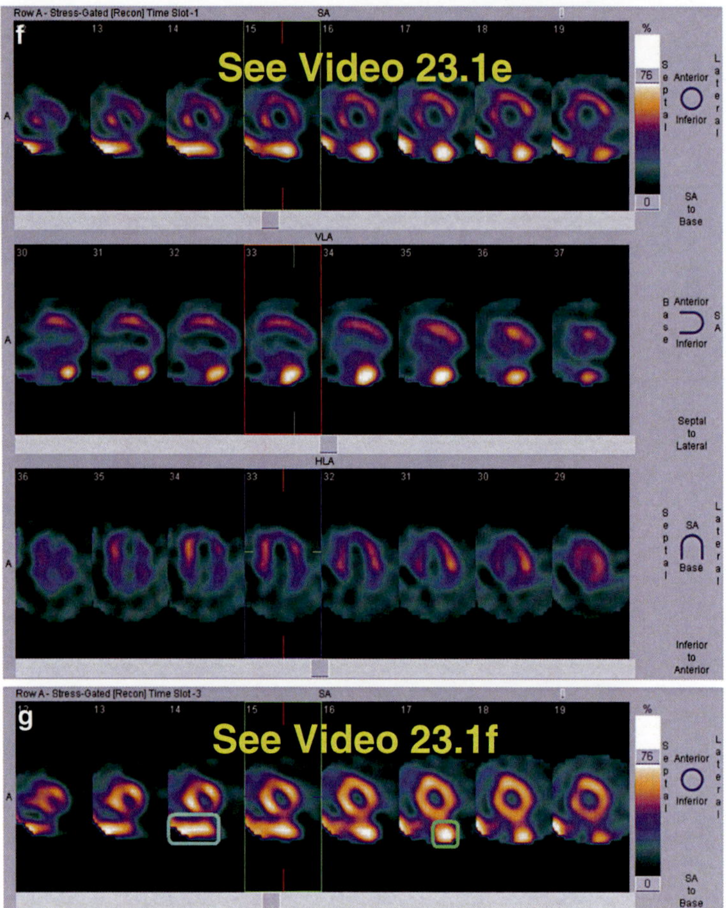

Fig 23.1 (continued)

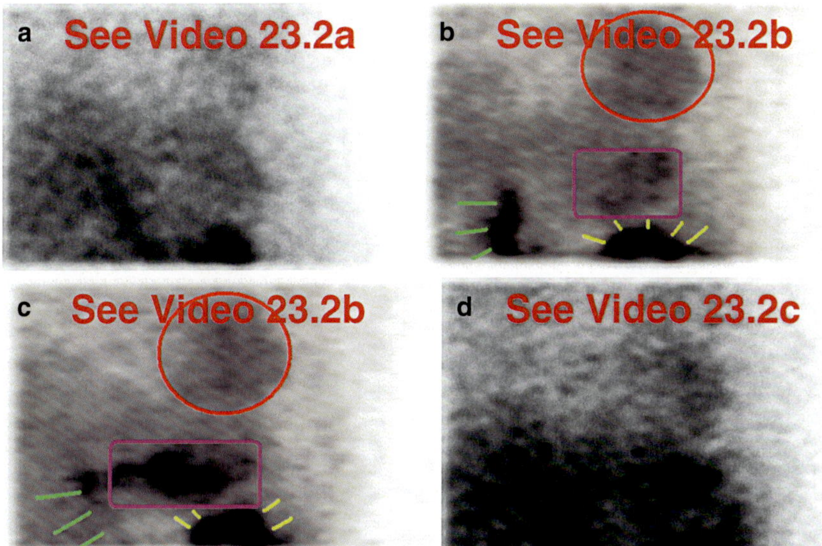

Fig 23.2   Active duodenogastric reflux. During image acquisition, duodenogastric reflux was captured dynamically (**a–c**). Excreted activity from the liver clearly moves from the duodenum into the stomach (compare **b** to **c**); activity also fills the jejunum as expected (compare **b** to **c**). The 40-year-old male has end-stage renal failure and a family history of coronary artery disease. Note that the significant duodenogastric reflux was present 1 year earlier (**d**). There is significant breathing motion artifact on both examinations.

(**a**) Current: stress raw projection images (Video 23.2a, frame 1), ^{99m}Tc sestamibi. (**b**) Current: stress raw projection image (Video 23.2b, frame 13), ^{99m}Tc sestamibi, stomach (*pink box*), duodenum (*green lines*), jejunum (*yellow lines*), heart for reference (*red oval*). (**c**) Current: stress raw projection image (Video 23.2b, frame 16), ^{99m}Tc sestamibi, stomach (*pink box*), duodenum (*green lines*), jejunum (*yellow lines*), heart for reference (*red oval*). (**d**) One year ago: stress raw projection images (Video 23.2c, frame 1), ^{99m}Tc sestamibi

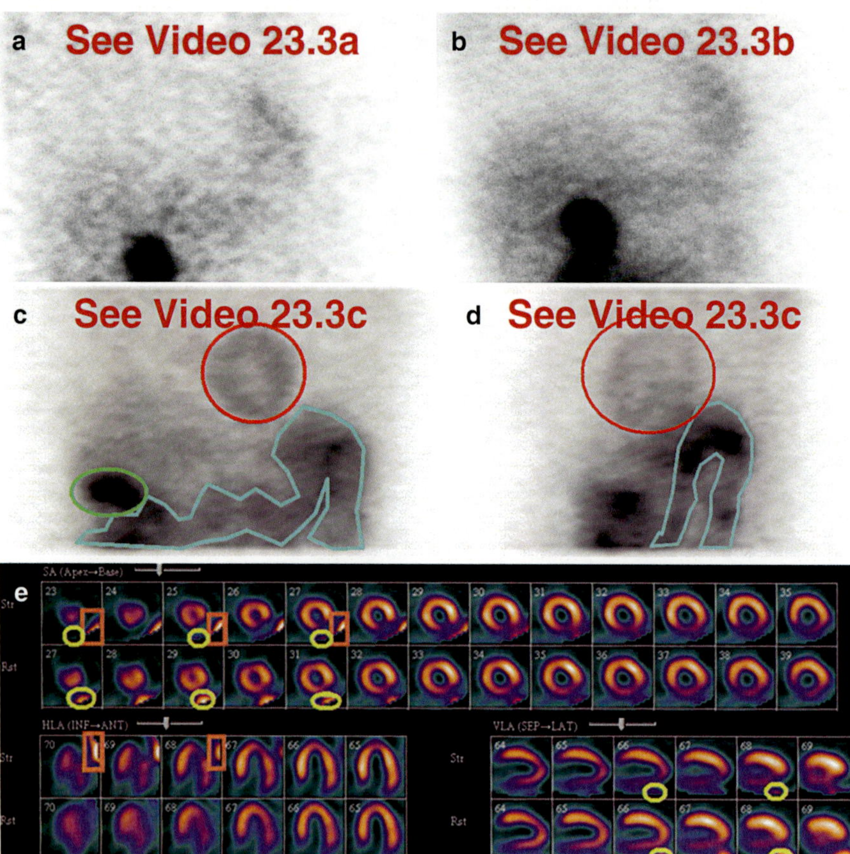

Fig. 23.3 Visualization of transverse colon and splenic flexure of large intestine. On the rest images (**a**) obtained 3.5 h after injection in a 46-year-old female, there is refluxed bile visualized in the stomach immediately inferior to the heart. On the stress images (**b–d**) acquired at 2 h after stress injection (5.5 h after the rest injection), there is less gastric activity, but the transverse and splenic flexure of the large intestine are well visualized. On the processed images (**e**), there is a small, partially reversible inferolateral defect, which might be caused, at least in part, by the adjacent "hot" splenic flexure. Note that the position of the stomach (identified by activity within it) is just medial to splenic flexure (**b, f**).

(**a**) Rest raw projection images (Video 23.3a, frame 1), ^{99m}Tc sestamibi. (**b**) Stress raw projection images (Video 23.3b, frame 1), ^{99m}Tc sestamibi. (**c**) Stress raw projection image (Video 23.3c, frame 29), ^{99m}Tc sestamibi, transverse colon and splenic flexure (*blue outline*), gallbladder (*green oval*), heart for reference (red oval). (**d**) Stress raw projection image (Video 23.3c, frame 45), ^{99m}Tc sestamibi, splenic flexure (*blue outline*), heart for reference (*red oval*). (**e**) Stress/rest processed SPECT images (SA, HLA, VLA), splenic flexure (*orange boxes*), stomach (*yellow ovals*) on selected images. (**f**) Coronal CT of abdomen at level of transverse colon (*pink line*), splenic flexure (*orange box*), and stomach (*yellow oval*)

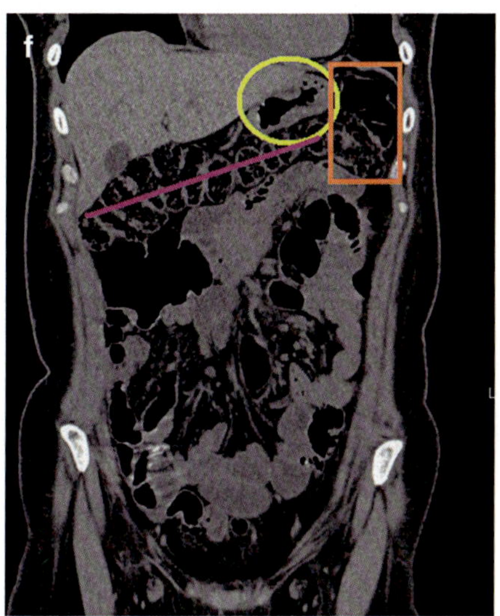

Fig 23.3 (continued)

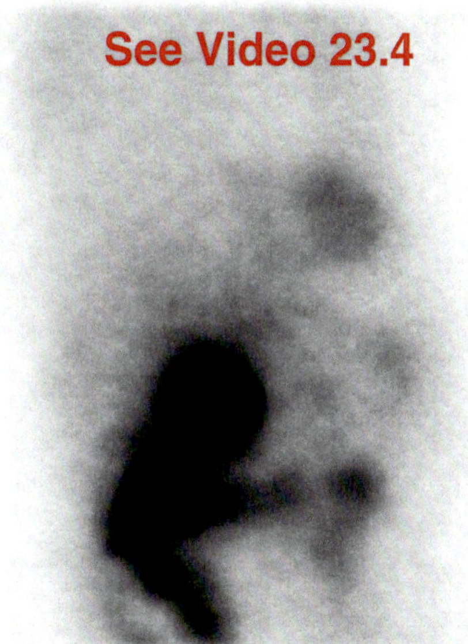

Fig. 23.4 Visualization of entire large intestine. On stress images obtained 2 h after stress injection and 3.5 h after rest injection, the entire large intestine—ascending, hepatic flexure (adjacent to "hot" gallbladder), transverse, splenic flexure (left upper quadrant closest to the heart), descending—is visualized. Note that there is no small intestinal activity; the intestinal activity resides in the large intestine due to the long interval between injection and imaging and intestinal peristalsis. A normal "hot" gallbladder is seen; minimal gastric activity likely represents duodenogastric reflux. Depending on a gamma camera detector's field-of-view, more or less of the large intestine will be included; there is considerable anatomic variability in the shape and position of the large bowel.

(**a**) Stress raw projection images (Video 23.4a, frame 1), ^{99m}Tc sestamibi

problematic. Infrequently, in selected cases, one might choose to issue a report as follows:

On the stress images, normal excreted activity is identified throughout the large intestine, likely due to rapid gastrointestinal transit. This activity is problematic because the splenic flexure overlies the heart in this patient who has an elevated left hemidiaphragm, and, as such, it limits evaluation of the inferolateral myocardial wall. Despite waiting and re-imaging, the activity did not clear sufficiently for complete evaluation.

Key Points
- The small intestine is always visualized due to the normal hepatobiliary clearance of the ^{99m}Tc MPI radiopharmaceuticals.
- Duodenogastric reflux of radioactive bile and "hot" jejunal activity can cause reconstruction processing artifacts.
- The large intestine may be seen if intestinal motility is relatively rapid, or there is a long interval between injection and imaging.

Adrenal Glands

24

The adrenal glands are not normally visualized on SPECT MPI. Differential diagnosis is quite limited (Table 24.1). However, adrenal masses are space occupying and, if large enough, can displace other abdominal organs and appear "cold" (Fig. 24.1). Finding an unknown abdominal mass always warrants direct personal communication.

Electronic supplementary material The online version of this chapter (doi:10.1007/978-3-319-25436-4_24) contains supplementary material, which is available to authorized users.

© Springer International Publishing Switzerland 2017

M.E. Oates, V.L. Sorrell, *Myocardial Perfusion Imaging - Beyond the Left Ventricle: Pathology, Artifacts and Pitfalls in the Chest and Abdomen*, DOI 10.1007/978-3-319-25436-4_24

Table 24.1 Differential diagnosis of "hot" and "cold" imaging findings related to the adrenal glands

Organ system	"Hot" finding	"Cold" finding	References
Adrenal glands	Not reported	Cyst *Neoplasm, primary* *Neoplasm, metastasis*	Not applicable

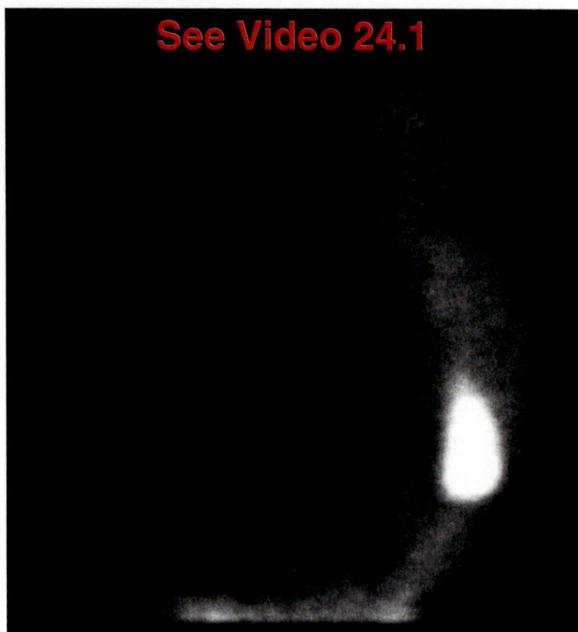

Fig. 24.1 Adrenocortical carcinoma. A very large, well-defined "cold" region displacing liver, gallbladder, and small intestine (note active peristalsis) into the left abdomen is due to a 37 cm × 25 cm × 17 cm malignant neoplasm arising from the right adrenal gland. Note a normal left kidney in the posterior mid-abdomen; there is excreted urinary activity in the catheter tubing outside the left lower abdomen.

(**a**) Stress raw projection images (Video 24.1a, frame 1), ^{99m}Tc tetrofosmin

Key Points
- The adrenal glands are not normally visualized on SPECT MPI.
- An unexpected abdominal mass, possibly of adrenal origin, warrants a notification to the referring physician.

Kidneys and Female Reproductive System

25

A wide variety of diffuse and focal, unilateral and bilateral renal conditions may be detected on review of the raw SPECT MPI data (Table 25.1) (Shih et al. 2002, 2005). A normal adult kidney measures approximately 11 cm in length. The size of the kidney can be quickly compared to the heart, and it should be slightly larger than a non-dilated heart. Increased visualization of the kidneys may be seen in liver failure as the kidneys are the alternate route of elimination (Fig. 25.1).

The left kidney is generally included in the field-of-view (Chamarthy and Travin 2010). Non-visualization of the left kidney (the right kidney is difficult to appreciate on a 180°acquisition) is abnormal and may be related to end-stage renal disease

Table 25.1 Differential diagnosis of "hot" and "cold" imaging findings related to the kidneys and female reproductive system

Organ system	"Hot" finding	"Cold" finding	References
Kidneys and female reproductive system	Retention of excreted radioactivity in dilated collecting system Stone disease Urinary catheters Physiologic in hepatic failure	Congenital absence/nephrectomy Ptotic or small kidney Atrophy/end-stage renal disease Scar/pyelonephritis Cyst/polycystic disease *Neoplasm, primary (kidney, uterine leiomyoma)* *Neoplasm, metastasis*	Chamarthy and Travin (2010) Garg et al. (2013) Gedik et al. (2007) Ghanbarinia et al. (2008) Howarth et al. (1996) Raza et al. (2005b) Shih et al. (2002) Shih et al. (2005)

Electronic supplementary material The online version of this chapter (doi:10.1007/978-3-319-25436-4_25) contains supplementary material, which is available to authorized users.

© Springer International Publishing Switzerland 2017

M.E. Oates, V.L. Sorrell, *Myocardial Perfusion Imaging - Beyond the Left Ventricle: Pathology, Artifacts and Pitfalls in the Chest and Abdomen*, DOI 10.1007/978-3-319-25436-4_25

(Fig. 25.2) (Shih et al. 2002). In a series of 566 patients who received ⁹⁹ᵐTc tetrofosmin, 2% had renal abnormalities, including absence, atrophy, and cysts as causes for "cold" findings (Shih et al. 2005). Cases of polycystic kidney disease have been reported. Displacement of other organs may occur when they are markedly enlarged. Focal "cold" lesions may be neoplastic (Chamarthy and Travin 2010; Gedik et al. 2007). Authors recommend correlative imaging and "whole-field-of-view reconstruction" for optimal characterization of abnormal kidneys (Ghanbarinia et al. 2008; Raza et al. 2005b).

In the pelvis, urinary catheters can be visualized if they contain radioactive urine (refer to Fig. 24.1) (Howarth et al. 1996). Regarding the female reproductive system, a massive "cold" uterine leiomyoma displacing small intestine and urinary bladder has been reported (Garg et al. 2013).

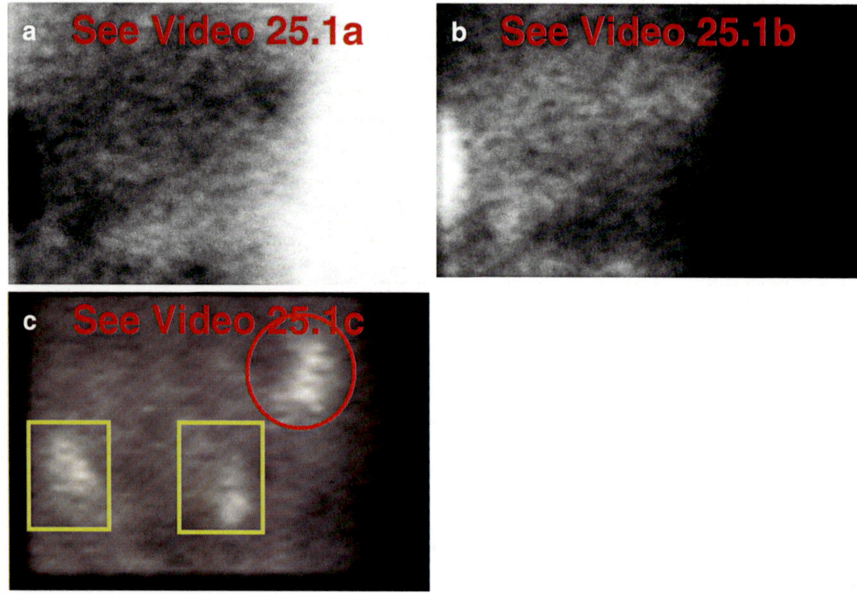

Fig. 25.1 "Hot" kidneys in liver disease. The 64-year-old female has elevated bilirubin and ascites. The liver is not seen, and there is virtually no intestinal activity—this is an extremely unusual circumstance. When the primary hepatobiliary route of clearance is impaired, the alternate urinary route becomes predominant (**a–c**). Note how different color rendering enhances recognition of this vicarious excretory pattern (**c**). There is normal myocardial perfusion (**d**).

(**a**) Stress "black-on-white" raw projection images (Video 25.1a, frame 1), ⁹⁹ᵐTc sestamibi. (**b**) Stress "white-on-black" raw projection images (Video 25.1b, frame 1), ⁹⁹ᵐTc sestamibi. (**c**) Stress "white-on-black" raw projection image (Video 25.1c, frame 19, Anterior), ⁹⁹ᵐTc sestamibi, kidneys (*yellow boxes*), heart for reference (*red oval*). (**d**) Stress/rest processed SPECT images (SA, HLA, VLA) (without and with AC)

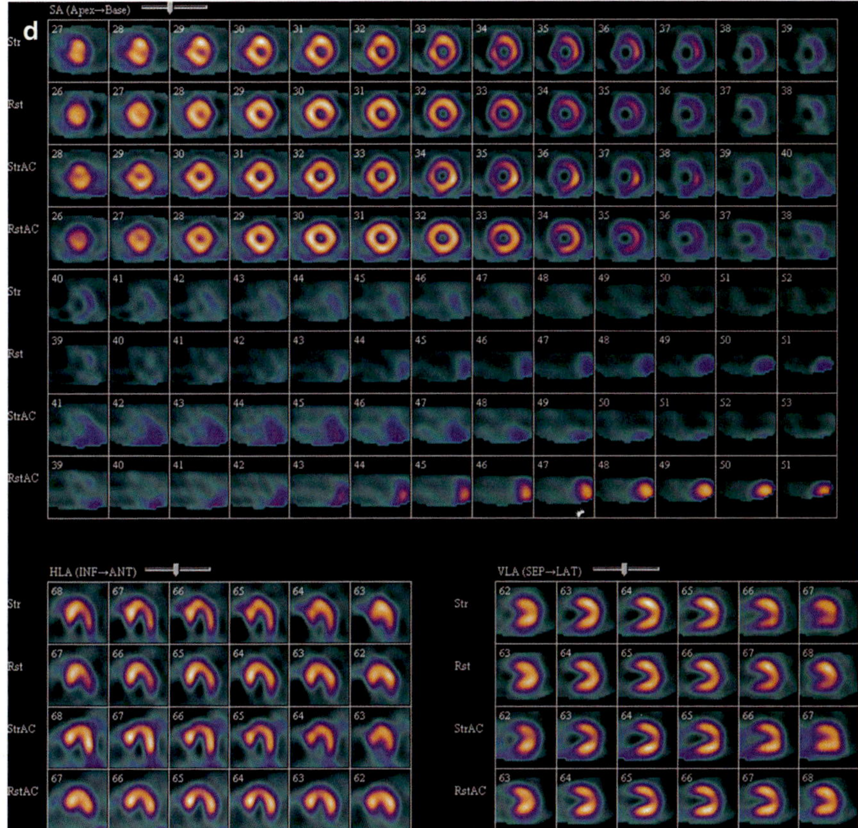

Fig. 25.1 (continued)

Renal abnormalities should be reported. For example,

The left kidney appears small; this appearance is in keeping with chronic renal disease in this dialysis-dependent patient.

Alternatively,

There is a large "cold" defect in the upper pole of the left kidney incidentally detected on review of the raw projection data. The differential diagnosis includes malignancy. No correlative imaging is available. The referring physician has been notified by telephone at the time of this report.

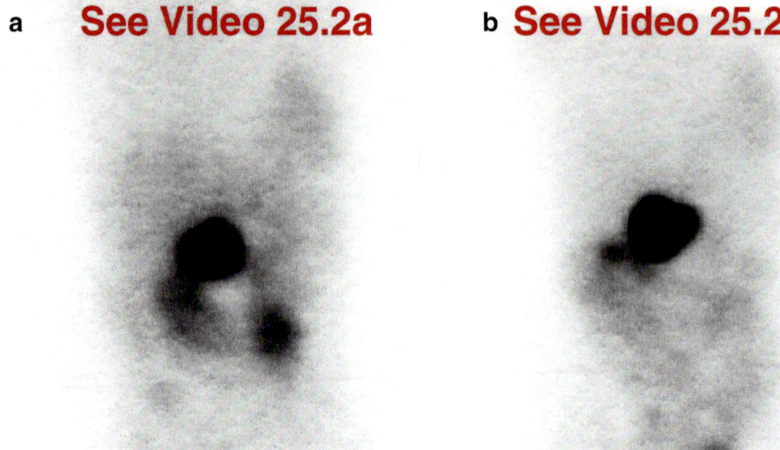

Fig. 25.2 Non-visualization of the kidneys. This 64-year-old female has end-stage kidney disease and is awaiting transplant. Note a normal gallbladder and normal peristalsis of the small intestine (**a**, **b**).

(**a**) Rest raw projection images (Video 25.2a, frame 1), ^{99m}Tc sestamibi. (**b**) Stress raw projection images (Video 25.2b, frame 1), ^{99m}Tc sestamibi

Key Points
- A least a portion of the left kidney is generally included in the field-of-view and readily visualized; the right kidney is often difficult to visualize on a 180° acquisition.
- Increased renal activity is associated with liver failure because the kidneys are the secondary route of clearance of the ^{99m}Tc MPI radiopharmaceuticals.
- "Hot" or "cold" defects within the kidneys are abnormal and require correlative imaging.
- Displacement of neighboring organs can result from large renal or pelvic masses.

Vascular System

26

Vascular-related imaging artifacts in the abdomen are similar to those in the chest and are listed in Table 26.1. The injection site might overlie the abdomen; it might appear focal (Fig. 26.1) or may be more linear if radiopharmaceutical is retained in catheter tubing or if extravasation occurred (Fig. 26.2). Care should be given to ensure that the injection site and the arms are moved away from the body to avoid subsequent processing artifacts (Chamarthy and Travin 2010; Gentili et al. 1994; Strauss et al. 2008). Except to qualify the diagnostic quality of the examination, reporting vascular system findings is generally not clinically warranted.

Electronic supplementary material The online version of this chapter (doi:10.1007/978-3-319-25436-4_26) contains supplementary material, which is available to authorized users.

© Springer International Publishing Switzerland 2017

M.E. Oates, V.L. Sorrell, *Myocardial Perfusion Imaging - Beyond the Left Ventricle: Pathology, Artifacts and Pitfalls in the Chest and Abdomen,* DOI 10.1007/978-3-319-25436-4_26

Table 26.1 Differential diagnosis of "hot" and "cold" imaging findings related to the vascular system

Organ system	"Hot" finding	"Cold" finding	References
Vascular system	Contamination from injection/ extravasation at injection site	Not reported	Chamarthy and Travin (2010) Gentili et al. (1994) Strauss et al. (2008)

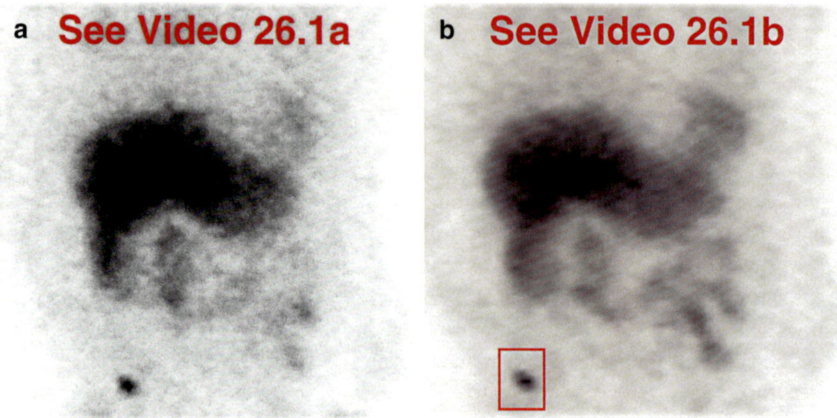

Fig. 26.1 "Hot" vascular injection site in right hand. This "hot" focus appears on the rest acquisition (**a, b**). Note that both arms are positioned along the patient's sides, creating corresponding "cold" defects. Another explanation for such a finding would be contamination from the radiopharmaceutical or excreted urine. Consultation with the technologist usually clarifies the etiology.

(**a**) Rest raw projection images (Video 26.1a, frame 1), ^{99m}Tc sestamibi. (**b**) Rest raw projection image (Video 26.1b, frame 4), ^{99m}Tc sestamibi, "hot focus" (*red box*)

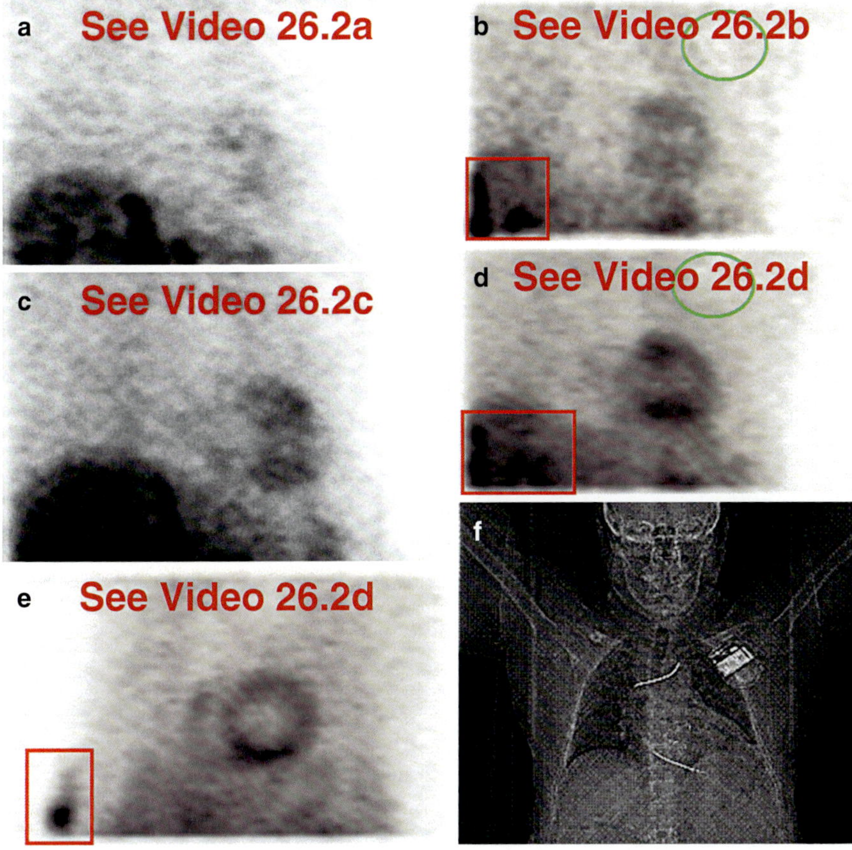

Fig. 26.2 Serpentine "hot" vascular injection site and likely extravasation on right forearm. On both rest (**a**, **b**) and stress (**c–e**) acquisitions, the extravasation probably occurred at rest because it appears more intense. Note the superficial position the more LAO projection (**e**) (the heart is in the best septal orientation relative to the detector—this is a clue to the freeze frame projection). CT (**f**) confirms that a pacemaker is the reason for the subtle "cold" defect in the left upper chest wall— did you catch this finding?

(**a**) Rest raw projection images (Video 26.2a, frame 1), ^{99m}Tc sestamibi. (**b**) Rest raw projection image (Video 26.2b, frame 14), ^{99m}Tc sestamibi, vascular activity (*red box*), "cold" pacemaker (*green oval*). (**c**) Stress raw projection images (Video 26.2c, frame 1), ^{99m}Tc sestamibi. (**d**) Stress raw projection image (Video 26.2d, frame 17), ^{99m}Tc sestamibi, vascular activity (*red box*), "cold" pacemaker (*green oval*). (**e**) Stress raw projection image (Video 26.2d, frame 35), ^{99m}Tc sestamibi, vascular activity (*red box*). (**f**) Chest CT scout image

Key Points
- To avoid potential sources of artifact related to the injection site, position the patient such that the injection site is not included in the imaging field-of-view (arms raised).

Part IV

Case Challenges: A Self-Assessment Tool

Self-Assessment Cases: Basic

____

Electronic supplementary material The online version of this chapter (doi:10.1007/978-3-319-25436-4_27) contains supplementary material, which is available to authorized users.

© Springer International Publishing Switzerland 2017
M.E. Oates, V.L. Sorrell, *Myocardial Perfusion Imaging - Beyond the Left Ventricle: Pathology, Artifacts and Pitfalls in the Chest and Abdomen,*
DOI 10.1007/978-3-319-25436-4_27

27.1   Case Challenge #1

27.1.1   Problem

Clinical Highlights

A 58-year-old male undergoes evaluation for chest pain after coronary artery stenting.

Images for Review

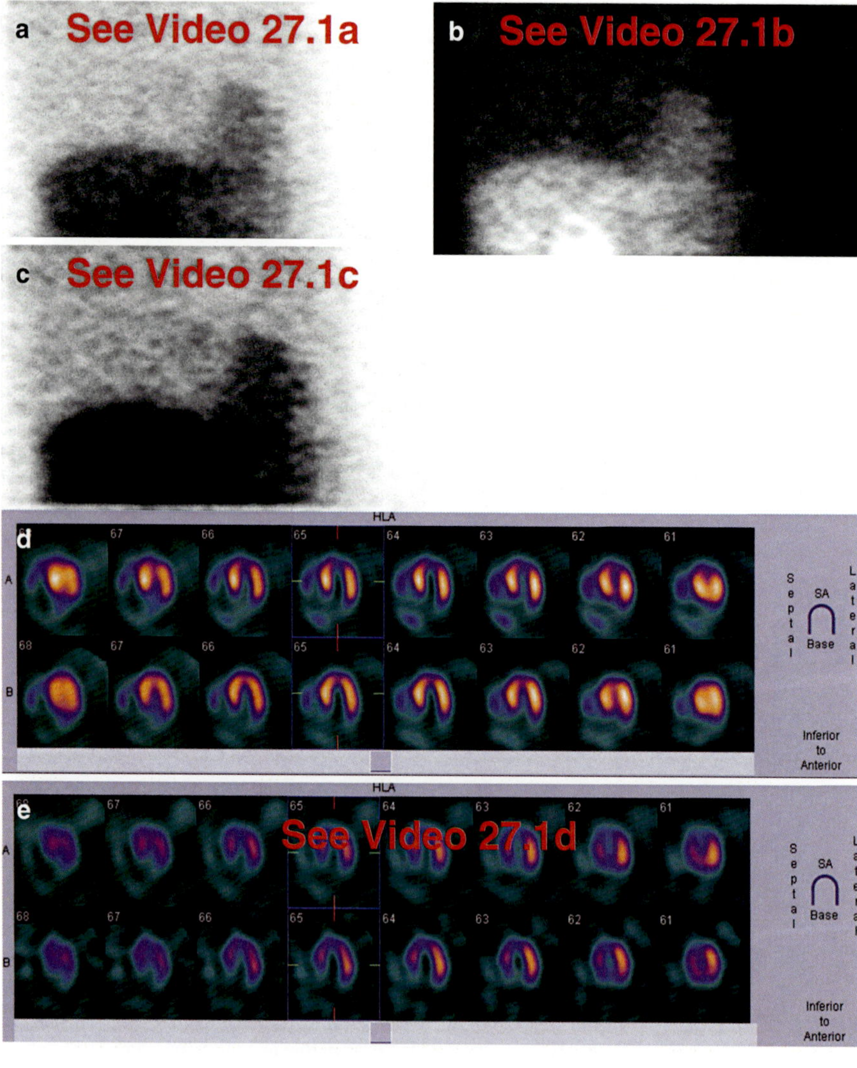

Fig. 27.1

(**a**) Stress "black-on-white" raw projection images at usual contrast setting for heart (Video 27.1a, frame 1), ^{99m}Tc sestamibi

(**b**) Stress "white-on-black" raw projection images at usual contrast setting for heart (Video 27.1b, frame 1), ^{99m}Tc sestamibi

(**c**) Stress "black-on-white" raw projection images with enhanced contrast setting (Video 27.1c, frame 1), ^{99m}Tc sestamibi

(**d**) Stress/rest processed SPECT images (HLA)

(**e**) Stress and rest gated SPECT images (Video 27.1d, frame 1) (HLA)

Characterize the Pertinent Finding(s)

- Chest
    - Thyroid gland: □ hot □ cold
    - Pleura: □ hot □ cold
    - Lungs: □ hot □ cold
    - Myocardium and pericardium: □ hot □ cold
    - Right atrium and right ventricle: □ hot □ cold
    - Vascular system: □ hot □ cold
- Abdomen
    - Abdominal wall: □ hot □ cold
    - Peritoneum: □ hot □ cold
    - Liver: □ hot □ cold
    - Spleen: □ hot □ cold
    - Stomach: □ hot □ cold
    - Kidneys and female reproductive system: □ hot □ cold

State Your Relevant Diagnosis(es)

- Chest
    - Thyroid gland: □ normal □ multinodular goiter
    - Pleura: □ normal □ effusion
    - Lungs: □ normal □ tuberculosis
    - Myocardium and pericardium: □ normal □ pericardial effusion
    - Right atrium and right ventricle: □ normal (right auricular appendage) □ abnormal (right auricular appendage)
    - Vascular system: □ normal □ extravasation at injection site
- Abdomen
    - Abdominal wall: □ normal □ cracked crystal
    - Peritoneum: □ normal □ peritoneal dialysate
    - Liver: □ normal □ post-thermal ablation cyst
    - Spleen: □ normal □ cyst
    - Stomach: □ normal □ chronic distension
    - Kidneys and female reproductive system: □ normal □ end-stage kidneys

27.1.2   Solution

Additional Annotated Images

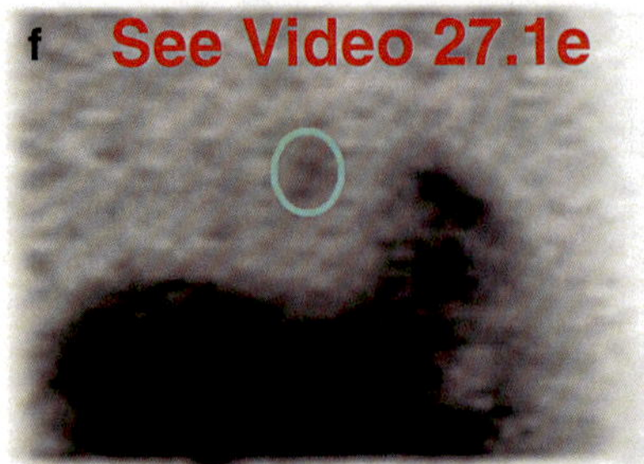

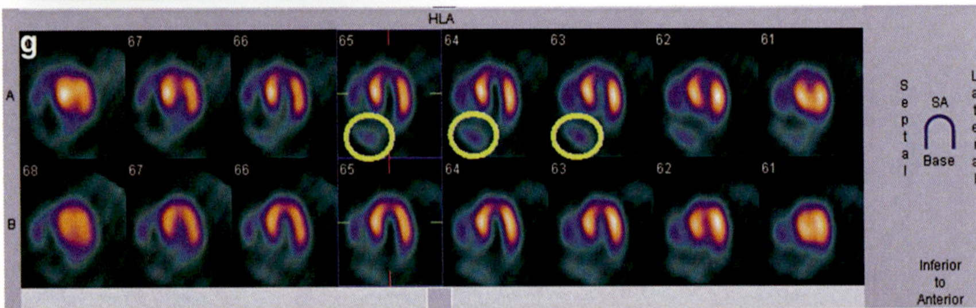

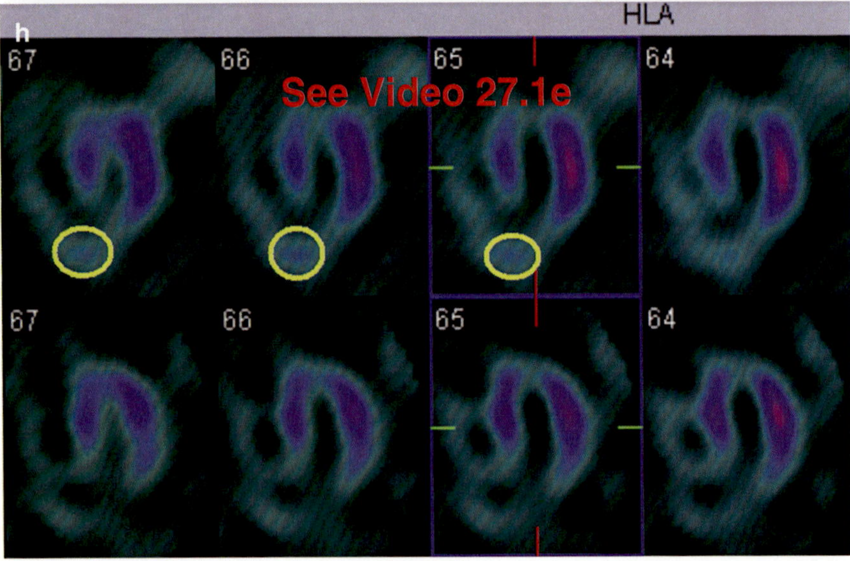

(**f**) Stress "black-on-white" raw projection image with enhanced contrast (Video 27.1e, frame 7), ^{99m}Tc sestamibi, "hot" right atrial focus (*blue oval*)

(**g**) Stress/rest processed SPECT images (HLA), "hot" right atrial focus (*yellow ovals*)

(**h**) Stress and rest gated SPECT image (Video 27.1f, frame 7) (HLA), "hot" right atrial focus (*yellow ovals* on representative images)

The Pertinent Findings

- Chest:
  - Right atrium and right ventricle: ■ hot □ cold
- Abdomen
  - Not applicable

The Relevant Diagnosis(es)

- Chest:
  - Right atrium and right ventricle: ■ normal (right auricular appendage)
- Abdomen
  - Not applicable

Discussion

Chest

There is a discrete focus of radiopharmaceutical localization in the region of the right atrium. It has an appearance characteristic of right auricular appendage, a common and normal finding seen on the raw projection data (a, b, c, f). Note its superior and deep location. It is enhanced by altering the color presentation (compare b to c and to f). The processed SPECT images (d, g) and the gated SPECT images (e, h) confirm its location and provide the key clue to its etiology and, thus, its clinical significance as a normal finding. It should not be misconstrued as a pathologic mediastinal mass. The small, mild, fixed apical defect is normal apical thinning. Incidental note of "septal rocking" (e) of unclear etiology (no history or left bundle branch block (LBBB) nor cardiac surgery).

The thyroid gland and injection sites (arms up) are not included in the field-of-view.

Abdomen

There is no abnormality.

Relevant Chapter(s)

Chapter 13

27.2 Case Challenge #2

27.2.1 Problem

Clinical Highlights

A 56-year-old female was found to have elevated calcium and parathormone (PTH) levels. Parathyroid SPECT scintigraphy is performed to identify and localize the culprit hyperfunctioning parathyroid gland as the cause of primary hyperparathyroidism.

Images for Review

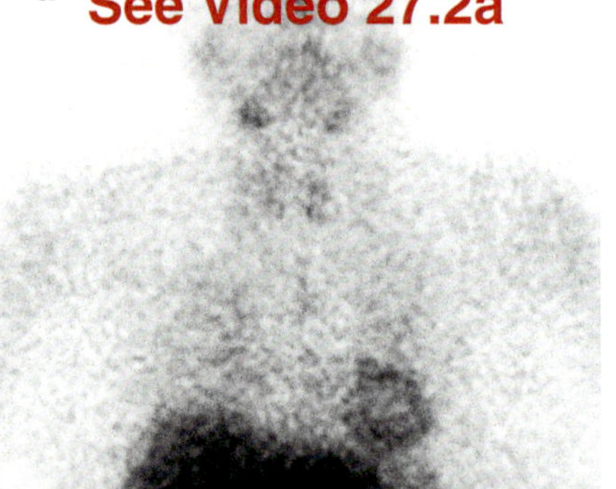

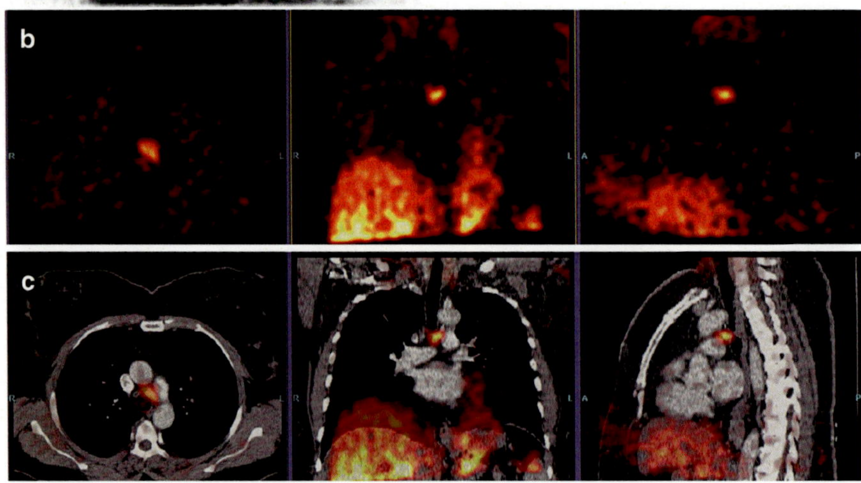

Fig. 27.2

(**a**) Raw projection images (360° Video 27.2a, frame 1), ^{99m}Tc sestamibi

(**b**) Axial, coronal, sagittal SPECT images

(**c**) Axial, coronal, sagittal fused SPECT/CT images

Characterize the Pertinent Finding(s)

- Chest
  - Thyroid gland: □ hot □ cold
  - Parathyroid glands: □ hot □ cold
  - Breasts: □ hot □ cold
  - Chest wall: □ hot □ cold
  - Pleura: □ hot □ cold
  - Vascular system: □ hot □ cold
- Abdomen
  - Abdominal wall: □ hot □ cold
  - Liver: □ hot □ cold
  - Biliary system and gallbladder: □ hot □ cold
  - Spleen: □ hot □ cold
  - Stomach: □ hot □ cold
  - Small intestine and large intestine: □ hot □ cold

State Your Relevant Diagnosis(es)

- Chest
  - Thyroid gland: □ normal □ diffuse toxic goiter
  - Parathyroid glands: □ normal □ parathyroid adenoma, ectopic
  - Breasts: □ normal □ malignant mass
  - Chest wall: □ normal □ contamination artifact
  - Pleura: □ normal □ effusion
  - Vascular system: □ normal □ extravasation at injection site
- Abdomen
  - Abdominal wall: □ normal □ malfunctioning photomultiplier tube
  - Liver: □ normal □ hepatocellular malignancy
  - Biliary system and gallbladder □ normal □ biliary stricture with obstruction
  - Spleen: □ normal □ malignant mass
  - Stomach: □ normal □ free ^{99m}Tc pertechnetate
  - Small intestine and large intestine: □ normal □ barium

27.2.2   Solution

Additional Annotated Images

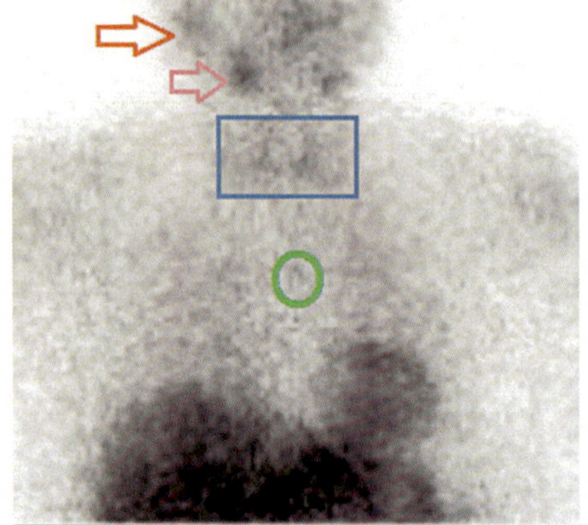

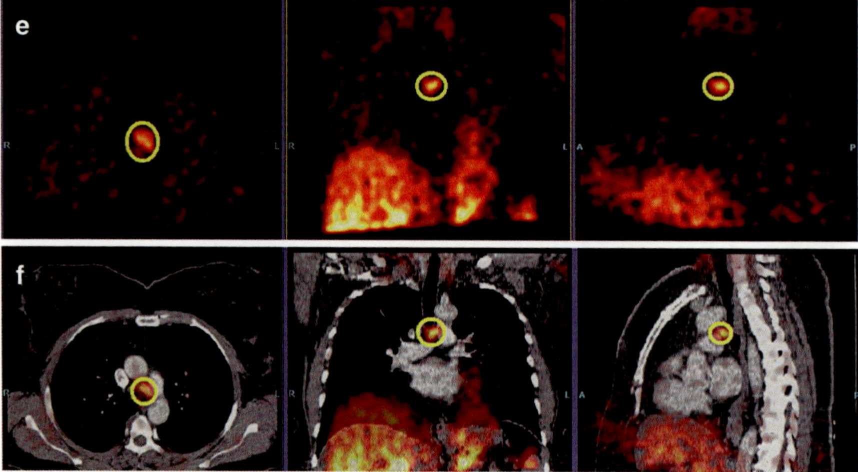

(**d**) Raw projection image (Video 27.2b, frame 6), ^{99m}Tc sestamibi, deep mediastinal focus (*green circle*), right parotid gland (*orange arrow*), right submandibular gland (*pink arrow*), thyroid gland (*blue box*)

(**e**) Axial, coronal, sagittal SPECT images, deep mediastinal focus (*yellow ovals*)

(**f**) Axial, coronal, sagittal fused SPECT/CT images, deep mediastinal focus (*yellow ovals*)

The Pertinent Findings

- Chest
    - Thyroid gland: ■ hot □ cold
    - Parathyroid glands: ■ hot □ cold
    - Breasts: □ hot ■ cold
- Abdomen
    - Liver: ■ hot □ cold

The Relevant Diagnosis(es)

- Chest
    - Thyroid gland: ■ normal
    - Parathyroid glands: ■ parathyroid adenoma, ectopic
    - Breasts: ■ normal
- Abdomen
    - Liver: ■ normal

Discussion

Chest

On the images of the chest, the visualized salivary glands and thyroid gland are normal (a, d). There is subtle but definite focal radiopharmaceutical localization deep in the midline chest superior to the heart (a, d). The SPECT and SPECT/CT images (the latter created with fusion software) localize the focus to the middle mediastinum situated between the anterolateral aspect of the trachea and the great vessels (b, c, e, f). The final diagnosis is ectopic parathyroid adenoma deep in the mediastinum as cause of primary hyperparathyroidism.

Why is this case presented in a book on SPECT MPI? Because this condition can be discovered on SPECT MPI, and one should be aware of its presentation. As in this case, fusion can be performed with software if there is a previous chest CT or MRI. Also, in contradistinction to 27.1, this lesion is not related to the right atrium and should not be misinterpreted as a normal finding.

Note that the relatively photopenic ("cold") normal breast tissue does not compromise the examination.

Abdomen

The liver is seen because imaging commenced shortly after radiopharmaceutical administration according to the parathyroid imaging protocol, and the ^{99m}Tc sestamibi has not yet cleared through the normal physiologic mechanism (a, d).

Relevant Chapter(s)

Chapters 4, 5, 6, and 19

27.3   Case Challenge #3

27.3.1   Problem

Clinical Highlights

A 65-year-old female presents with acute worsening of chronic dyspnea.

Images for Review

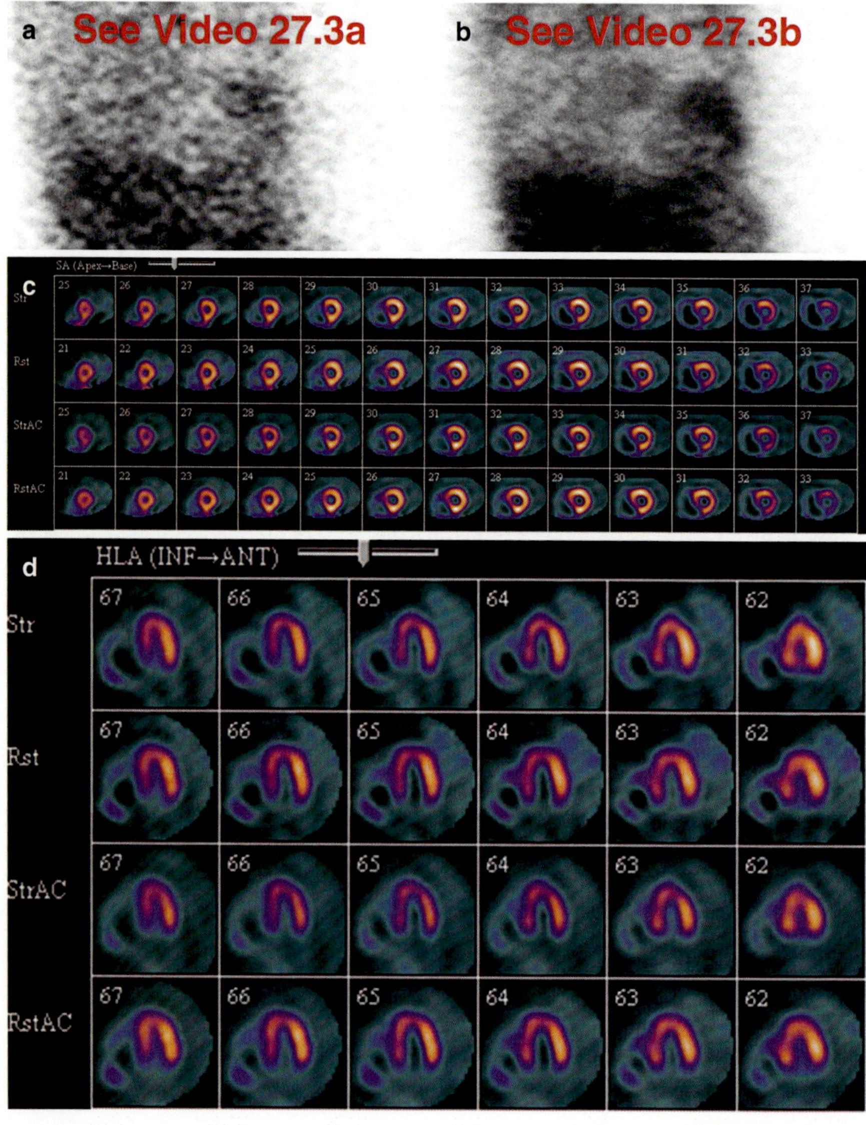

Fig. 27.3

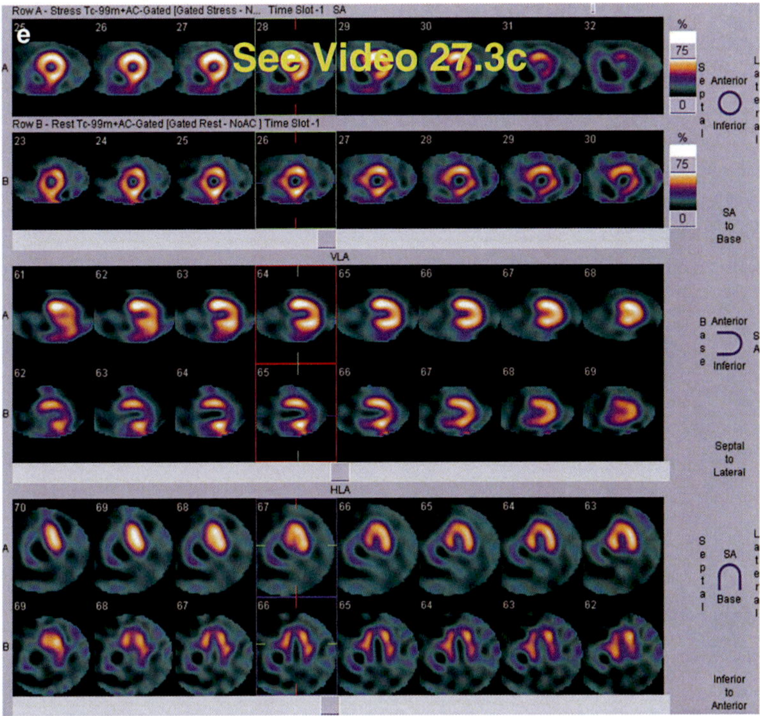

Fig. 27.3 (continued)

(**a**) Rest raw projection images (Video 27.3a, frame 1), ^{99m}Tc sestamibi
(**b**) Stress raw projection images (Video 27.3b, frame 1), ^{99m}Tc sestamibi
(**c**) Stress/rest processed SPECT images (SA) (with and without AC)
(**d**) Stress/rest processed SPECT images (HLA) (with and without AC)
(**e**) Stress and rest gated SPECT images (Video 27.3c, frame 1) (SA, VLA, HLA)

Characterize the Pertinent Finding(s)

- Chest
    - Chest wall: □ hot □ cold
    - Skeleton: □ hot □ cold
    - Pleura: □ hot □ cold
    - Lungs: □ hot □ cold
    - Mediastinum: □ hot □ cold
    - Right atrium and right ventricle: □ hot □ cold
- Abdomen
    - Abdominal wall: □ hot □ cold
    - Peritoneum: □ hot □ cold
    - Liver: □ hot □ cold
    - Spleen: □ hot □ cold
    - Stomach: □ hot □ cold
    - Adrenal glands: □ hot □ cold

State Your Relevant Diagnosis(es)

- Chest
    - Chest wall: ☐ normal ☐ malignant soft-tissue mass
    - Skeleton: ☐ normal ☐ metastases
    - Pleura: ☐ normal ☐ effusion
    - Lungs: ☐ normal ☐ hyperexpansion/diffuse process
    - Mediastinum: ☐ normal ☐ malignant mass
    - Right atrium and right ventricle: ☐ normal ☐ enlargement/hypertrophy
- Abdomen
    - Abdominal wall: ☐ normal ☐ metallic artifact
    - Peritoneum: ☐ normal ☐ ascites
    - Liver: ☐ normal ☐ cystic mass
    - Spleen: ☐ normal ☐ enlargement
    - Stomach: ☐ normal ☐ duodenogastric reflux
    - Adrenal glands: ☐ normal ☐ malignant mass

27.3.2 Solution

Additional Annotated Images

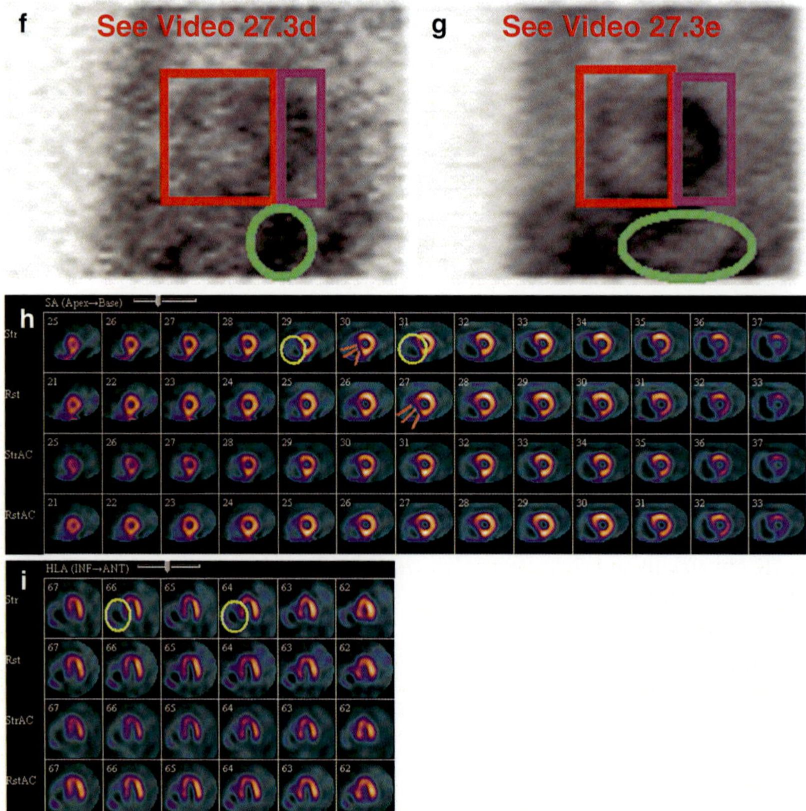

(f) Rest raw projection image (Video 27.3d, frame 33), ^{99m}Tc sestamibi, right ventricle (*red box*), left ventricle (*pink box*), stomach (*green oval*)

(g) Stress raw projection image (Video 27.3e, frame 35),), ^{99m}Tc sestamibi, right ventricle (*red box*), left ventricle (*pink box*), stomach (*green oval*)

(h) Stress/rest processed SPECT images (SA) (with and without AC), right ventricle (*yellow ovals*), septal wall (*orange lines*)

(i) Stress/rest processed SPECT images (HLA) (with and without AC), right ventricle (*yellow ovals*)

The Pertinent Findings

- Chest
  - Lungs: ■ hot □ cold
  - Right atrium and right ventricle: ■ hot ■ cold
- Abdomen
  - Stomach: ■ hot ■ cold

The Relevant Diagnosis(es)

- Chest
  - Lungs: ■ hyperexpansion/diffuse process
  - Right atrium and right ventricle: ■ enlargement/hypertrophy
- Abdomen
  - Stomach: ■ duodenogastric reflux

Discussion

Chest

The upper lungs are diffusely "hot," while the lower lungs are more normal in their uptake pattern; the diaphragms are flattened indicating hyperexpanded lungs (a, b).

There is an extremely enlarged right ventricular cavity on the raw data (a, b, f, g) distorting the shape of the heart on the processed images (c, d, h, i). The right ventricular myocardium appears thickened and "hotter" than normal (a, b). Note the flattened septum evident on the raw data (a, b) as well as on the processed data (c, d, h, i). The left ventricle appears normal in size and has a normal perfusion pattern (c, d). The left ventricular function is normal with a normal ejection fraction of 53 %; note the enlarged right ventricle on gated SPECT images (e). The final diagnosis is a huge right ventricle related to pulmonary hypertension due to underlying chronic lung disease.

Abdomen

On rest raw images (a, f), the stomach is "hot" but clears with fluid, appearing "cold" on stress raw images (b, g). This is due to duodenogastric reflux, a common finding. The gastric activity does not impact on the interpretation of the reconstructed images (c, d).

Relevant Chapter(s)

Chapters 10, 13, and 22

27.4   Case Challenge #4

27.4.1   Problem

Clinical Highlights

A 55-year-old male, a longtime smoker, has a history of tuberculosis.

Images for Review

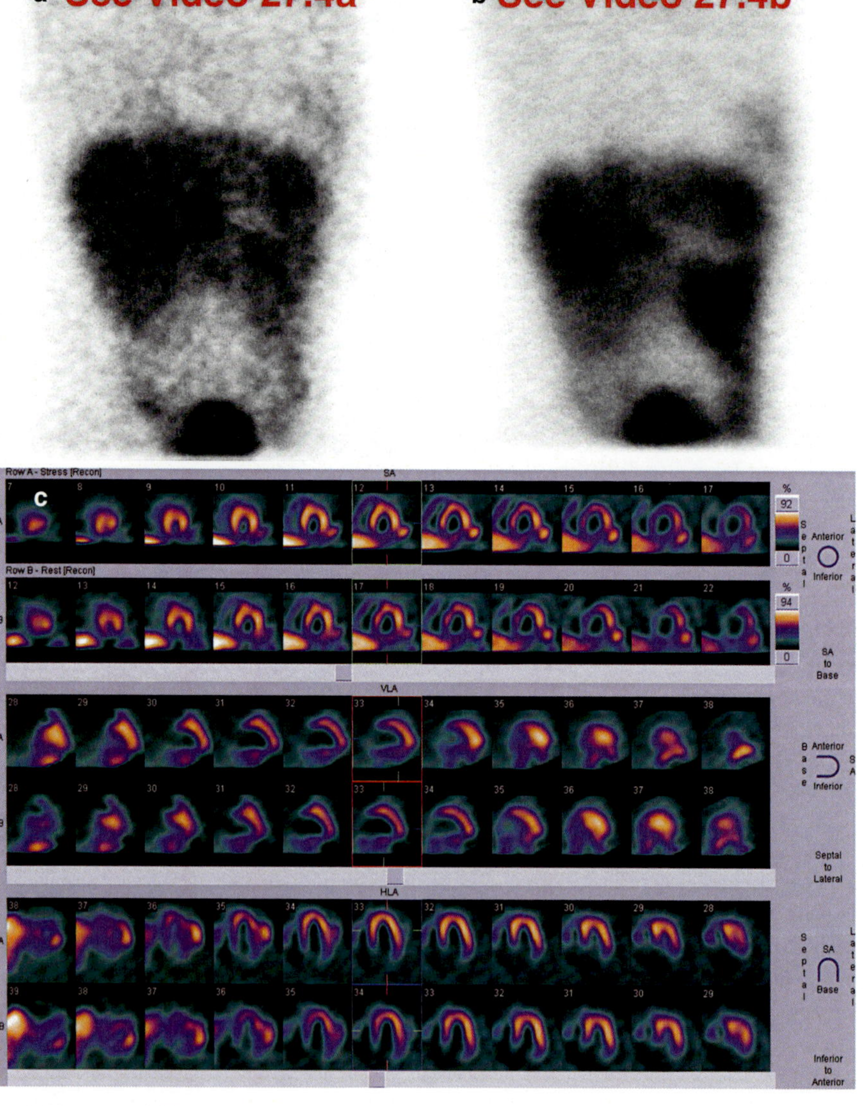

Fig. 27.4

(**a**) Rest raw projection images (Video 27.4a, frame 1), ^{99m}Tc sestamibi
(**b**) Stress raw projection images (Video 27.4b, frame 1), ^{99m}Tc sestamibi
(**c**) Stress/rest processed SPECT images (SA, VLA, HLA)
(**d**) Stress and rest gated SPECT images (Video 27.4c, frame 1) (SA, VLA, HLA)

Characterize the Pertinent Finding(s)

- Chest
  - Thyroid gland: □ hot □ cold
  - Breasts: □ hot □ cold
  - Pleura: □ hot □ cold
  - Lungs: □ hot □ cold
  - Right atrium and right ventricle: □ hot □ cold
  - Diaphragm: □ hot □ cold
- Abdomen
  - Abdominal wall: □ hot □ cold
  - Peritoneum: □ hot □ cold
  - Liver: □ hot □ cold
  - Stomach: □ hot □ cold
  - Adrenal glands: □ hot □ cold
  - Vascular system: □ hot □ cold

State Your Relevant Diagnosis(es)

- Chest
  - Thyroid gland: □ normal □ benign tumor
  - Breasts: □ normal □ malignant primary tumor
  - Pleura: □ normal □ effusion
  - Lungs: □ normal □ hyperinflation and volume loss with mediastinal shift
  - Right atrium and right ventricle: □ normal □ enlargement
  - Diaphragm: □ normal □ flattening
- Abdomen
  - Abdominal wall: □ normal □ belt buckle
  - Peritoneum: □ normal □ ascites
  - Liver: □ normal □ hepatomegaly with retention in left lobe
  - Stomach: □ normal □ duodenogastric reflux into fundus
  - Adrenal glands: □ normal □ benign tumor
  - Vascular system: □ normal □ contamination related to injection

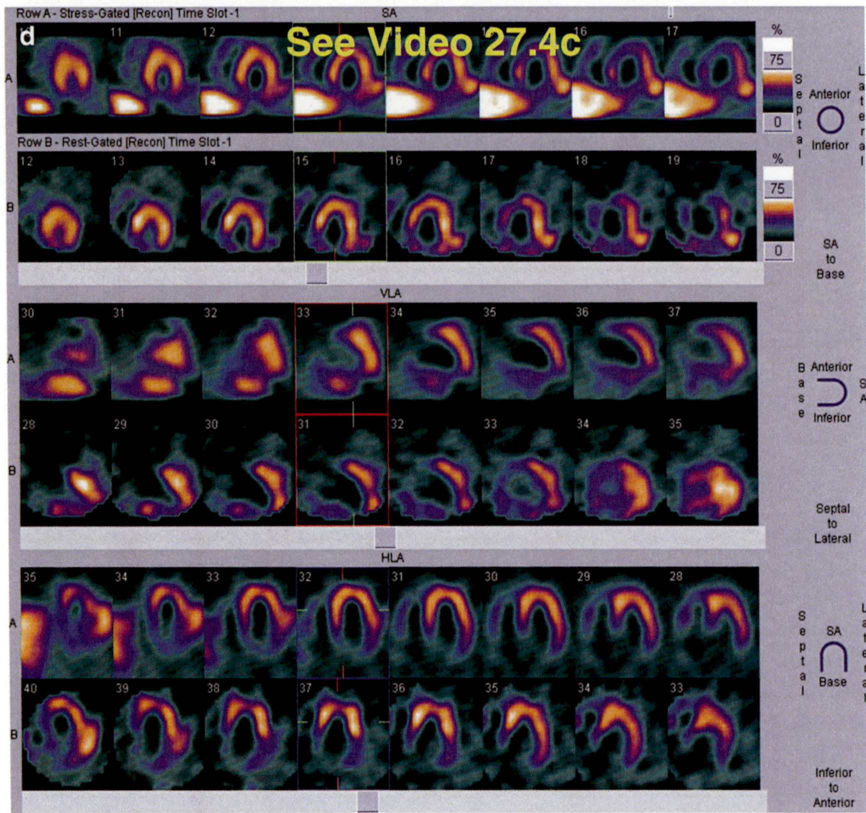

Fig. 27.4 (continued)

27.4.2   Solution

Additional Images
(**e**) AP chest radiograph
(**f**) CT of the chest at level of heart and lung bases at lung window setting

The Pertinent Findings
- Chest
  - Lungs: □ hot ■ cold
  - Right atrium and right ventricle: ■ hot ■ cold
  - Diaphragm: □ hot ■ cold
- Abdomen
  - Liver: ■ hot □ cold
  - Stomach: ■ hot □ cold

The Relevant Diagnosis(es)

- Chest
    - Lungs: ■ hyperinflation and volume loss with mediastinal shift
    - Right atrium and right ventricle: ■ enlargement
    - Diaphragm: ■ flattening
- Abdomen
    - Liver: ■ hepatomegaly with retention in left lobe
    - Stomach: ■ duodenogastric reflux into fundus

Discussion

Chest

There is marked mediastinal shift to the left (a, b) confirmed by radiography (e) and CT scan (f). The right lung is markedly hyperinflated with cystic bronchiectasis with a flattened right hemidiaphragm, while there is almost complete replacement of the left lung with cysts and cavitation. There is such striking volume loss that the entire mediastinum, including the heart, is shifted to the left. The malposition of the heart is evident on the projection data (a, b).

There is an enlarged right ventricle related to the associated pulmonary hypertension (a, b, c, d). Right ventricular function is reduced (d). Global and regional left ventricular function is normal with LVEF of 53 %.

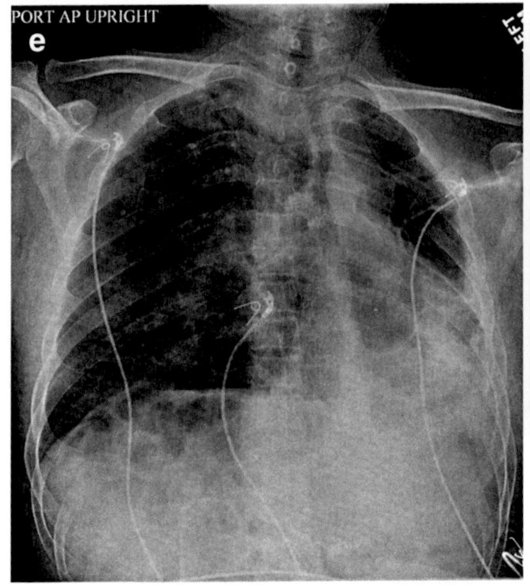

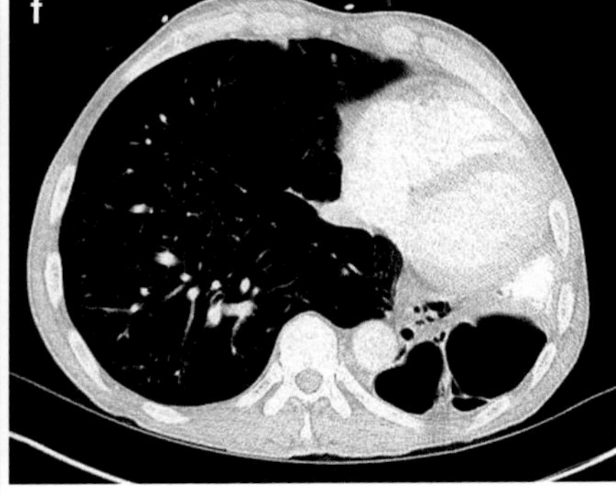

Abdomen

There is an enlarged liver with a prominent left lobe demonstrating marked retention of radiopharmaceutical; its location immediately adjacent to the heart creates a processing artifact affecting the inferior wall. The gastric fundus is also "hot," creating a similar effect on the inferolateral myocardium. The affected inferior wall myocardium is located between the "hot" left hepatic lobe and the "hot" gastric fundus (a, b, c). There is normal wall motion and thickening in this region (d). Diaphragmatic attenuation and the unusual position of the heart may contribute to the fixed inferior wall perfusion defect, likely artifactual.

Relevant Chapter(s)

Chapters 10, 13, 16, 19, and 22

27.5 Case Challenge #5

27.5.1 Problem

Clinical Highlights

A 47-year-old obese female presents with chest pain. Her regadenoson stress test is normal.

Images for Review

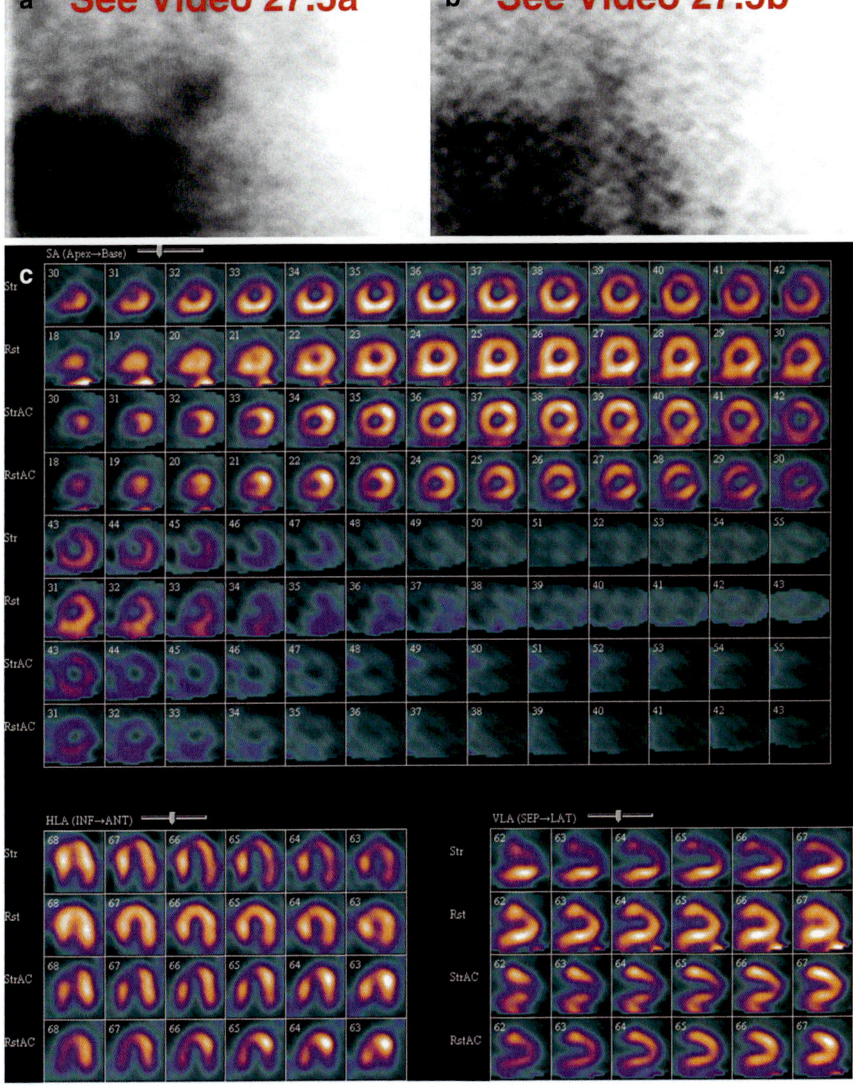

Fig. 27.5

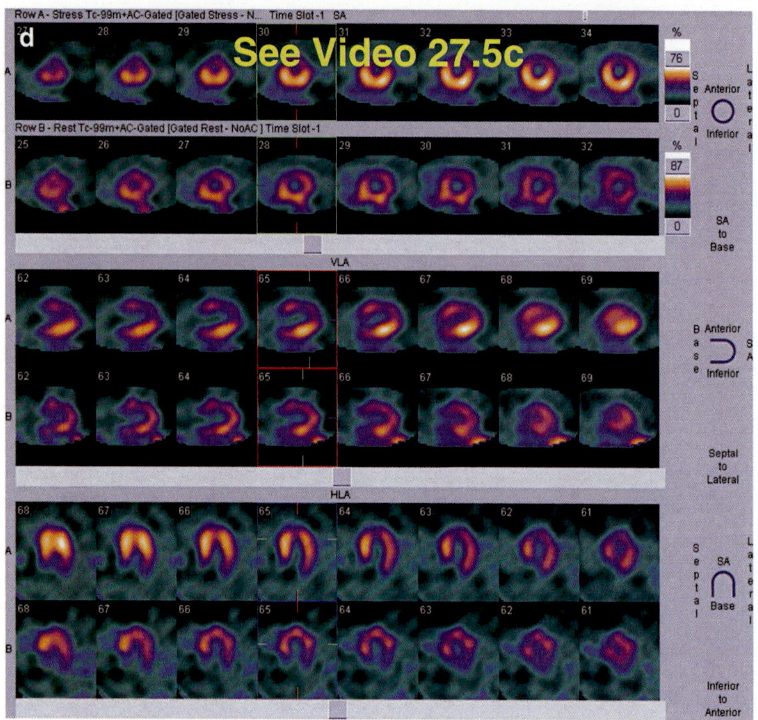

Fig. 27.5 (continued)

(**a**) Day 1: stress raw projection images (Video 27.5a, frame 1), ^{99m}Tc sestamibi
(**b**) Day 2: rest raw projection images (Video 27.5b, frame 1), ^{99m}Tc sestamibi
(**c**) Stress/rest processed SPECT images (SA, HLA, VLA) (with and without AC)
(**d**) Stress and rest gated SPECT images (Video 27.5c, frame 1) (SA, VLA, HLA)

Characterize the Pertinent Finding(s)

- Chest
    - Breasts: □ hot □ cold
    - Chest wall: □ hot □ cold
    - Pleura: □ hot □ cold
    - Vascular system: □ hot □ cold
    - Lymphatic system: □ hot □ cold
    - Diaphragm: □ hot □ cold
- Abdomen
    - Abdominal wall: □ hot □ cold
    - Peritoneum: □ hot □ cold
    - Liver: □ hot □ cold
    - Spleen: □ hot □ cold
    - Adrenal glands: □ hot □ cold
    - Kidneys and female reproductive system: □ hot □ cold

State Your Relevant Diagnosis(es)

- Chest
    - Breasts: ☐ normal ☐ fibroadenoma
    - Chest wall: ☐ normal ☐ contamination artifact
    - Pleura: ☐ normal ☐ effusion
    - Vascular system: ☐ normal ☐ extravasation at injection site
    - Lymphatic system: ☐ normal ☐ left axillary nodes
    - Diaphragm: ☐ normal ☐ flattening
- Abdomen
    - Abdominal wall: ☐ normal ☐ contamination artifact
    - Peritoneum: ☐ normal ☐ ascites
    - Liver: ☐ normal ☐ primary hepatocellular carcinoma
    - Spleen: ☐ normal ☐ enlargement
    - Adrenal glands: ☐ normal ☐ malignant mass
    - Kidneys and female reproductive system: ☐ normal ☐ scarred left kidney

27.5.2   Solution

Additional Annotated Images

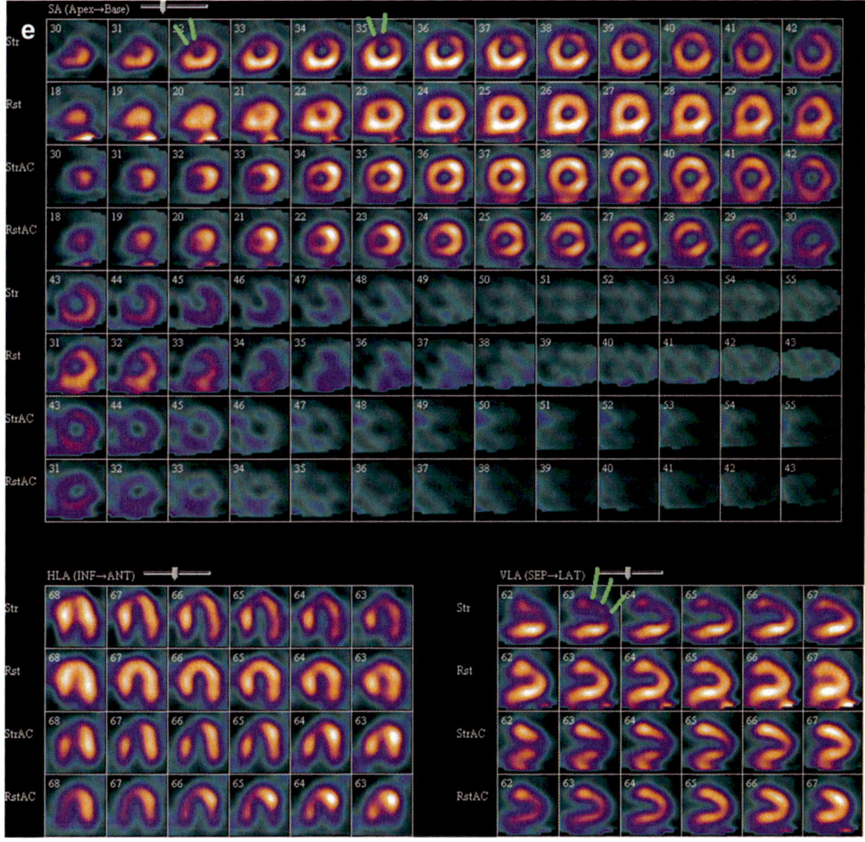

27.6   Case Challenge #6

27.6.1   Problem

Clinical Highlights

A 66-year-old female presents for evaluation of chest pain. She undergoes a 1-day rest/stress MPI.

Images for Review

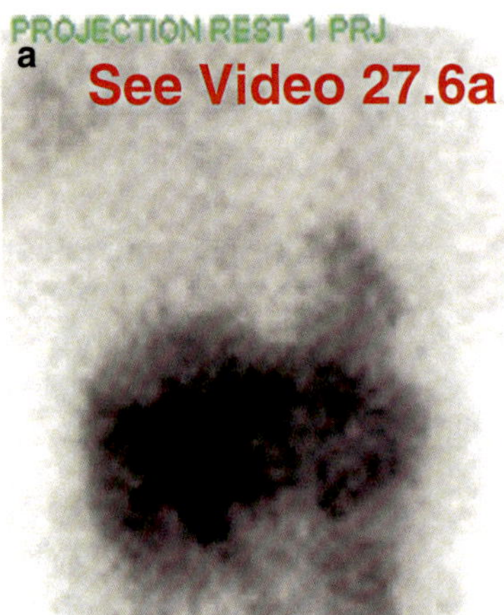

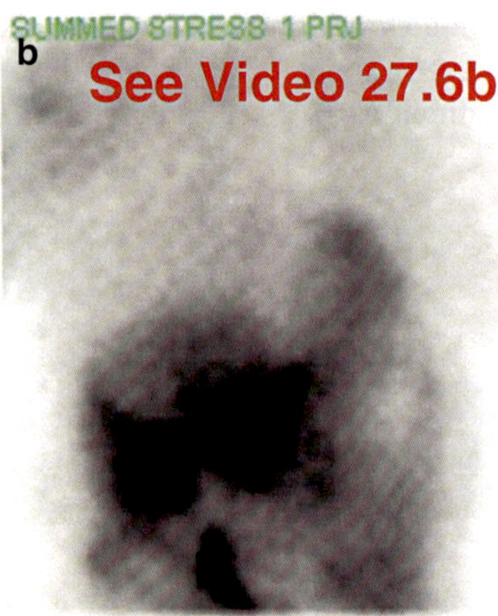

Fig. 27.6

(**a**) Rest raw projection images (Video 27.6a, frame 1), ^{99m}Tc sestamibi
(**b**) Stress raw projection images (Video 27.6b, frame 1), ^{99m}Tc sestamibi

Characterize the Pertinent Finding(s)
- Chest
    - Thyroid gland: ☐ hot ☐ cold
    - Parathyroid glands: ☐ hot ☐ cold
    - Breasts: ☐ hot ☐ cold
    - Mediastinum: ☐ hot ☐ cold
    - Vascular system: ☐ hot ☐ cold
    - Diaphragm: ☐ hot ☐ cold
- Abdomen
    - Abdominal wall: ☐ hot ☐ cold
    - Peritoneum: ☐ hot ☐ cold
    - Liver: ☐ hot ☐ cold
    - Biliary system and gallbladder: ☐ hot ☐ cold
    - Spleen: ☐ hot ☐ cold
    - Stomach: ☐ hot ☐ cold

State Your Relevant Diagnosis(es)

- Chest
  - Thyroid gland: □ normal □ substernal goiter
  - Parathyroid glands: □ normal □ substernal parathyroid adenoma
  - Breasts: □ normal □ source of attenuation artifact
  - Mediastinum: □ normal □ esophageal malignancy
  - Vascular system: □ normal □ extravasation at injection site
  - Diaphragm: □ normal □ flattening
- Abdomen
  - Abdominal wall: □ normal □ contamination artifact during injection
  - Peritoneum: □ normal □ ascites
  - Liver: □ normal □ cirrhosis
  - Biliary system and gallbladder: □ normal □ inadequate fasting state
  - Spleen: □ normal □ enlargement
  - Stomach: □ normal □ duodenogastric reflux with clearance

27.6.2 Solution

Additional Annotated Images

None

The Relevant Diagnosis(es)

- Chest
  - Breasts: ■ source of attenuation artifact
  - Vascular system: ■ extravasation at injection site
- Abdomen
  - Biliary system and gallbladder: ■ normal/physiologic
  - Stomach: ■ duodenogastric reflux with clearance

Discussion

Chest

The right breast overlies the dome of the liver and creates an attenuation artifact (a, b). The left breast is also evident on the raw data, but because the left arm is raised in the standard position for imaging, the position and shape of the left breast appears different compared to the right breast with the patient's right arm by her side.

There is extravasation in the right antecubital fossa that occurred at rest (a); note that the right arm is positioned by the patient's side for both rest (a) and stress (b) acquisitions permitting its identification. The extravasation is still present but appears less intense on the later same-day stress raw images (b). If the extravasation had occurred during the stress test, this would have raised concern about achieving the appropriate threefold ratio of administered activity between stress and rest injections.

Abdomen

The "hot" distended gallbladder and the "hot" stomach that are quite apparent on the rest raw images (a) appear partially contracted and distended ("cold"), respectively, on the later same-day stress raw images (b) after ingestion of food and drink. These represent expected physiologic changes in the stomach and gallbladder. The technologist can aid the physician's interpretation by recording these details in the stress test record.

Relevant Chapter(s)

Chapters 6, 14, 20, and 22

27.7   Case Challenge #7

27.7.1   Problem

Clinical Highlights

A 75-year-old male presents for evaluation of recurring chest pain.

Images for Review

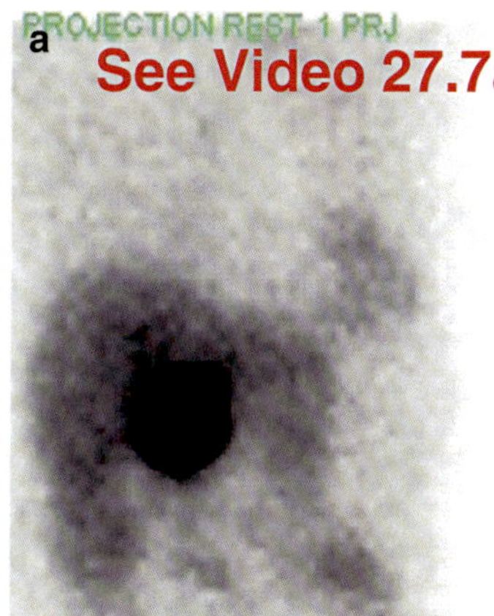

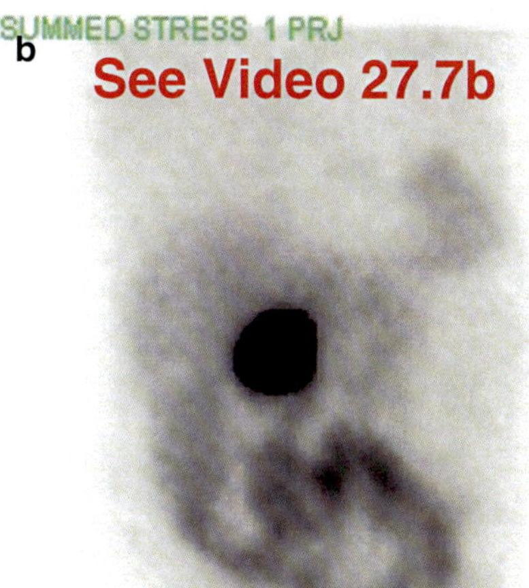

Fig. 27.7

(**a**) Rest raw projection images (Video 27.7a, frame 1), ^{99m}Tc sestamibi
(**b**) Stress raw projection images (Video 27.7b, frame 1, ^{99m}Tc sestamibi

Characterize the Pertinent Finding(s)
- Chest
    - Parathyroid glands: ☐ hot ☐ cold
    - Breasts: ☐ hot ☐ cold
    - Chest wall: ☐ hot ☐ cold
    - Skeleton: ☐ hot ☐ cold
    - Vascular system: ☐ hot ☐ cold
    - Lymphatic system: ☐ hot ☐ cold
- Abdomen
    - Biliary system and gallbladder: ☐ hot ☐ cold
    - Spleen: ☐ hot ☐ cold
    - Stomach: ☐ hot ☐ cold
    - Small intestine and large intestine: ☐ hot ☐ cold
    - Adrenal glands: ☐ hot ☐ cold
    - Kidneys and female reproductive system: ☐ hot ☐ cold

State Your Relevant Diagnosis(es)

- Chest
  - Parathyroid glands: □ normal □ parathyroid adenoma
  - Breasts: □ normal □ malignant mass
  - Chest wall: □ normal □ external source artifact ("cross talk")
  - Skeleton: □ normal □ fracture
  - Vascular system: □ normal □ extravasation at injection site
  - Lymphatic system: □ normal □ left axillary lymph nodes, pathologic
- Abdomen
  - Biliary system and gallbladder: □ normal □ acute cholecystitis
  - Spleen: □ normal □ enlargement
  - Stomach: □ normal □ gastropathy
  - Small intestine and large intestine: □ normal □ stasis
  - Adrenal glands: □ normal □ malignant mass
  - Kidneys and female reproductive system: □ normal □ absent left kidney

27.7.2   Solution

Additional Images

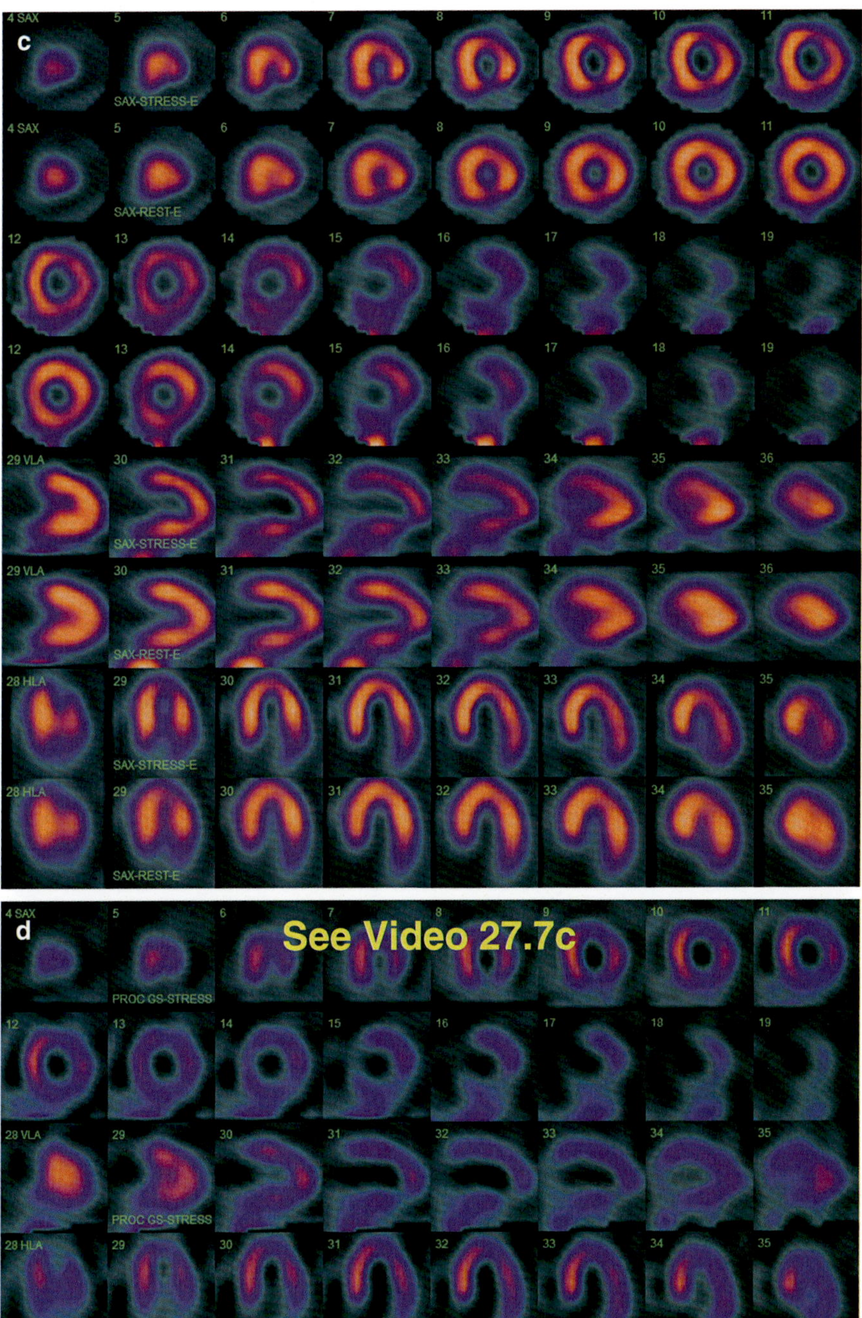

(**c**) Stress/rest processed SPECT images (SA, VLA, HLA)
(**d**) Stress gated SPECT (Video 27.7c, frame 1) (SA, VLA, HLA)

The Pertinent Findings
- Chest
    - Chest wall: ■ hot □ cold
- Abdomen
    - Biliary system and gallbladder: ■ hot □ cold
    - Kidneys and female reproductive system: ■ hot □ cold

The Relevant Diagnosis(es)
- Chest
    - Chest wall: ■ external source artifact ("cross talk")
- Abdomen
    - Biliary system and gallbladder: ■ normal
    - Kidneys and female reproductive system: ■ normal

Discussion
Chest
On two frames of the raw rest image data (a), external activity appears to surround the patient's body; this activity is related to an extraneous radioactive source which emanated from another patient who was injected with ^{99m}Tc sestamibi on the treadmill during this patient's image acquisition. Note that this finding is not present on the raw stress (b) images. This artifact does not affect the processed SPECT data (c, d) but should be noted to initiate operational quality improvement. Where is the treadmill relative to the gamma camera? How are the detectors oriented relative to other potential sources of radioactivity?

The MPI (c, d) shows a small, severe, fixed inferoapical defect with associated akinesis (scar) and a medium-size, moderately severe, reversible anterior/anterolateral defect with normal wall motion and wall thickening (ischemia). LVEF is normal at 50 %. Did you notice that the LV cavity size is larger on the post-stress images compared to the rest images? This pattern is referred to as TID (transient ischemic dilatation), a finding that correlates with multivessel CAD and confers a high-risk prognosis.

Abdomen
The gallbladder appears to be "beating" due to patient motion artifact on both acquisitions (a, b). A normal-size left kidney is clearly visible (a, b).

Relevant Chapter(s)
Chapters 7, 20, and 25

27.8   Case Challenge #8

27.8.1   Problem

Clinical Highlights
A 57-year-old male presents with a cardiac history and liver disease.

Images for Review

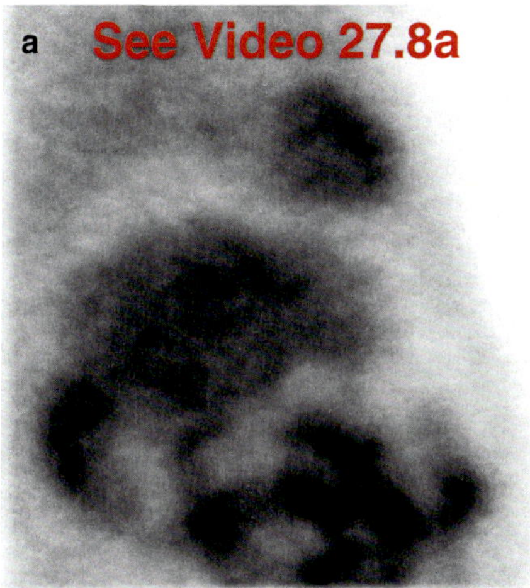

Fig. 27.8

(**a**) Stress raw projection images (Video 27.8a, frame 1), ^{99m}Tc sestamibi

Characterize the Pertinent Finding(s)
- Chest
    - Chest wall: ☐ hot ☐ cold
    - Skeleton: ☐ hot ☐ cold
    - Pleura: ☐ hot ☐ cold
    - Lungs: ☐ hot ☐ cold
    - Vascular system: ☐ hot ☐ cold
    - Diaphragm: ☐ hot ☐ cold
- Abdomen
    - Abdominal wall: ☐ hot ☐ cold
    - Peritoneum: ☐ hot ☐ cold
    - Biliary system and gallbladder: ☐ hot ☐ cold
    - Spleen: ☐ hot ☐ cold
    - Small intestine and large intestine: ☐ hot ☐ cold
    - Kidneys and female reproductive system: ☐ hot ☐ cold

State Your Relevant Diagnosis(es)

- Chest
    - Chest wall: ▢ normal ▢ metallic object (pacemaker)
    - Skeleton: ▢ normal ▢ anemia
    - Pleura: ▢ normal ▢ effusion
    - Lungs: ▢ normal ▢ low lung volumes
    - Vascular system: ▢ normal ▢ extravasation at injection site
    - Diaphragm: ▢ normal ▢ elevation
- Abdomen
    - Abdominal wall: ▢ normal ▢ metallic object (jewelry)
    - Peritoneum: ▢ normal ▢ ascites
    - Biliary system and gallbladder: ▢ normal ▢ cholecystectomy
    - Spleen: ▢ normal ▢ enlargement
    - Small intestine and large intestine: ▢ normal ▢ obstruction
    - Kidneys and female reproductive system: ▢ normal ▢ hyperfunctioning renal system (hepatic failure)

27.8.2   Solution

Additional Annotated Images

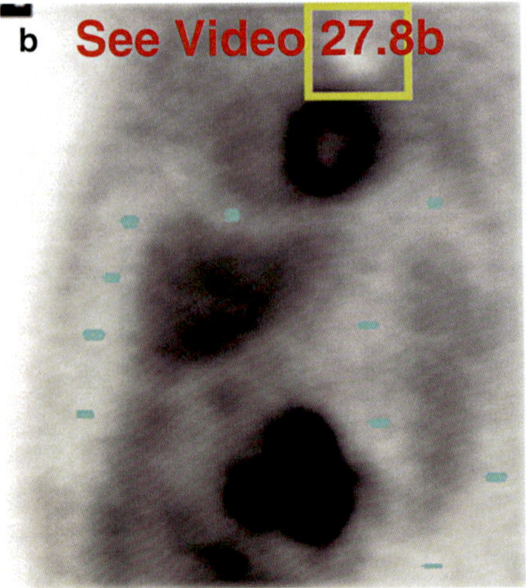

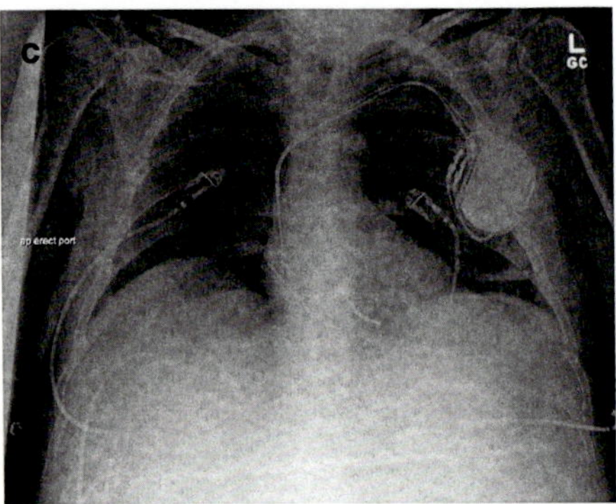

(**b**) Stress raw projection image (Video 27.8b, frame 33), ^{99m}Tc sestamibi, pacemaker (*yellow box*), ascites (*blue dots*)

(**c**) AP portable chest radiograph

The Pertinent Findings
- Chest
  - Chest wall: □ hot ■ cold
  - Lungs: □ hot ■ cold
  - Diaphragm: ■ hot □ cold
- Abdomen
  - Peritoneum: □ hot ■ cold
  - Biliary system and gallbladder: □ hot ■ cold
  - Spleen: ■ hot □ cold
  - Small intestine and large intestine: ■ hot □ cold
  - Kidneys and female reproductive system: ■ hot □ cold

The Relevant Diagnosis(es)
- Chest
  - Chest wall: ■ metallic object (pacemaker)
  - Lungs: ■ low lung volumes
  - Diaphragm: ■ elevation
- Abdomen
  - Peritoneum: ■ ascites
  - Biliary system and gallbladder: ■ cholecystectomy
  - Spleen: ■ enlargement
  - Small intestine and large intestine: ■ normal
  - Kidneys and female reproductive system: ■ hyperfunctioning renal system (hepatic failure)

Discussion
Chest
There is a well-defined circular "cold" defect in the left chest separate from and superior to the heart (a, b); this defect is confirmed to be a metallic implanted pacemaker when correlated with chest radiograph (c). The diaphragms are elevated by the ascites (a, c) and there are low lung volumes (a, c).

Abdomen
Diffuse photopenia throughout the abdomen represents large volume ascites (a, b). The small intestine floats centrally (a). Note that the gallbladder is not visualized, consistent with known cholecystectomy (a); differential diagnosis would include acute or chronic cholecystitis, or non-fasting state. The spleen is slightly enlarged, representing modest splenomegaly. Both kidneys are relatively well seen, suggesting greater renal excretion in the setting of liver dysfunction (a).

Relevant Chapter(s)
Chapters 7, 10, 16, 18, 20, 21, 23, and 25

27.9   Case Challenge #9

27.9.1   Problem

Clinical Highlights

A 50-year-old male presents for evaluation of chest pain.

Images for Review

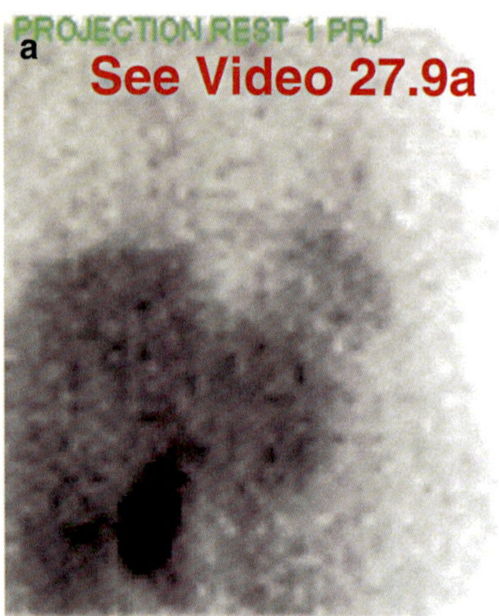

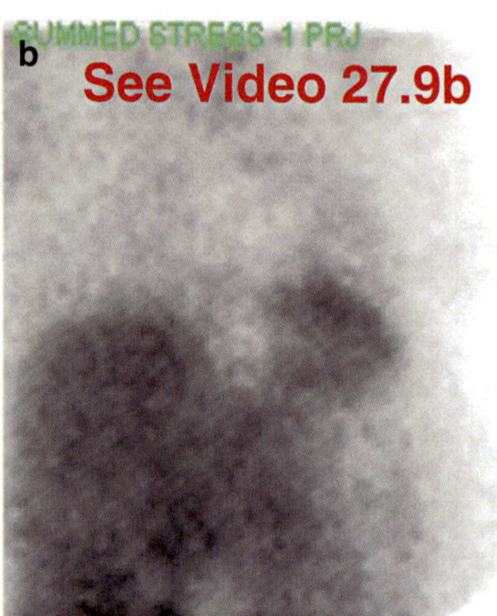

Fig. 27.9

(**a**) Rest raw projection images (Video 27.9a, frame 1), ^{99m}Tc sestamibi
(**b**) Stress raw projection images (Video 27.9b, frame 1), ^{99m}Tc sestamibi

Characterize the Pertinent Finding(s)
- Chest
    - Chest wall: ☐ hot ☐ cold
    - Pleura: ☐ hot ☐ cold
    - Lungs: ☐ hot ☐ cold
    - Mediastinum: ☐ hot ☐ cold
    - Myocardium and pericardium: ☐ hot ☐ cold
    - Right atrium and right ventricle: ☐ hot ☐ cold
- Abdomen
    - Peritoneum: ☐ hot ☐ cold
    - Biliary system and gallbladder: ☐ hot ☐ cold
    - Spleen: ☐ hot ☐ cold
    - Stomach: ☐ hot ☐ cold
    - Small intestine and large intestine: ☐ hot ☐ cold
    - Vascular system: ☐ hot ☐ cold

State Your Relevant Diagnosis(es)

- Chest
  - Chest wall: ☐ normal ☐ artifact due to another patient ("cross talk")
  - Pleura: ☐ normal ☐ effusion
  - Lungs: ☐ normal ☐ emphysema
  - Mediastinum: ☐ normal ☐ dilated esophagus
  - Myocardium and pericardium: ☐ normal ☐ effusion
  - Right atrium and right ventricle: ☐ normal ☐ dilatation, hypertrophy
- Abdomen
  - Peritoneum: ☐ normal ☐ ascites
  - Biliary system and gallbladder: ☐ normal ☐ intermittent gallbladder
  - Spleen: ☐ normal ☐ surgically absent
  - Stomach: ☐ normal ☐ postprandial state
  - Small intestine and large intestine: ☐ normal ☐ absent bile excretion
  - Vascular system: ☐ normal ☐ central port injection site

27.9.2 Solution

Additional Images

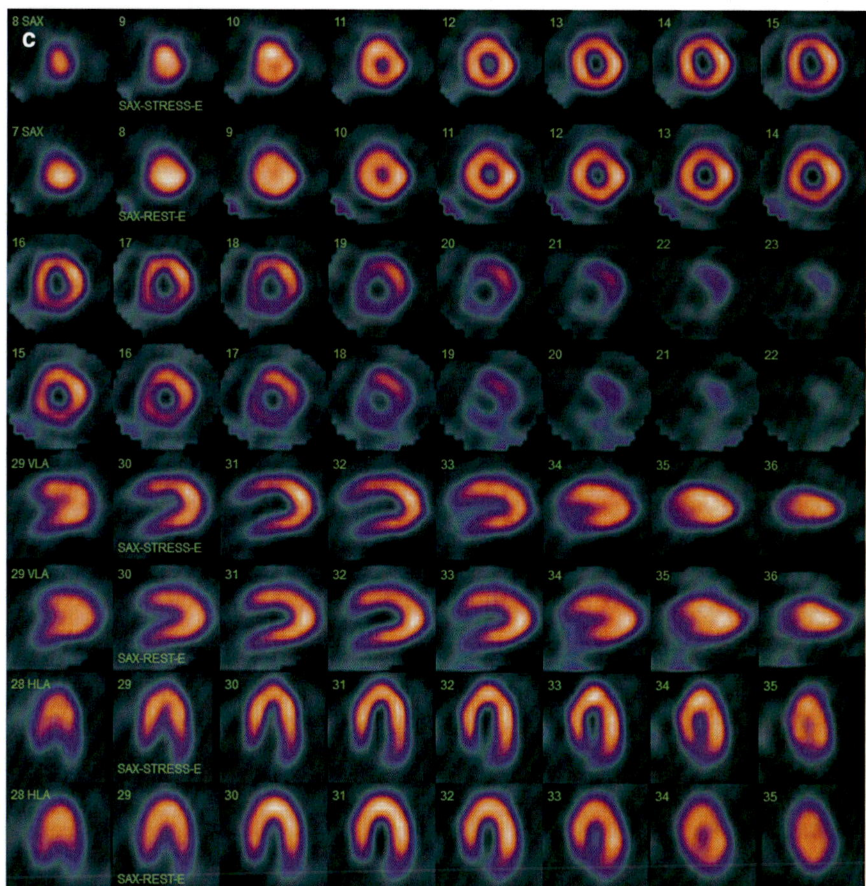

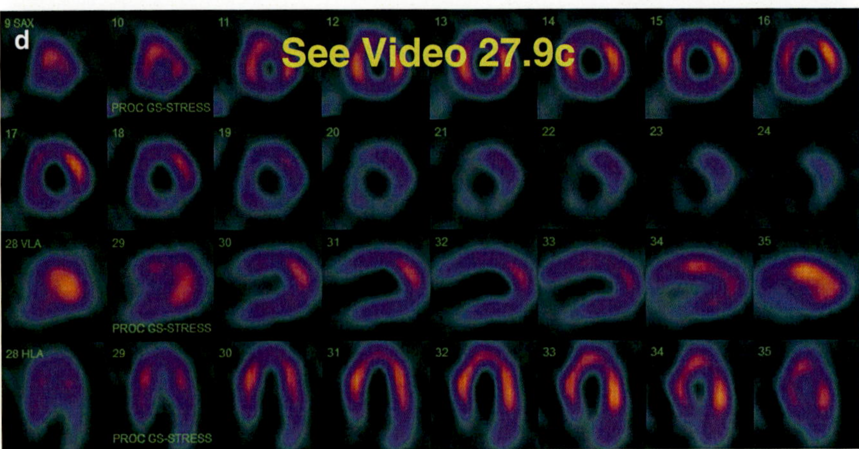

(**c**) Stress/rest processed SPECT images (SA, VLA, HLA)

(**d**) Stress gated SPECT (Video 27.9c, frame 1) (SA, VLA, HLA)

The Pertinent Findings

- Chest
  - Chest wall: ■ hot □ cold
- Abdomen
  - Biliary system and gallbladder: ■ hot ■ cold
  - Stomach: □ hot ■ cold

The Relevant Diagnosis(es)

- Chest
  - Chest wall: ■ artifact due to another patient ("cross talk")
- Abdomen
  - Biliary system and gallbladder: ■ intermittent gallbladder
  - Stomach: ■ postprandial state

Discussion

Chest

On frames 45–46 of the rest raw (a) data, external activity appears adjacent to the patient's right chest; this activity is related to an extraneous radioactive source which emanated from another patient who was injected with ^{99m}Tc sestamibi while on the treadmill during this patient's image acquisition. Note that this finding is not present on the stress raw (b) images. This example is much less apparent than Case 27.7. In neither case did this extraneous activity affect the processed SPECT images (c, d). Perfusion is normal (c); function is normal with LVEF = 67 % (d). However, as mentioned in Case 27.7, there might be opportunity for evaluating the operational layout of the facility.

Note the normal activity about the shoulders. The thyroid gland is just inside the top of the field-of-view on stress raw images.

Abdomen

A normally distended radiopharmaceutical-filled gallbladder is seen on the rest raw images (a), but it has emptied substantially on the stress raw images (b). Note the "cold" stomach on the stress images (b) indicating that the patient ate between the rest and stress images and the stomach is distended. Food stimulates gallbladder contraction, and the gallbladder should empty. The spleen is not enlarged.

Relevant Chapter(s)

Chapters 7, 20, and 22

27.10　Case Challenge #10

27.10.1　Problem

Clinical Highlights
48-year-old female presents with chest pain.

Images for Review

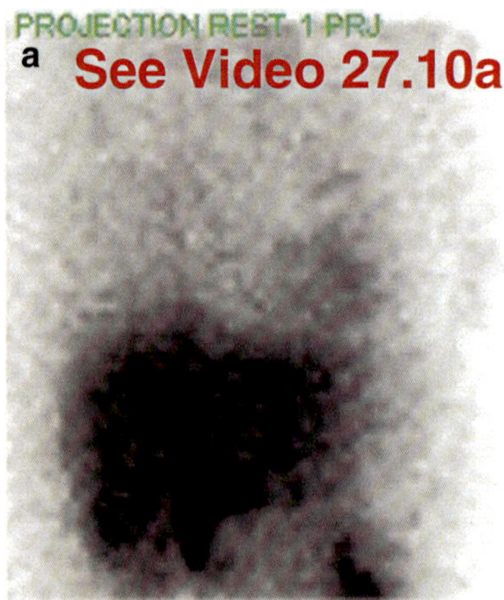

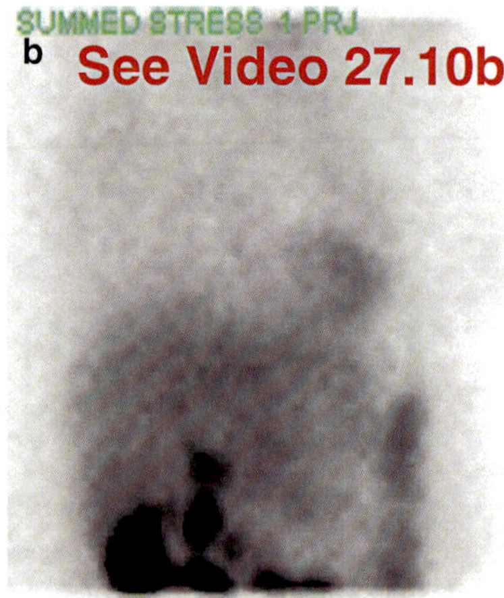

Fig. 27.10

(**a**) Rest raw projection images (Video 27.10a, frame 1), ^{99m}Tc sestamibi
(**b**) Stress raw projection images (Video 27.10b, frame 1), ^{99m}Tc sestamibi

Characterize the Pertinent Finding(s)
- Chest
    - Chest wall: ☐ hot ☐ cold
    - Skeleton: ☐ hot ☐ cold
    - Lungs: ☐ hot ☐ cold
    - Mediastinum: ☐ hot ☐ cold
    - Right atrium and right ventricle: ☐ hot ☐ cold
    - Lymphatic system: ☐ hot ☐ cold
- Abdomen
    - Abdominal wall: ☐ hot ☐ cold
    - Peritoneum: ☐ hot ☐ cold
    - Liver: ☐ hot ☐ cold
    - Biliary system and gallbladder: ☐ hot ☐ cold
    - Spleen: ☐ hot ☐ cold
    - Small intestine and large intestine: ☐ hot ☐ cold

State Your Relevant Diagnosis(es)

- Chest
  - Chest wall: ☐ normal ☐ metallic artifact
  - Skeleton: ☐ normal ☐ Paget disease
  - Lungs: ☐ normal ☐ congestive heart failure
  - Mediastinum: ☐ normal ☐ gastroesophageal reflux
  - Right atrium and right ventricle: ☐ normal ☐ brown adipose tissue
  - Lymphatic system: ☐ normal ☐ sarcoidosis
- Abdomen
  - Abdominal wall: ☐ normal ☐ metallic artifact
  - Peritoneum: ☐ normal ☐ ascites
  - Liver: ☐ normal ☐ infarcted tumor after therapeutic intervention
  - Biliary system and gallbladder: ☐ normal ☐ non-visualization
  - Spleen: ☐ normal ☐ enlargement
  - Small intestine and large intestine: ☐ normal ☐ fast motility

27.10.2 Solution

Additional Annotated Images

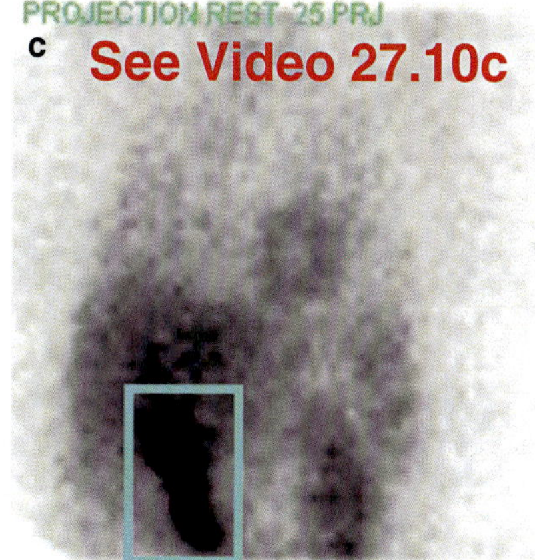

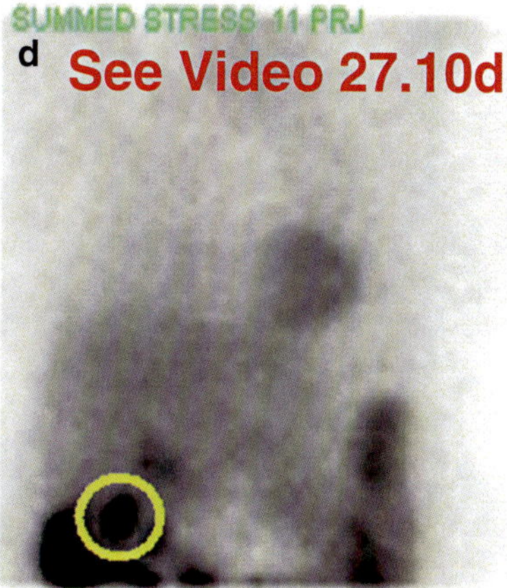

(**c**) Rest raw projection image (Video 27.10c, frame 25), ^{99m}Tc sestamibi, duodenal activity (*blue box*)

(**d**) Stress raw projection image (Video 27.10d, frame 11), ^{99m}Tc sestamibi, hepatic flexure not gallbladder (*yellow circle*)

The Pertinent Findings

- Chest
  - Not applicable
- Abdomen
  - Biliary system and gallbladder: ☐ hot ■ cold
  - Small intestine and large intestine: ■ hot ☐ cold

The Relevant Diagnosis(es)

- Chest
  - Not applicable
- Abdomen
  - Biliary system and gallbladder: ■ non-visualization
  - Small intestine and large intestine: ■ fast motility

Discussion

Chest

There are no abnormalities.

Abdomen

Non-visualization of the gallbladder on both image sets (a, b) suggests surgical history of cholecystectomy vs. underlying gallbladder disease. By carefully comparing the position of the duodenum (c) and the hepatic flexure of the large intestine (d) on the two raw data sets (a, b), one can avoid a gallbladder mimicker. Visualization of the large intestine is not uncommon and should be considered physiologic. Check the patient's history and/or review correlative imaging.

Relevant Chapter(s)

Chapters 20 and 23

27.11 Case Challenge #11

27.11.1 Problem

Clinical Highlights

A 54-year-old male requires a preoperative evaluation.

Images for Review

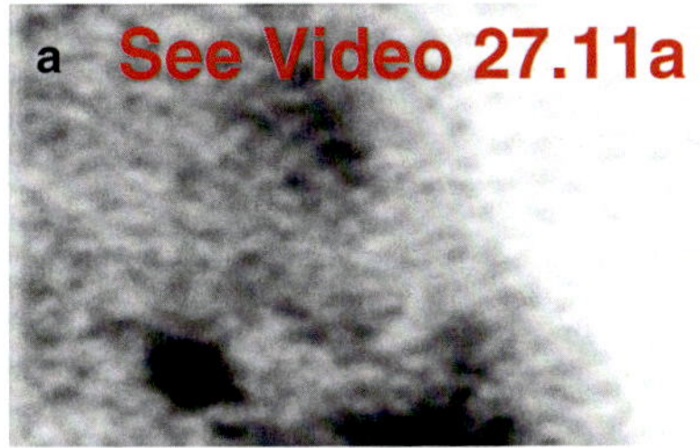

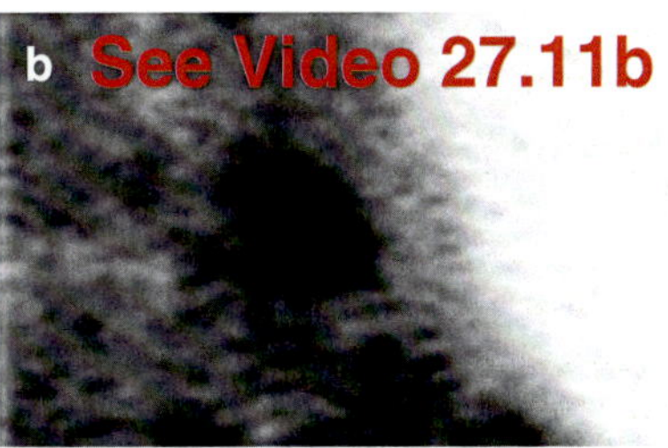

Fig. 27.11

(**a**) Rest raw projection images (Video 27.11a, frame 1), ^{99m}Tc sestamibi
(**b**) Stress raw projection images (Video 27.11b, frame 1), ^{99m}Tc sestamibi

Characterize the Pertinent Finding(s)
- Chest
  - Chest wall: ☐ hot ☐ cold
  - Skeleton: ☐ hot ☐ cold
  - Pleura: ☐ hot ☐ cold
  - Lungs: ☐ hot ☐ cold
  - Myocardium and pericardium: ☐ hot ☐ cold
  - Right atrium and right ventricle: ☐ hot ☐ cold
- Abdomen
  - Abdominal wall: ☐ hot ☐ cold
  - Peritoneum: ☐ hot ☐ cold
  - Liver: ☐ hot ☐ cold
  - Biliary system and gallbladder: ☐ hot ☐ cold
  - Spleen: ☐ hot ☐ cold
  - Stomach: ☐ hot ☐ cold

State Your Relevant Diagnosis(es)
- Chest
  - Chest wall: ☐ normal ☐ urine contamination
  - Skeleton: ☐ normal ☐ anemia
  - Pleura: ☐ normal ☐ effusion
  - Lungs: ☐ normal ☐ emphysema
  - Myocardium and pericardium: ☐ normal ☐ effusion
  - Right atrium and right ventricle: ☐ normal ☐ hypertrophy

- Abdomen
  - Abdominal wall: □ normal □ urine contamination
  - Peritoneum: □ normal □ ascites
  - Liver: □ normal □ cirrhosis
  - Biliary system and gallbladder: □ normal □ acute cholecystitis
  - Spleen: □ normal □ splenomegaly
  - Stomach: □ normal □ gastropathy

27.11.2 Solution

Additional Annotated Images

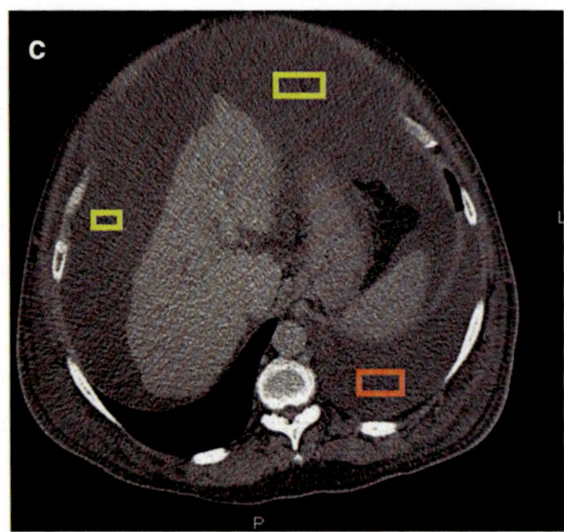

(**c**) CT image of lower chest/upper abdomen, ascites (*yellow boxes*), left pleural effusion (*orange box*)

The Pertinent Findings

- Chest
  - Skeleton: ■ hot □ cold
  - Pleura: □ hot ■ cold
- Abdomen
  - Peritoneum: □ hot ■ cold
  - Liver: □ hot ■ cold
  - Biliary system and gallbladder: ■ hot □ cold
  - Spleen: ■ hot □ cold
  - Stomach: ■ hot □ cold

The Relevant Diagnosis(es)

- Chest
  - Skeleton: ■ anemia
  - Pleura: ■ effusion
- Abdomen
  - Peritoneum: ■ ascites
  - Liver: ■ cirrhosis
  - Biliary system and gallbladder: ■ normal
  - Spleen: ■ splenomegaly
  - Stomach: ■ gastropathy

Discussion

Chest

Both sets of images (a, b) demonstrate a "cold" left hemithorax. Left pleural fluid is confirmed by CT (c).

Abdomen

Both sets of images (a, b) demonstrate a "cold" protuberant abdomen; ascites is confirmed by CT (c). Note the small liver, normal gallbladder, large spleen, and "hot" stomach (cirrhosis-associated gastropathy). Due to the large volume ascites, the stomach appears more horizontally oriented (a, b).

Relevant Chapter(s)

Chapters 8, 9, 18, 19, 20, 21, and 22

27.12 Case Challenge #12

27.12.1 Problem

Clinical Highlights

A 59-year-old female has chest pain, hypertension, and hyperlipidemia. She exercised on the treadmill for 4 minutes, achieving 7 METS, and had no symptoms nor ECG changes.

Images for Review

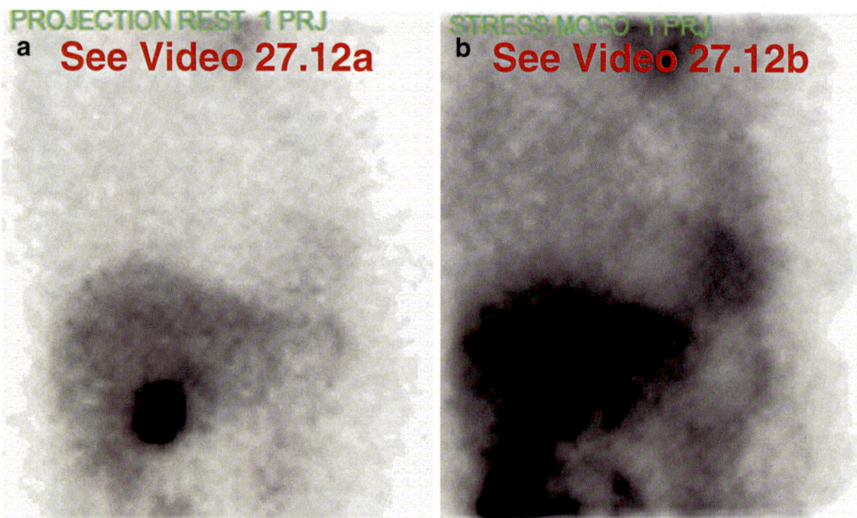

Fig. 27.12

(**a**) Rest raw projection images (Video 27.12a, frame 1), ^{99m}Tc sestamibi
(**b**) Stress raw projection images (Video 27.12b, frame 1), ^{99m}Tc sestamibi

Characterize the Pertinent Finding(s)
- Chest
    - Thyroid gland: ☐ hot ☐ cold
    - Parathyroid glands: ☐ hot ☐ cold
    - Breasts: ☐ hot ☐ cold
    - Lungs: ☐ hot ☐ cold
    - Myocardium and pericardium: ☐ hot ☐ cold
    - Vascular system: ☐ hot ☐ cold

- Abdomen
    - Liver: □ hot □ cold
    - Biliary system and gallbladder: □ hot □ cold
    - Spleen: □ hot □ cold
    - Stomach: □ hot □ cold
    - Small intestine and large intestine: □ hot □ cold
    - Vascular system: □ hot □ cold

State Your Relevant Diagnosis(es)

- Chest
    - Thyroid gland: □ normal □ multinodular goiter
    - Parathyroid glands: □ normal □ cystic adenoma
    - Breasts: □ normal □ soft-tissue attenuation
    - Lungs: □ normal □ pneumonia
    - Myocardium and pericardium: □ normal □ effusion
    - Vascular system: □ normal □ retention in central venous catheter
- Abdomen
    - Liver: □ normal □ cirrhosis
    - Biliary system and gallbladder: □ normal □ chronic cholecystitis
    - Spleen: □ normal □ splenomegaly
    - Stomach: □ normal □ duodenogastric reflux
    - Small intestine and large intestine: □ normal □ hyperperistalsis
    - Vascular system: □ normal □ extravasation at injection site

27.12.2 Solution

Additional Annotated Images

None

The Pertinent Findings

- Chest
    - Thyroid gland: ■ hot □ cold
    - Breasts: □ hot ■ cold
- Abdomen
    - Stomach: ■ hot ■ cold

The Relevant Diagnosis(es)

- Chest
    - Thyroid gland: ■ multinodular goiter
    - Breasts: ■ soft-tissue attenuation
- Abdomen
    - Stomach: ■ duodenogastric reflux

Discussion
Chest
There is a prominent, enlarged thyroid gland at the top of the field-of-view (a, b). The left lobe appears larger than the right. Medical record review confirmed known euthyroid multinodular goiter evaluated by ultrasonography with biopsies of the larger nodules 4 years ago. The left breast creates the usual attenuation artifact on the heart. The processed SPECT MPI images (not shown) are normal.

Abdomen
The stomach lumen appears "hot" on the rest images and "cold" on the stress images after water ingestion to clear duodenogastric activity (a, b). Incidental note is made of a physiologically normal gallbladder (a, b).

Relevant Chapter(s)
Chapters 4, 6, and 22

____

Electronic supplementary material The online version of this chapter (doi:10.1007/978-3-319-25436-4_28) contains supplementary material, which is available to authorized users.

© Springer International Publishing Switzerland 2017
M.E. Oates, V.L. Sorrell, *Myocardial Perfusion Imaging - Beyond the Left Ventricle: Pathology, Artifacts and Pitfalls in the Chest and Abdomen,*
DOI 10.1007/978-3-319-25436-4_28

28.1   Case Challenge #13

28.1.1 Problem

Clinical Highlights

A 59-year-old male presents for preoperative risk assessment.

Images for Review

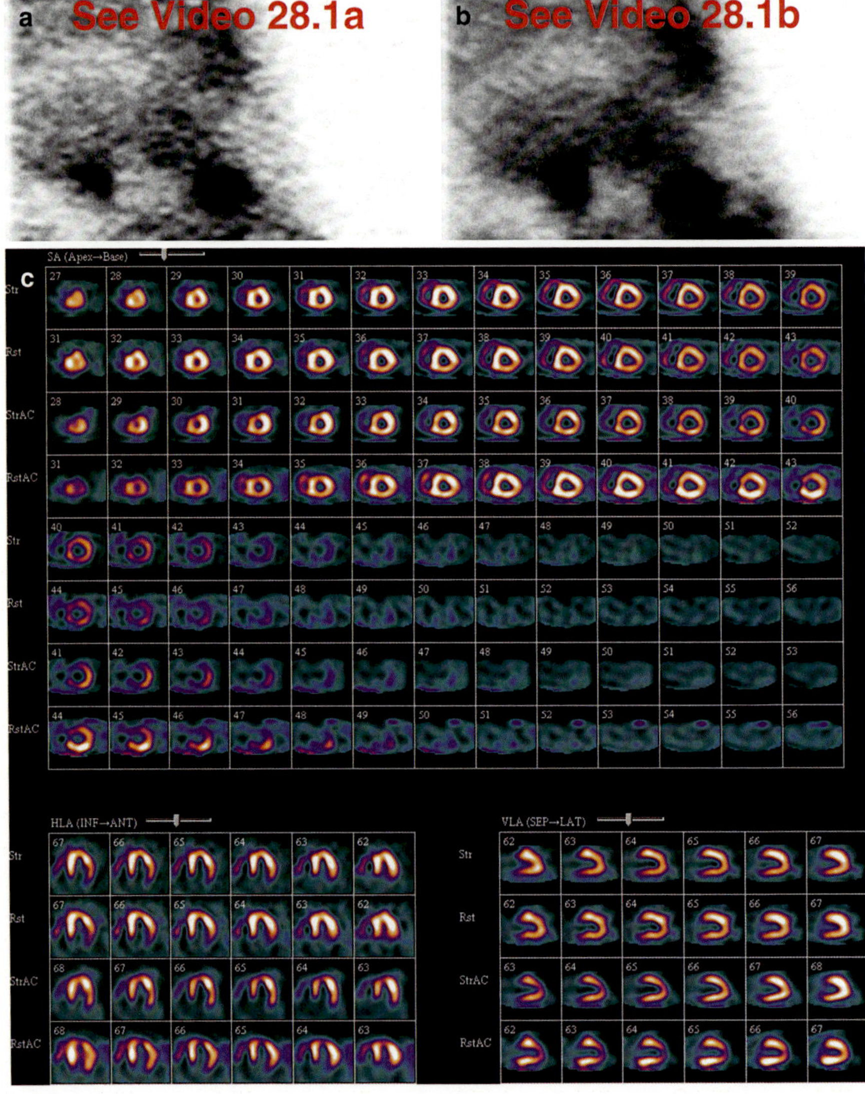

Fig. 28.1

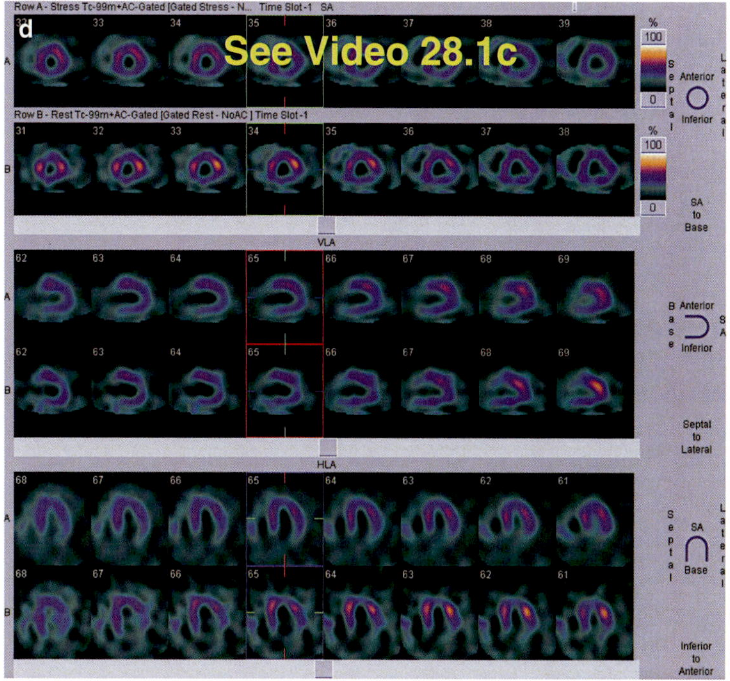

Fig. 28.1 (continued)

(**a**) Rest raw projection images (Video 28.1a, frame 1), ^{99m}Tc sestamibi
(**b**) Stress raw projection images (Video 28.1b, frame 1), ^{99m}Tc sestamibi
(**c**) Stress/rest processed SPECT images (SA, HLA, VLA) (without and with AC)
(**d**) Stress and rest gated SPECT images (Video 28.1c, frame 1) (SA, VLA, HLA)

Characterize the Pertinent Finding(s)

- Chest
    - Parathyroid glands: ☐ hot ☐ cold
    - Breasts: ☐ hot ☐ cold
    - Chest wall: ☐ hot ☐ cold
    - Skeleton: ☐ hot ☐ cold
    - Pleura: ☐ hot ☐ cold
    - Lungs: ☐ hot ☐ cold
    - Mediastinum: ☐ hot ☐ cold
    - Myocardium and pericardium: ☐ hot ☐ cold
    - Right atrium and right ventricle: ☐ hot ☐ cold

- Abdomen
    - Peritoneum: □ hot □ cold
    - Liver: □ hot □ cold
    - Biliary system and gallbladder: □ hot □ cold
    - Spleen: □ hot □ cold
    - Stomach: □ hot □ cold
    - Small intestine and large intestine: □ hot □ cold
    - Adrenal glands: □ hot □ cold
    - Kidneys and female reproductive system: □ hot □ cold

State Your Relevant Diagnosis(es)

- Chest
    - Parathyroid glands: □ normal □ mediastinal adenoma
    - Breasts: □ normal □ malignancy
    - Chest wall: □ normal □ arms by sides
    - Skeleton: □ normal □ anemia
    - Pleura: □ normal □ effusion
    - Lungs: □ normal □ emphysema
    - Mediastinum: □ normal □ malignancy
    - Myocardium and pericardium: □ normal □ effusion
    - Right atrium and right ventricle: □ normal □ pulmonary hypertension
- Abdomen
    - Peritoneum: □ normal □ ascites
    - Liver: □ normal □ cirrhosis
    - Biliary system and gallbladder: □ normal □ prolonged fasting
    - Spleen: □ normal □ splenomegaly
    - Stomach: □ normal □ gastropathy
    - Small intestine and large intestine: □ normal □ large intestine across upper abdomen
    - Adrenal glands: □ normal □ malignancy
    - Kidneys and female reproductive system: □ normal □ polycystic disease

28.1.2 Solution

Additional Annotated Images

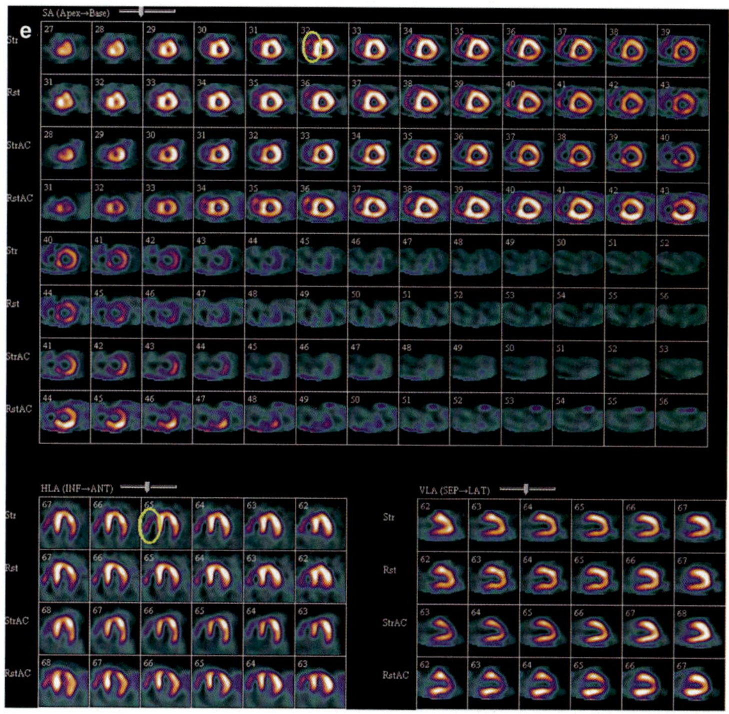

(**e**) Stress/rest processed SPECT images (SA, HLA, VLA) (without and with AC), right ventricle (*yellow ovals*) on selected SA and HLA images

The Pertinent Findings

- Chest
    - Skeleton: ■ hot □ cold
    - Right atrium and right ventricle: ■ hot ■ cold
- Abdomen
    - Peritoneum: □ hot ■ cold
    - Liver: □ hot ■ cold
    - Biliary system and gallbladder: ■ hot □ cold
    - Spleen: ■ hot □ cold
    - Stomach: ■ hot □ cold

The Relevant Diagnosis(es)

- Chest
  - Skeleton: ■ anemia
  - Right atrium and right ventricle: ■ pulmonary hypertension
- Abdomen
  - Peritoneum: ■ ascites
  - Liver: ■ cirrhosis
  - Biliary system and gallbladder: ■ normal
  - Spleen: ■ splenomegaly
  - Stomach: ■ gastropathy

Discussion

Chest

The right ventricle is enlarged and has a thickened "hot" wall (a, b, c, d, e). Note the flattened septum and D-shaped left ventricle. Function is preserved (d). The skeleton is slightly prominent, consistent with liver disease-related anemia.

Abdomen

The abdomen demonstrates the classical constellation of findings of advanced liver disease and portal hypertension: small liver, "cold" ascites, "hot" spleen, and "hot" stomach. Note the normally filled gallbladder. Most often, even in cirrhosis, the gallbladder will be visualized.

The intestinal tract and left kidney are not included in the field-of-view and cannot be evaluated.

Relevant Chapter(s)

8, 13, 18, 19, 20, 21, and 22

28.2 Case Challenge #14

28.2.1 Problem

Clinical Highlights
A 62-year-old female has chest pain.

Images for Review

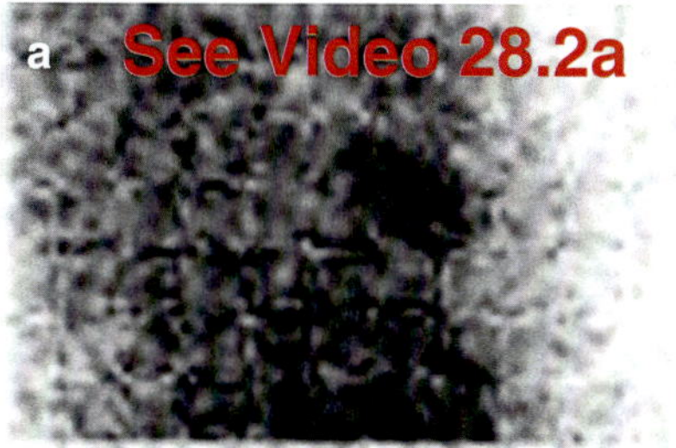

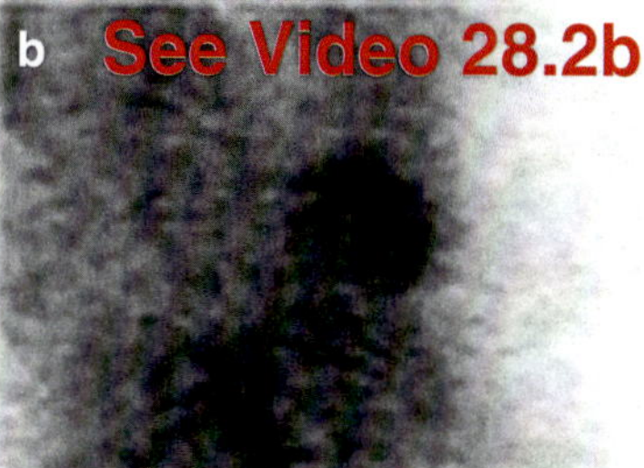

Fig. 28.2

(**a**) Rest raw projection images (Video 28.2a, frame 1), ^{99m}Tc sestamibi
(**b**) Stress raw projection images (Video 28.2b, frame 1), ^{99m}Tc sestamibi

Characterize the Pertinent Finding(s)
- Chest
    - Breasts: □ hot □ cold
    - Chest wall: □ hot □ cold
    - Skeleton: □ hot □ cold
    - Pleura: □ hot □ cold
    - Lungs: □ hot □ cold
    - Mediastinum: □ hot □ cold
    - Myocardium and pericardium: □ hot □ cold
    - Right atrium and right ventricle: □ hot □ cold
    - Vascular system: □ hot □ cold
- Abdomen
    - Peritoneum: □ hot □ cold
    - Liver: □ hot □ cold
    - Biliary system and gallbladder: □ hot □ cold
    - Spleen: □ hot □ cold
    - Stomach: □ hot □ cold
    - Small intestine and large intestine: □ hot □ cold
    - Adrenal glands: □ hot □ cold
    - Kidneys and female reproductive system: □ hot □ cold

State Your Relevant Diagnosis(es)
- Chest
  - Breasts: □ normal □ mastectomy
  - Chest wall: □ normal □ contamination artifact
  - Skeleton: □ normal □ anemia
  - Pleura: □ normal □ effusion
  - Lungs: □ normal □ pneumonectomy
  - Mediastinum: □ normal □ hilar mass
  - Myocardium and pericardium: □ normal □ myocardial mass
  - Right atrium and right ventricle: □ normal □ enlargement
  - Vascular system: □ normal □ port injection site
- Abdomen
  - Peritoneum: □ normal □ ascites
  - Liver: □ normal □ cirrhosis
  - Biliary system and gallbladder: □ normal □ cholecystectomy
  - Spleen: □ normal □ splenectomy
  - Stomach: □ normal □ gastropathy
  - Small intestine and large intestine: □ normal □ ileus
  - Adrenal glands: □ normal □ mass
  - Kidneys and female reproductive system: □ normal □ renal cyst

28.2.2 Solution

Additional Annotated Images
None.

The Pertinent Findings
- Chest
  - Not applicable
- Abdomen
  - Peritoneum: □ hot ■ cold
  - Liver: □ hot ■ cold
  - Biliary system and gallbladder: □ hot ■ cold
  - Spleen: □ hot ■ cold
  - Stomach: ■ hot □ cold

The Relevant Diagnosis(es)
- Chest
  - Not applicable
- Abdomen
  - Peritoneum: ■ ascites
  - Liver: ■ cirrhosis
  - Biliary system and gallbladder: ■ cholecystectomy
  - Spleen: ■ splenectomy
  - Stomach: ■ gastropathy

Discussion
Chest
There are no abnormalities.

Abdomen
There is photopenia due to ascites throughout the abdomen (a, b). The liver is small, consistent with cirrhosis, and the stomach is diffusely "hot," consistent with gastropathy. This constellation is characteristic of the sequelae of cirrhosis. The unusual feature to this case is absence of the spleen rather than the expected splenomegaly; according to the medical record, the spleen is surgically absent from unrelated trauma in the past. The gallbladder is also surgically absent. The left kidney is present.

Relevant Chapter(s)
18, 19, 20, 21, and 22

28.3 Case Challenge #15

28.3.1 Problem

Clinical Highlights

A 50-year-old male awaits renal transplant; he provides a previous surgical history.

Images for Review

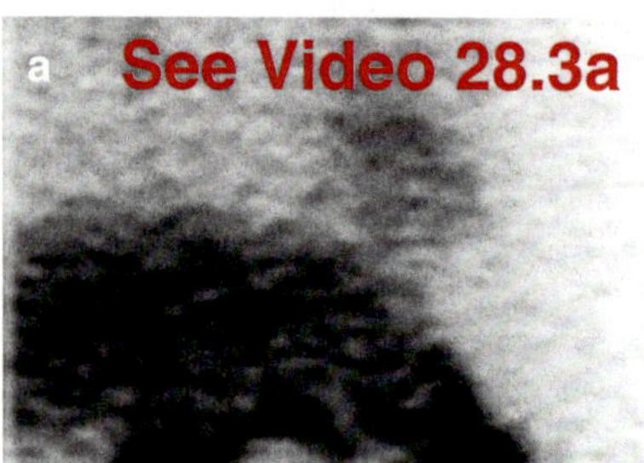

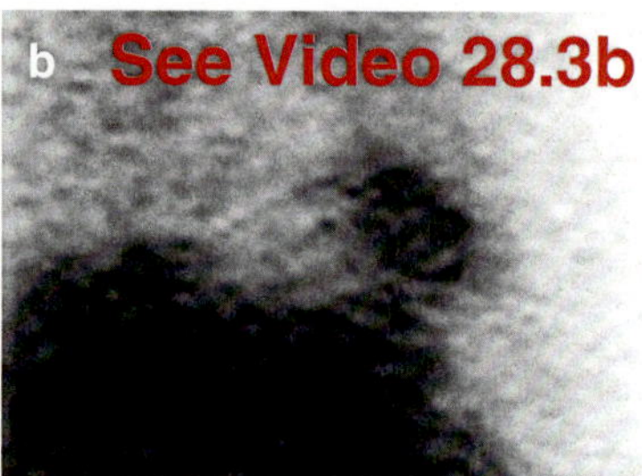

Fig. 28.3

(**a**) Current: stress raw projection images (Video 28.3a, frame 1), ^{99m}Tc sestamibi (75 minutes after injection)

(**b**) Two years previously: stress raw projection images (Video 28.3b, frame 1), ^{99m}Tc sestamibi

Characterize the Pertinent Finding(s)
- Chest
    - Breasts: ☐ hot ☐ cold
    - Chest wall: ☐ hot ☐ cold
    - Skeleton: ☐ hot ☐ cold
    - Pleura: ☐ hot ☐ cold
    - Lungs: ☐ hot ☐ cold
    - Mediastinum: ☐ hot ☐ cold
    - Myocardium and pericardium: ☐ hot ☐ cold
    - Right atrium and right ventricle: ☐ hot ☐ cold
    - Vascular system: ☐ hot ☐ cold
- Abdomen
    - Abdominal wall: ☐ hot ☐ cold
    - Peritoneum: ☐ hot ☐ cold
    - Liver: ☐ hot ☐ cold
    - Biliary system and gallbladder: ☐ hot ☐ cold
    - Spleen: ☐ hot ☐ cold
    - Stomach: ☐ hot ☐ cold
    - Small intestine and large intestine: ☐ hot ☐ cold
    - Adrenal glands: ☐ hot ☐ cold

State Your Relevant Diagnosis(es)

- Chest
    - Breasts: ☐ normal ☐ gynecomastia
    - Chest wall: ☐ normal ☐ pacemaker
    - Skeleton: ☐ normal ☐ metastatic disease
    - Pleura: ☐ normal ☐ mesothelioma
    - Lungs: ☐ normal ☐ emphysema
    - Mediastinum: ☐ normal ☐ metastatic disease
    - Myocardium and pericardium: ☐ normal ☐ effusion
    - Right atrium and right ventricle: ☐ normal ☐ pulmonary hypertension
    - Vascular system: ☐ normal ☐ injection site
- Abdomen
    - Abdominal wall: ☐ normal ☐ patient's arm and hand
    - Peritoneum: ☐ normal ☐ ascites
    - Liver: ☐ normal ☐ transplant for cirrhosis
    - Biliary system and gallbladder: ☐ normal ☐ cholecystectomy
    - Spleen: ☐ normal ☐ enlargement
    - Stomach: ☐ normal ☐ gastric outlet obstruction
    - Small intestine and large intestine: ☐ normal ☐ large bowel visualization
    - Adrenal glands: ☐ normal ☐ metastatic lung cancer

28.3.2 Solution

Additional Images

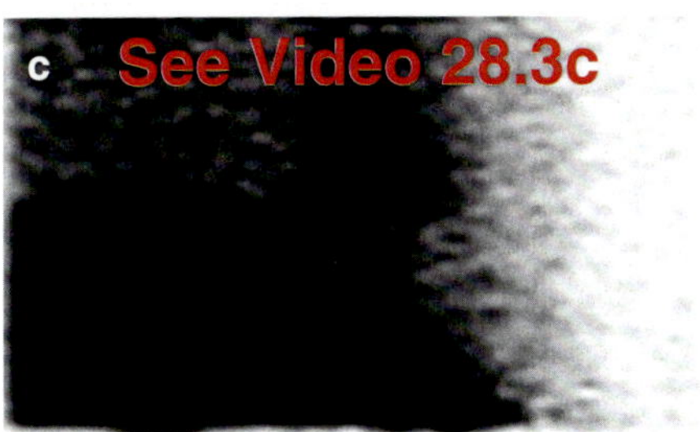

(**c**) Current: stress raw projection images, contrast adjusted for breasts (Video 28.3c, frame 1), ^{99m}Tc sestamibi (75 minutes after injection)

The Pertinent Findings

- Chest
    - Breasts: ■ hot ☐ cold
- Abdomen
    - Liver: ■ hot ☐ cold
    - Biliary system and gallbladder: ☐ hot ■ cold
    - Spleen: ■ hot ☐ cold
    - Small intestine and large intestine: ■ hot ☐ cold

The Relevant Diagnosis(es)
- Chest
    - Breasts: ■ gynecomastia
- Abdomen
    - Liver: ■ transplant for cirrhosis
    - Biliary system and gallbladder: ■ cholecystectomy
    - Spleen: ■ enlargement
    - Stomach: ■ normal
    - Small intestine and large intestine: ■ large bowel visualization

Discussion
Chest
There is subtle, symmetric uptake in the areolar breast tissue in this male patient who underwent liver transplant for cirrhosis; this suggests gynecomastia (a, b, c).

Abdomen
The liver appears normal on the current examination (a), but it was distinctly abnormal on the previous examination before the transplant (b). Note difference in liver size, shape, and uptake pattern – and he no longer has a gallbladder! The enlarged spleen (a, b) persists after transplant (a, b). Prominent large intestinal activity on the current examination (a) could be mistaken for a normal gallbladder; follow the activity on the cinematic display.

Relevant Chapter(s)
6, 19, 20, 21, and 23

28.4   Case Challenge #16

28.4.1 Problem

Clinical Highlights

A 58-year-old diabetic female with known coronary artery disease undergoes stress testing to exclude inducible ischemia. She has chronic obstructive pulmonary disease and provides a past surgical history following a motor vehicle accident.

Images for Review

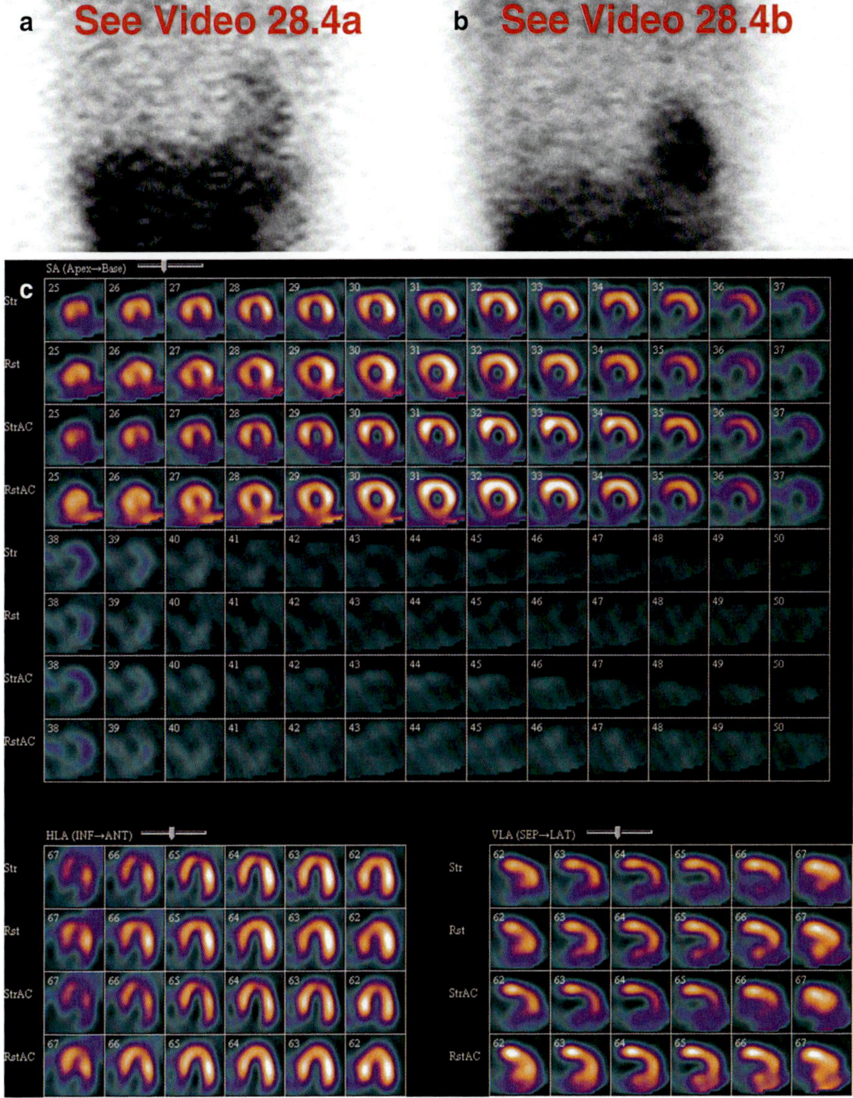

Fig. 28.4

(**a**) Rest raw projection images (Video 28.4a, frame 1), ^{99m}Tc sestamibi
(**b**) Stress raw projection images (Video 28.4b, frame 1), ^{99m}Tc sestamibi
(**c**) Stress/rest processed SPECT images (SA, HLA, VLA) (with and without AC)

Characterize the Pertinent Finding(s)

- Chest
    - Thyroid gland: ☐ hot ☐ cold
    - Breasts: ☐ hot ☐ cold
    - Chest wall: ☐ hot ☐ cold
    - Pleura: ☐ hot ☐ cold
    - Lungs: ☐ hot ☐ cold
    - Mediastinum: ☐ hot ☐ cold
    - Myocardium and pericardium: ☐ hot ☐ cold
    - Right atrium and right ventricle: ☐ hot ☐ cold
    - Diaphragm: ☐ hot ☐ cold
- Abdomen
    - Abdominal wall: ☐ hot ☐ cold
    - Liver: ☐ hot ☐ cold
    - Biliary system and gallbladder: ☐ hot ☐ cold
    - Spleen: ☐ hot ☐ cold
    - Stomach: ☐ hot ☐ cold
    - Small intestine and large intestine: ☐ hot ☐ cold
    - Kidneys and female reproductive system: ☐ hot ☐ cold
    - Vascular system: ☐ hot ☐ cold

State Your Relevant Diagnosis(es)

- Chest
    - Thyroid gland: ☐ normal ☐ substernal goiter
    - Breasts: ☐ normal ☐ soft-tissue attenuation artifact
    - Chest wall: ☐ normal ☐ pacemaker
    - Pleura: ☐ normal ☐ effusion
    - Lungs: ☐ normal ☐ emphysema
    - Mediastinum: ☐ normal ☐ cystic mass
    - Myocardium and pericardium: ☐ normal ☐ effusion
    - Right atrium and right ventricle: ☐ normal ☐ right auricular appendage and pulmonary hypertension
    - Diaphragm: ☐ normal ☐ flattening
- Abdomen
    - Abdominal wall: ☐ normal ☐ urinary contamination artifact
    - Liver: ☐ normal ☐ polycystic disease
    - Biliary system and gallbladder: ☐ normal ☐ dilated intrahepatic ducts with stasis
    - Spleen: ☐ hot ☐ cold
    - Stomach: ☐ normal ☐ fluid filled after ingestion of fluids
    - Small intestine and large intestine: ☐ normal ☐ internal hernia
    - Kidneys and female reproductive system: ☐ normal ☐ hydronephrotic obstructed left kidney
    - Vascular system: ☐ normal ☐ extravasation

28.4.2 Solution

Additional Annotated Images

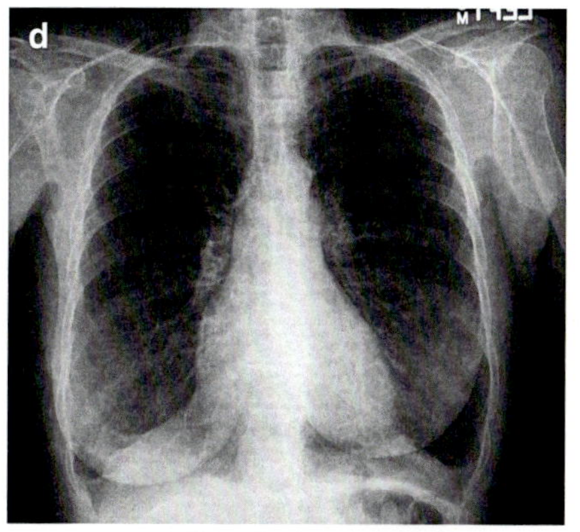
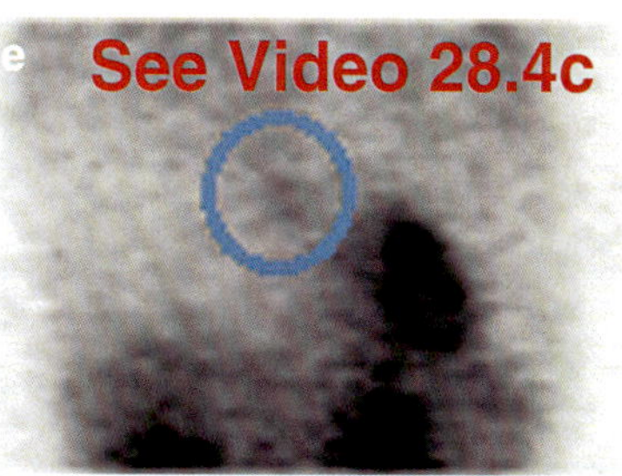

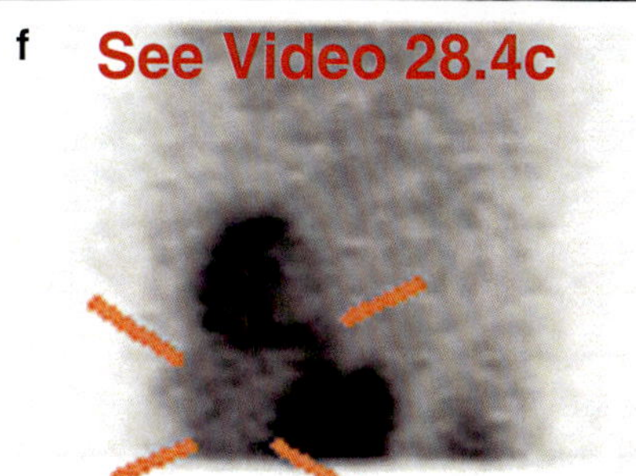

(**d**) PA chest radiograph

(**e**) Stress raw projection image (Video 28.4c, frame 9, Anterior, image 9), ^{99m}Tc sestamibi, right auricular appendage (*blue oval*)

(**f**) Stress raw projection image (Video 28.4c, frame 60, left lateral, image 60), ^{99m}Tc sestamibi, "cold" stomach with "hot" wall (*orange lines*)

The Pertinent Findings

- Chest
    - Breasts: ☐ hot ■ cold
    - Lungs: ☐ hot ■ cold
    - Right atrium and right ventricle: ■ hot ■ cold
    - Diaphragm: ☐ hot ■ cold
- Abdomen
    - Spleen: ☐ hot ■ cold
    - Stomach: ■ hot ■ cold

The Relevant Diagnosis(es)

- Chest
  - Breasts: ▪ soft-tissue attenuation artifact
  - Lungs: ▪ emphysema
  - Right atrium and right ventricle: ▪ right auricular appendage and pulmonary hypertension
  - Diaphragm: ▪ flattening
- Abdomen
  - Spleen: ▪ splenectomy
  - Stomach: ▪ fluid filled after ingestion of fluids

Discussion

Chest

There is superimposed "cold" breast tissue (a, b) which creates slight breast attenuation artifact in the anterior wall of the left ventricle (c). There are hyperexpanded "cold" lungs, especially involving the lower lobes, with flattened diaphragms (a, b); radiography is confirmatory (d).

The right ventricle is enlarged with prominent right ventricular myocardial uptake (a, b, e), consistent with pulmonary hypertension in the setting of advanced obstructive pulmonary disease; there is a normal right auricular appendage (a, b, e). There is a large reversible perfusion defect in the inferior wall consistent with right coronary artery ischemia (c).

Abdomen

The biliary system appears normal; a gallbladder is present but is not included in the field-of-view. The spleen is surgically absent, and the left kidney and small intestine occupy the left upper quadrant adjacent to the stomach (a, b). The stomach appears both "hot" and "cold," likely reflecting gastric wall uptake, plus a mixture of duodenogastric reflux and fluid ingestion (a, b, f). Given the history of diabetes mellitus, prolonged gastric distension can suggest gastroparesis.

Relevant Chapter(s)

6, 10, 13, 16, 21, and 22

28.5   Case Challenge #17

28.5.1 Problem

Clinical Highlights

A 33-year-old male undergoes preoperative planning. He complains of dyspnea. The regadenoson stress test is normal. Recent echocardiogram showed LVEF of 67 %. Calcified gallstones are noted on ultrasonography.

Images for Review

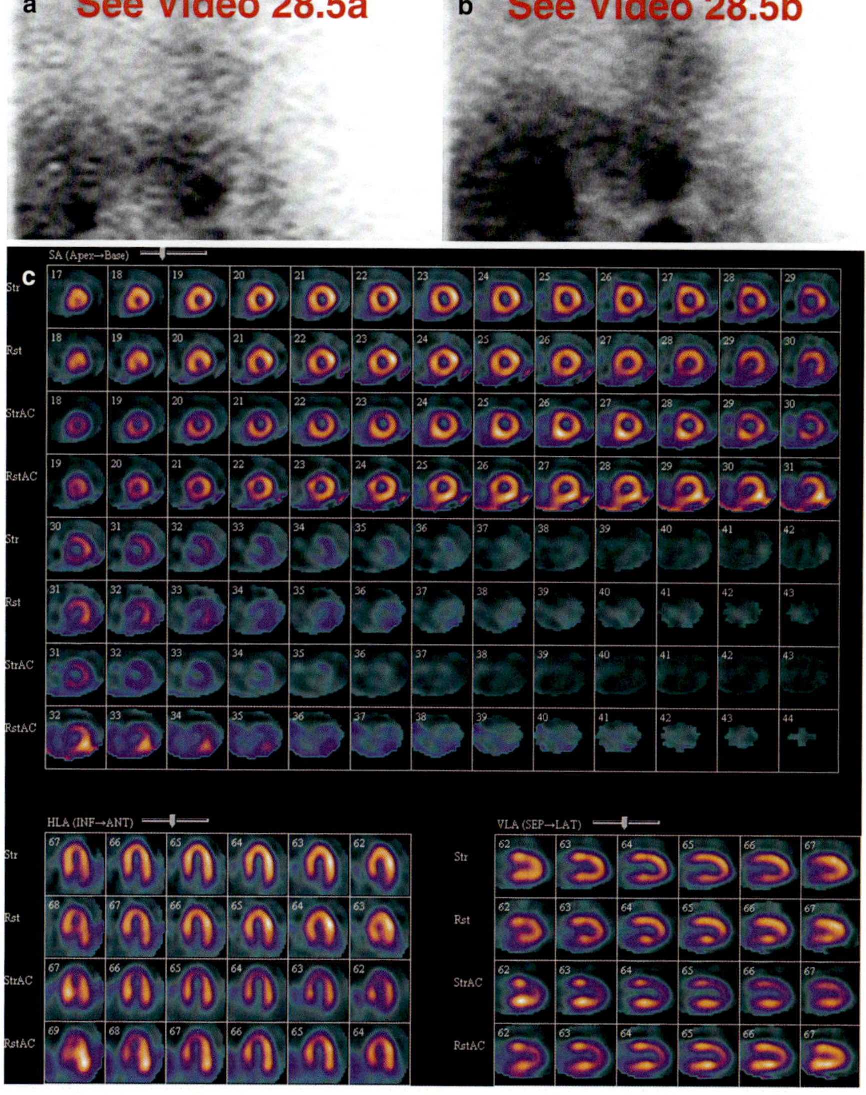

Fig. 28.5

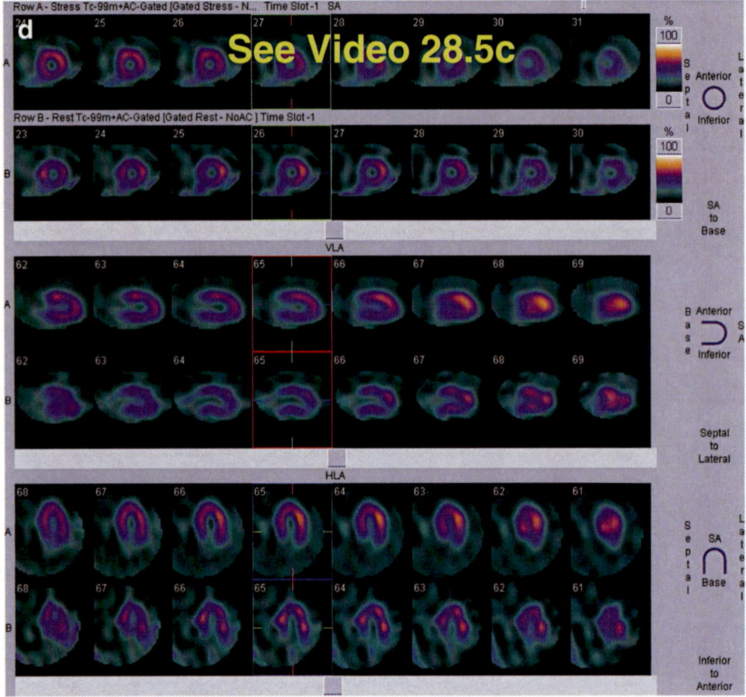

Fig. 28.5 (continued)

(**a**) Rest raw projection images (Video 28.5a, frame 1), ^{99m}Tc sestamibi

(**b**) Stress raw projection images (Video 28.5b, frame 1), ^{99m}Tc sestamibi

(**c**) Stress/rest processed SPECT images (SA, HLA, VLA) (without and with AC)

(**d**) Stress and rest gated SPECT images (Video 28.5c, frame 1) (SA, VLA, HLA)

Characterize the Pertinent Finding(s)

- Chest
  - Breasts: ☐ hot ☐ cold
  - Chest wall: ☐ hot ☐ cold
  - Pleura: ☐ hot ☐ cold
  - Lungs: ☐ hot ☐ cold
  - Mediastinum: ☐ hot ☐ cold
  - Right atrium and right ventricle: ☐ hot ☐ cold
  - Vascular system: ☐ hot ☐ cold
  - Lymphatic system: ☐ hot ☐ cold
  - Diaphragm: ☐ hot ☐ cold

- Abdomen
  - Abdominal wall: ☐ hot ☐ cold
  - Peritoneum: ☐ hot ☐ cold
  - Liver: ☐ hot ☐ cold
  - Biliary system and gallbladder: ☐ hot ☐ cold
  - Spleen: ☐ hot ☐ cold
  - Stomach: ☐ hot ☐ cold
  - Small intestine and large intestine: ☐ hot ☐ cold
  - Kidneys and female reproductive system: ☐ hot ☐ cold

State Your Relevant Diagnosis(es)

- Chest
  - Breasts: ☐ normal ☐ carcinoma
  - Chest wall: ☐ normal ☐ implanted defibrillator device
  - Pleura: ☐ normal ☐ effusion
  - Lungs: ☐ normal ☐ active granulomatous disease
  - Mediastinum: ☐ normal ☐ paravertebral mass (extramedullary hematopoiesis)
  - Right atrium and right ventricle: ☐ normal ☐ enlarged atrium
  - Vascular system: ☐ normal ☐ retention in central veins
  - Lymphatic system: ☐ normal ☐ metastatic breast carcinoma
  - Diaphragm: ☐ normal ☐ herniated small intestine
- Abdomen
  - Abdominal wall: ☐ normal ☐ metallic object
  - Peritoneum: ☐ normal ☐ ascites
  - Liver: ☐ normal ☐ cirrhosis
  - Biliary system and gallbladder: ☐ normal ☐ pathologic variability, gallbladder
  - Spleen: ☐ normal ☐ splenomegaly
  - Stomach: ☐ normal ☐ gastropathy
  - Small intestine and large intestine: ☐ normal ☐ ileus
  - Kidneys and female reproductive system: ☐ normal ☐ atrophy

28.5.2 Solution

Additional Annotated Images

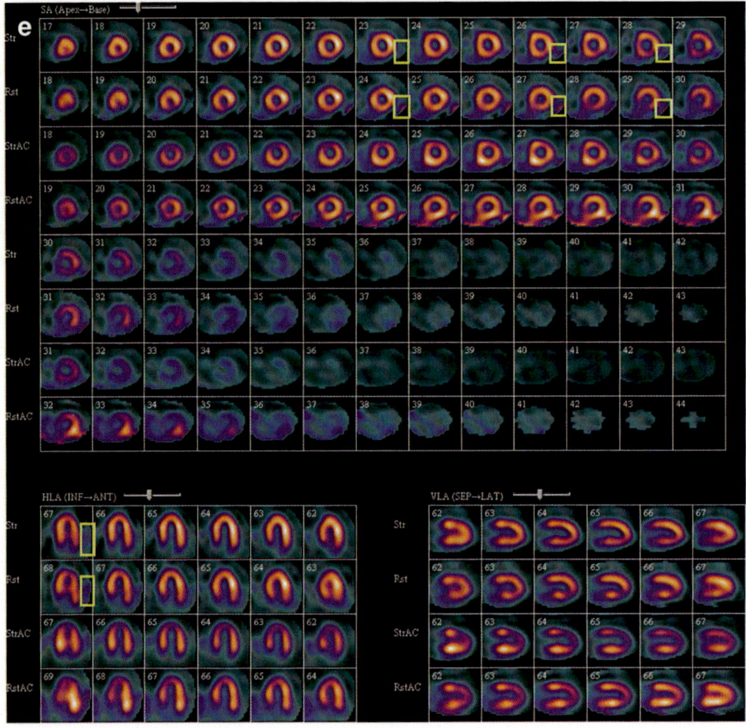

(**e**) Stress/rest processed SPECT images (SA, HLA, VLA) (without and with AC), splenic activity (*yellow boxes*) on selected non-AC and AC SA and HLA images

The Pertinent Findings
- Chest
  - Not applicable
- Abdomen
  - Peritoneum: □ hot ■ cold
  - Liver: □ hot ■ cold
  - Biliary system and gallbladder: ■ hot ■ cold
  - Spleen: ■ hot □ cold
  - Stomach: ■ hot □ cold

The Relevant Diagnosis(es)

- Chest
  - Not applicable
- Abdomen
  - Peritoneum: ▪ ascites
  - Liver: ▪ cirrhosis
  - Biliary system and gallbladder: ▪ pathologic variability, gallbladder
  - Spleen: ▪ splenomegaly
  - Stomach: ▪ gastropathy

Discussion

Chest

On rest raw images (a) performed first, the gallbladder appears small and contracted; the patient was fasting. On later same-day stress raw images (b), the gallbladder appears more distended with radioactive bile. Differential distension of the gallbladder signals chronic gallbladder disease. The patency of the cystic duct excludes acute cholecystitis. [Two months later, the patient developed acute cholecystitis requiring cholecystostomy tube placement.]

Abdomen

Note small liver, ascites, splenomegaly, and gastropathy (a, b). Neither the "high" spleen nor the "hot" stomach creates artifacts on the processed SPECT images (c, e) nor on the gated images (d).

Relevant Chapter(s)

18, 19, 20, 21, and 22

28.6 Case Challenge #18

28.6.1 Problem

Clinical Highlights

A 58-year-old male presents with shortness of breath and chest pain.

Images for Review

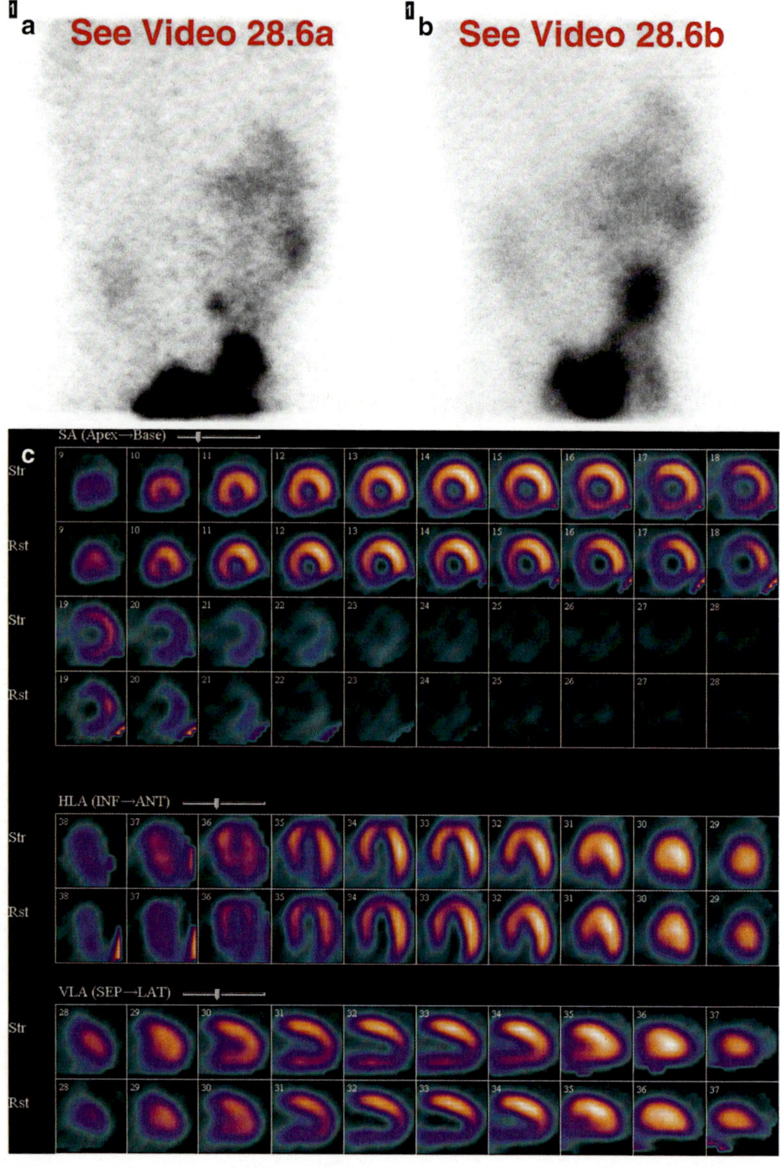

Fig. 28.6

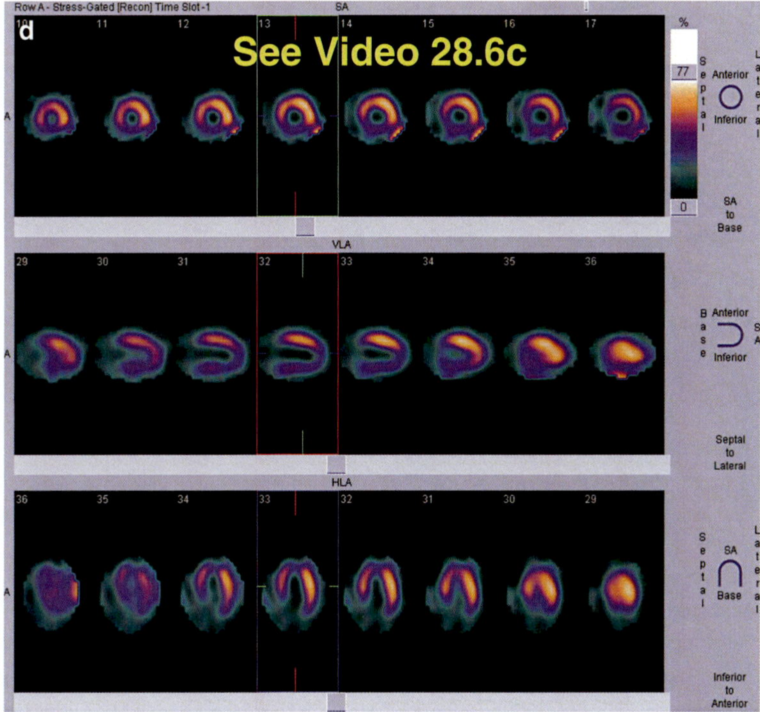

Fig. 28.6   (continued)

(**a**) Rest raw projection images (Video 28.6a, frame 1), ^{99m}Tc sestamibi
(**b**) Stress raw projection images (Video 28.6b, frame 1), ^{99m}Tc sestamibi
(**c**) Stress/rest processed SPECT images (SA, HLA, VLA)
(**d**) Stress gated SPECT images (Video 28.6c, frame 1) (SA, HLA, VLA)

Characterize the Pertinent Finding(s)

- Chest
    - Thyroid gland: ☐ hot ☐ cold
    - Parathyroid glands: ☐ hot ☐ cold
    - Breasts: ☐ hot ☐ cold
    - Lungs: ☐ hot ☐ cold
    - Mediastinum: ☐ hot ☐ cold
    - Myocardium and pericardium: ☐ hot ☐ cold
    - Right atrium and right ventricle: ☐ hot ☐ cold
    - Vascular system: ☐ hot ☐ cold
    - Lymphatic system: ☐ hot ☐ cold

- Abdomen
    - Abdominal wall: ☐ hot ☐ cold
    - Peritoneum: ☐ hot ☐ cold
    - Liver: ☐ hot ☐ cold
    - Biliary system and gallbladder: ☐ hot ☐ cold
    - Spleen: ☐ hot ☐ cold
    - Stomach: ☐ hot ☐ cold
    - Small intestine and large intestine: ☐ hot ☐ cold
    - Vascular system: ☐ hot ☐ cold

State Your Relevant Diagnosis(es)

- Chest
    - Thyroid gland: ☐ normal ☐ primary malignancy
    - Parathyroid glands: ☐ normal ☐ parathyroid adenoma
    - Breasts: ☐ normal ☐ breast cancer
    - Lungs: ☐ normal ☐ emphysema
    - Mediastinum: ☐ normal ☐ dilated esophagus with gastroesophageal reflux
    - Myocardium and pericardium: ☐ normal ☐ pericardial mass
    - Right atrium and right ventricle: ☐ normal ☐ dilatation
    - Vascular system: ☐ normal ☐ extravasation
    - Lymphatic system: ☐ normal ☐ venous extravasation resulting in axillary lymph node visualization
- Abdomen
    - Abdominal wall: ☐ normal ☐ metallic object
    - Peritoneum: ☐ normal ☐ ascites
    - Liver: ☐ normal ☐ rapid excretion
    - Biliary system and gallbladder: ☐ normal ☐ gallbladder non-visualization
    - Spleen: ☐ normal ☐ enlargement
    - Stomach: ☐ normal ☐ duodenogastric reflux
    - Small intestine and large intestine: ☐ normal ☐ active peristalsis
    - Vascular system: ☐ normal ☐ extravasation

28.6.2 Solution

Additional Images

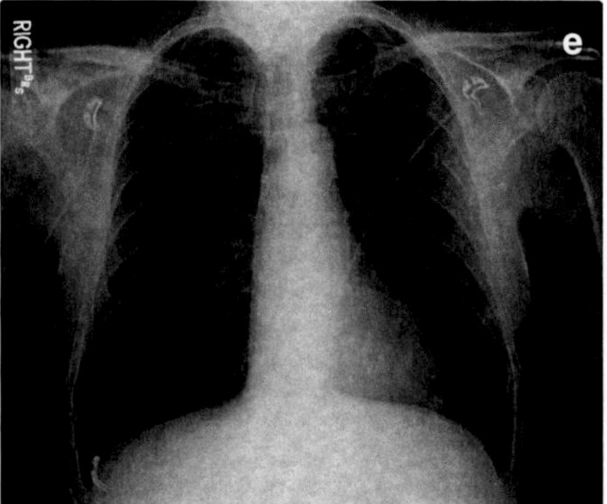

(e) PA chest radiograph

The Pertinent Findings

- Chest
  - Lungs: ☐ hot ■ cold
- Abdomen
  - Liver: ☐ hot ■ cold
  - Biliary system and gallbladder: ☐ hot ■ cold
  - Stomach: ■ hot ☐ cold
  - Small intestine and large intestine: ■ hot ■ cold

The Relevant Diagnosis(es)

- Chest
  - Lungs: ■ emphysema
- Abdomen
  - Liver: ■ rapid excretion
  - Biliary system and gallbladder: ■ gallbladder non-visualization
  - Stomach: ■ duodenogastric reflux
  - Small intestine and large intestine: ■ active peristalsis

Discussion

Chest

The "cold" lungs are due to emphysema (a, b); radiography (e) confirms hyperinflation and flattened diaphragms.

Abdomen

There is complete hepatic clearance on both image sets (a, b). The "hot" stomach is present on both sets of raw data (a, b), perhaps more pronounced on rest compared to stress. The stomach appears distended. On processed images (c), decreased uptake in the inferolateral-basal myocardial wall appears more pronounced on rest images compared to stress (a "reverse" fixed defect) (c); this may be related to the nearby gastric activity which is just visible at the lower right corner of some of the SA frames and the more inferior HLA frames. On gated SPECT images, the inferior wall has normal wall motion and wall thickening (d), favoring artifact rather than scar.

There is a curious focus of small intestinal activity located deep in the midline on the rest raw images (a); this focal activity clears by peristalsis on later stress raw images (a), confirming physiologic stasis with peristaltic clearance.

Relevant Chapter(s)

10, 19, 22, and 23

28.7   Case Challenge #19

28.7.1 Problem

Clinical Highlights

A 60-year-old male gives a history of surgery as a child. His mother told him he was a "blue baby." Regadenoson stress test is normal.

Images for Review

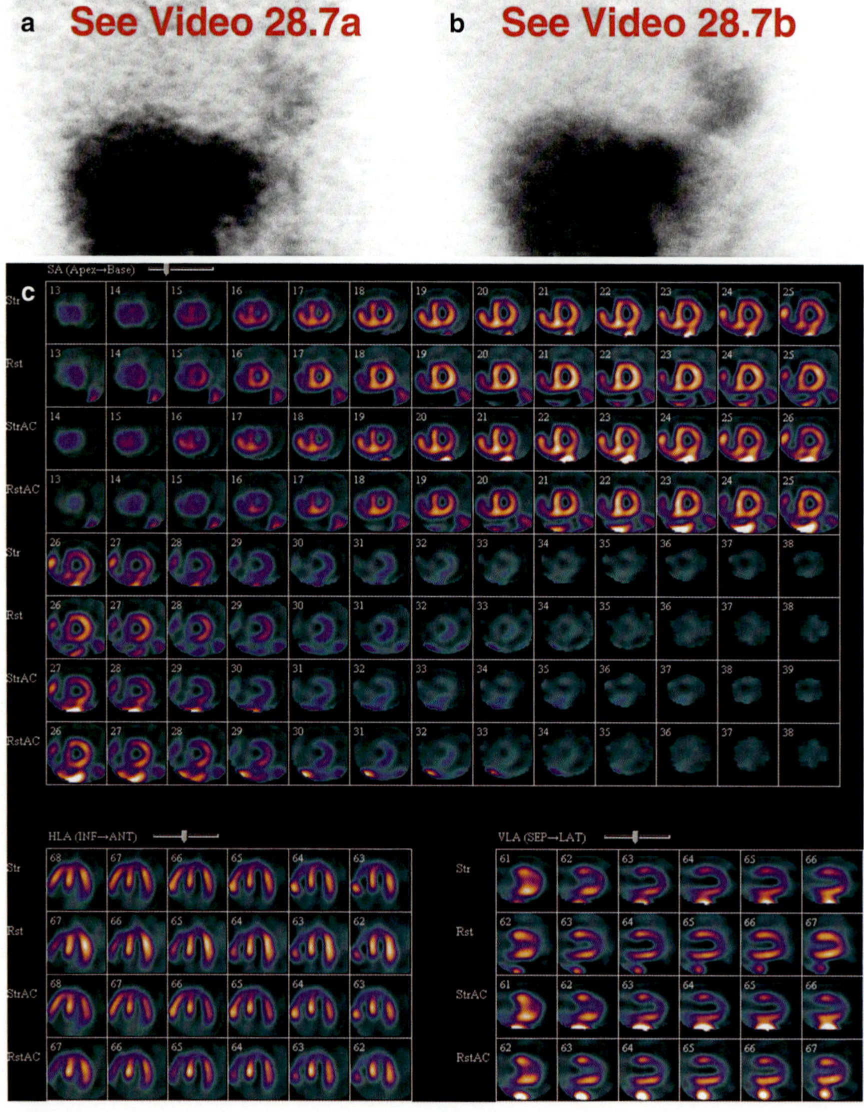

Fig. 28.7

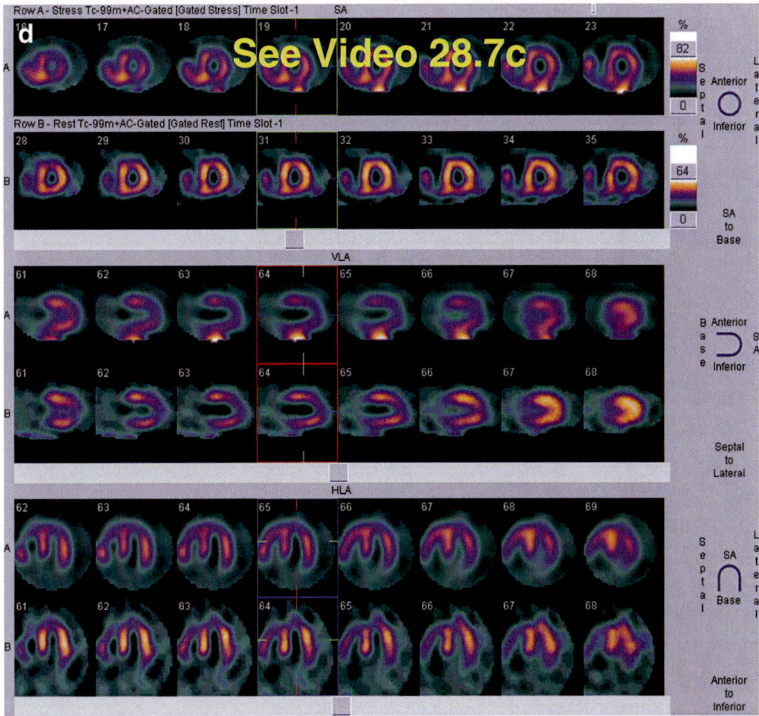

Fig. 28.7   (continued)

(**a**) Rest raw projection images (Video 28.7a, frame 1), ^{99m}Tc sestamibi
(**b**) Stress raw projection images (Video 28.7b, frame 1), ^{99m}Tc sestamibi
(**c**) Stress/rest processed SPECT images (SA, HLA, VLA) (without and with AC)
(**d**) Stress and rest gated SPECT images (Video 28.7c, frame 1) (SA, VLA, HLA)

Characterize the Pertinent Finding(s)

- Chest
  - Thyroid gland: ☐ hot ☐ cold
  - Parathyroid glands: ☐ hot ☐ cold
  - Breasts: ☐ hot ☐ cold
  - Chest wall: ☐ hot ☐ cold
  - Skeleton: ☐ hot ☐ cold
  - Pleura: ☐ hot ☐ cold
  - Lungs: ☐ hot ☐ cold
  - Right atrium and right ventricle: ☐ hot ☐ cold
  - Diaphragm: ☐ hot ☐ cold

- Abdomen
  - Abdominal wall: ☐ hot ☐ cold
  - Peritoneum: ☐ hot ☐ cold
  - Liver: ☐ hot ☐ cold
  - Biliary system and gallbladder: ☐ hot ☐ cold
  - Stomach: ☐ hot ☐ cold
  - Small intestine and large intestine: ☐ hot ☐ cold
  - Kidneys and female reproductive system: ☐ hot ☐ cold
  - Vascular system: ☐ hot ☐ cold

State Your Relevant Diagnosis(es)

- Chest
  - Thyroid gland : ☐ normal ☐ substernal goiter
  - Parathyroid glands: ☐ normal ☐ substernal adenoma
  - Breasts: ☐ normal ☐ gynecomastia
  - Chest wall: ☐ normal ☐ pacemaker
  - Skeleton: ☐ normal ☐ anemia
  - Pleura: ☐ normal ☐ effusion
  - Lungs: ☐ normal ☐ malignant mass
  - Right atrium and right ventricle: ☐ normal ☐ congenital heart disease, repaired
  - Diaphragm: ☐ normal ☐ flattening
- Abdomen
  - Abdominal wall: ☐ normal ☐ contamination
  - Peritoneum: ☐ normal ☐ peritoneal dialysate
  - Liver: ☐ normal ☐ postoperative
  - Biliary system and gallbladder: ☐ normal ☐ prominent biliary tree
  - Stomach: ☐ normal ☐ duodenogastric reflux
  - Small intestine and large intestine: ☐ normal ☐ peristalsis
  - Kidneys and female reproductive system: ☐ normal ☐ ptotic left kidney
  - Vascular system: ☐ normal ☐ injection site

28.7.2 Solution

Additional Images

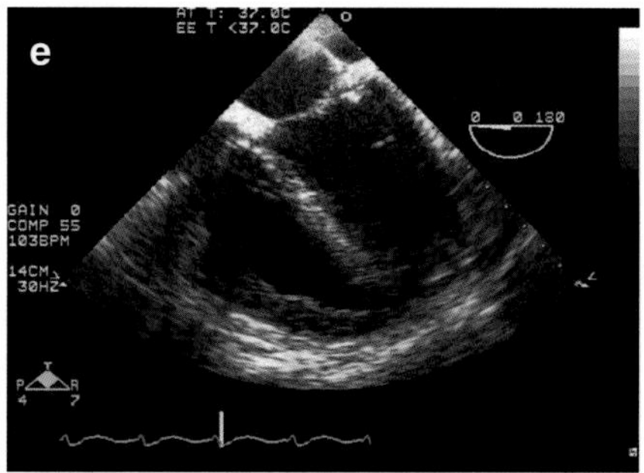

(**e**) 2D transesophageal echocardiogram (left atrium at *top*) with LV on right of display and RV on left of display

The Pertinent Findings

- Chest
  - Right atrium and right ventricle: ■ hot ■ cold
- Abdomen
  - Biliary system and gallbladder: ■ hot □ cold
  - Stomach: ■ hot □ cold
  - Small intestine and large intestine: ■ hot □ cold

The Relevant Diagnosis(es)

- Chest
  - Right atrium and right ventricle: ■ congenital heart disease, repaired
- Abdomen
  - Biliary system and gallbladder: ■ prominent biliary tree
  - Stomach: ■ duodenogastric reflux
  - Small intestine and large intestine: ■ normal

Discussion

Chest

The patient has a history of repaired tetralogy of Fallot and pulmonary artery atresia and known pulmonary hypertension. There is a markedly enlarged right ventricular cavity with a markedly thickened and prominent right ventricular wall (a, b, c, d), mimicking the letter "M" (the golden arches?). These findings are easier to appreciate on the more count-rich stress raw images (b). The right ventricle is dilated; there is right ventricular wall hypertrophy and reduced function by echocardiography (e). The right atrium also appears enlarged (a, b). The constellation is consistent with clinical history. The left ventricular cavity is normal in size, and perfusion and function are normal (c, d, e).

Abdomen

There are prominent intrahepatic and extrahepatic bile ducts, which is not necessarily abnormal. No gallbladder is visible. The changing gastric activity is evident on both the two sets of raw images and on the processed images (a, b, c). The duodenogastric reflux is actively occurring during imaging (b). The "hot" stomach creates a small fixed perfusion defect in the adjacent inferior myocardial wall (c, d).

Relevant Chapter(s)

13, 20, 22, and 23

28.8   Case Challenge #20

28.8.1 Problem

Clinical Highlights

A 64-year-old male presents for evaluation for organ transplant.

Images for Review

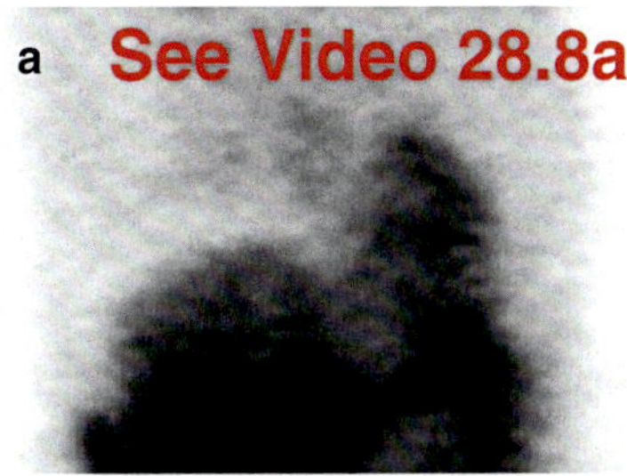

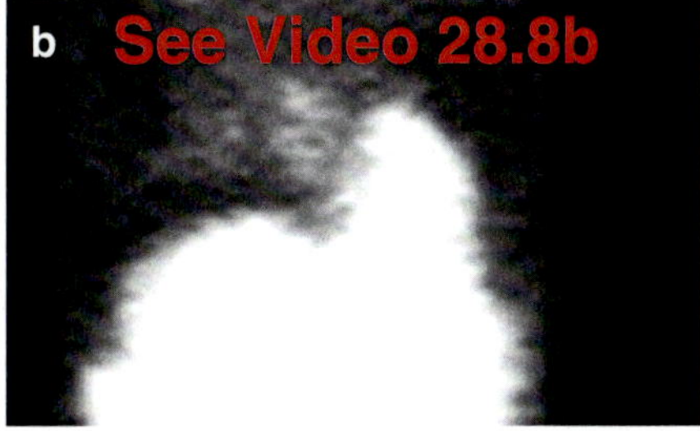

Fig. 28.8

(**a**) Stress "black-on-white" raw projection images (Video 28.8a, frame 1), ^{99m}Tc sestamibi, contrast adjusted for extracardiac structures

(**b**) Stress "white-on-black" raw projection images (Video 28.8b, frame 1), ^{99m}Tc sestamibi, contrast adjusted for extracardiac structures

Characterize the Pertinent Finding(s)

- Chest
  - Thyroid gland: □ hot □ cold
  - Chest wall: □ hot □ cold
  - Pleura: □ hot □ cold
  - Lungs: □ hot □ cold
  - Mediastinum: □ hot □ cold
  - Myocardium and pericardium: □ hot □ cold
  - Right atrium and right ventricle: □ hot □ cold
  - Lymphatic system: □ hot □ cold
  - Diaphragm: □ hot □ cold
- Abdomen
  - Abdominal wall: □ hot □ cold
  - Peritoneum: □ hot □ cold
  - Liver: □ hot □ cold
  - Biliary system and gallbladder: □ hot □ cold
  - Spleen: □ hot □ cold
  - Stomach: □ hot □ cold
  - Small intestine and large intestine: □ hot □ cold
  - Kidneys and female reproductive system: □ hot □ cold

State Your Relevant Diagnosis(es)

- Chest
    - Thyroid gland: ☐ normal ☐ primary malignancy
    - Chest wall: ☐ normal ☐ pacemaker
    - Pleura: ☐ normal ☐ effusion
    - Lungs: ☐ normal ☐ atelectasis
    - Mediastinum: ☐ normal ☐ malignant neoplasm
    - Myocardium and pericardium: ☐ normal ☐ effusion
    - Right atrium and right ventricle: ☐ normal ☐ dilatation
    - Lymphatic system: ☐ normal ☐ axillary lymphoma
    - Diaphragm: ☐ normal ☐ flattening
- Abdomen
    - Abdominal wall: ☐ normal ☐ urinary contamination
    - Peritoneum: ☐ normal ☐ ascites
    - Liver: ☐ normal ☐ cirrhosis
    - Biliary system and gallbladder: ☐ normal ☐ acute cholecystitis
    - Spleen: ☐ normal ☐ splenomegaly
    - Stomach: ☐ normal ☐ gastropathy
    - Small intestine and large intestine: ☐ normal ☐ hyperperistalsis
    - Kidneys and female reproductive system: ☐ normal ☐ absent left kidney

28.8.2 Solution

Additional Annotated Images

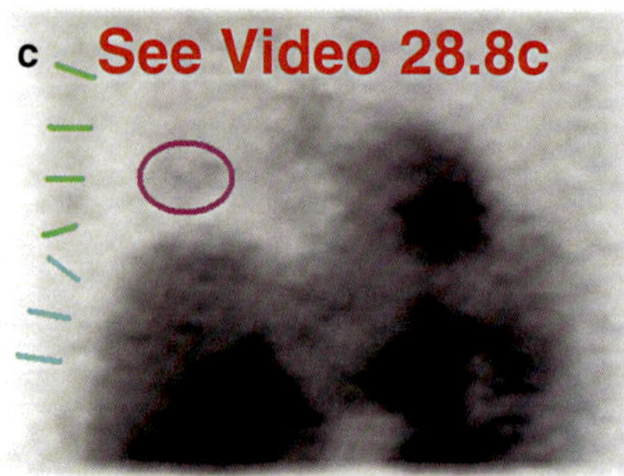

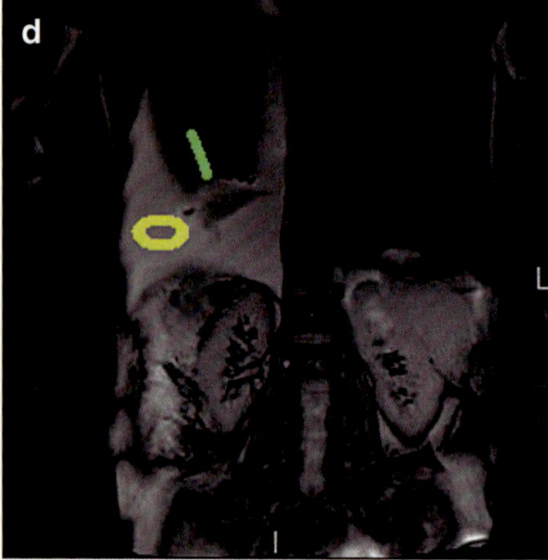

(**c**) Stress "black-on-white" raw projection image contrast-adjusted for extracardiac structures (Video 28.8c, frame 15), ^{99m}Tc sestamibi, pleural effusion (*green lines*), atelectasis (*pink oval*), and ascites (*blue lines*)

(**d**) Coronal MRI of posterior chest/upper abdomen, pleural effusion (*yellow oval*), and atelectasis (*green line*)

The Pertinent Findings

- Chest
    - Pleura: □ hot ■ cold
    - Lungs: ■ hot □ cold
- Abdomen
    - Peritoneum: □ hot ■ cold
    - Liver: □ hot ■ cold
    - Spleen: ■ hot □ cold
    - Stomach: ■ hot ■ cold
    - Kidneys and female reproductive system: ■ hot □ cold

The Relevant Diagnosis(es)

- Chest
    - Pleura: ■ effusion
    - Lungs: ■ atelectasis
- Abdomen
    - Peritoneum: ■ ascites
    - Liver: ■ cirrhosis
    - Spleen: ■ splenomegaly
    - Stomach: ■ gastropathy
    - Kidneys and female reproductive system: ■ normal

Discussion

Chest

The right hemithorax appears "cold" and there is focal increased uptake at the right lung base representing compressed atelectatic lung tissue (a, b, c). Right pleural fluid is confirmed on MRI (d).

Abdomen

The peritoneal cavity appears "cold" (a, b, c) due to abdominal ascites (d). There is a small liver, an enlarged spleen, and a diffusely "hot" stomach with a "cold" lumen (a, b). A normal left kidney is situated next to the spleen (c, d); it appears relatively "hot" on the raw data (a, b), likely related to greater urinary clearance of the radiopharmaceutical in the setting of liver dysfunction.

Relevant Chapter(s)

9, 10, 18, 19, 21, 22, and 25

28.9   Case Challenge #21

28.9.1 Problem

Clinical Highlights

A 67-year-old male is evaluated for possible cardiac sarcoidosis.

Images for Review

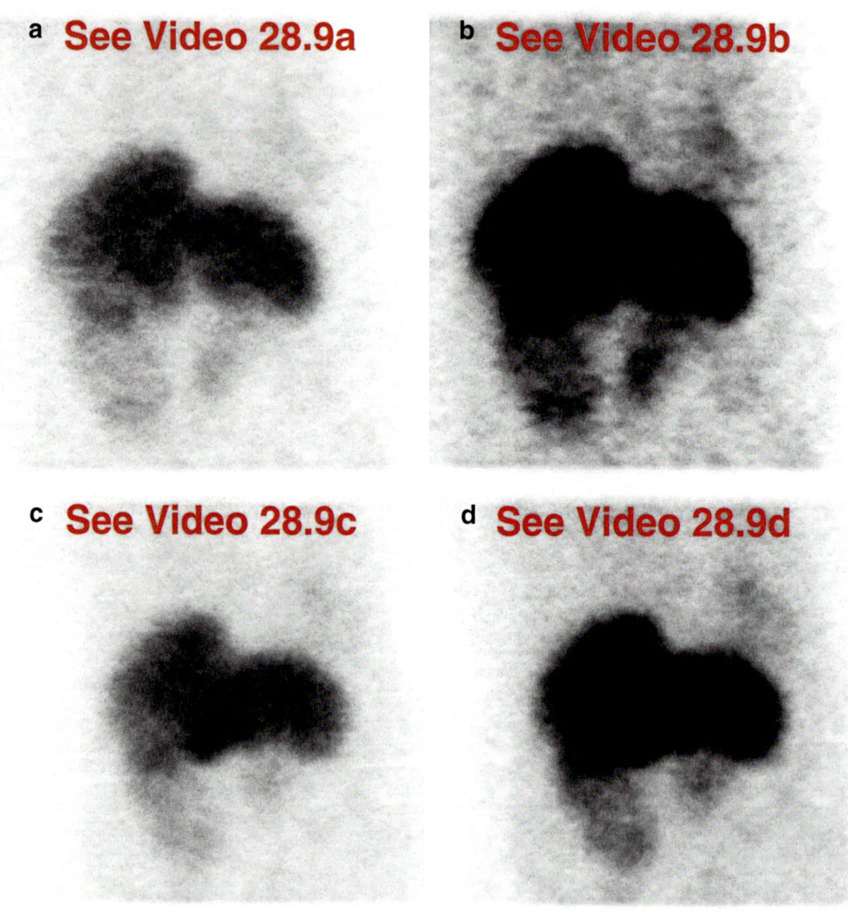

Fig. 28.9

(**a**) Rest raw projection images (Video 28.9a, frame 1) at usual setting to view heart, ^{99m}Tc sestamibi

(**b**) Rest raw projection images (Video 28.9b, frame 1) adjusted to view abdomen, ^{99m}Tc sestamibi

(**c**) Stress raw projection images (Video 28.9c, frame 1) at usual setting to view heart, ^{99m}Tc sestamibi

(**d**) Stress raw projection images (Video 28.9d, frame 1 adjusted to view abdomen, ^{99m}Tc sestamibi

Characterize the Pertinent Finding(s)

- Chest
  - Parathyroid glands: □ hot □ cold
  - Breasts: □ hot □ cold
  - Skeleton: □ hot □ cold
  - Lungs: □ hot □ cold
  - Mediastinum: □ hot □ cold
  - Myocardium and pericardium: □ hot □ cold
  - Right atrium and right ventricle: □ hot □ cold
  - Vascular system: □ hot □ cold
  - Diaphragm: □ hot □ cold
- Abdomen
  - Liver: □ hot □ cold
  - Biliary system and gallbladder: □ hot □ cold
  - Spleen: □ hot □ cold
  - Stomach: □ hot □ cold
  - Small intestine and large intestine: □ hot □ cold
  - Adrenal glands: □ hot □ cold
  - Kidneys and female reproductive system: □ hot □ cold
  - Vascular system: □ hot □ cold

State Your Relevant Diagnosis(es)

- Chest
  - Parathyroid glands: □ normal □ hyperplasia
  - Breasts: □ normal □ gynecomastia
  - Skeleton: □ normal □ osteomyelitis
  - Lungs: □ normal □ bronchial carcinoid tumor
  - Mediastinum: □ normal □ thymoma
  - Myocardium and pericardium: □ normal □ carcinoid tumor
  - Right atrium and right ventricle: □ normal □ valvular disease
  - Vascular system: □ normal □ extravasation during injection
  - Diaphragm: □ normal □ eventration
- Abdomen
  - Liver: □ normal □ cirrhosis
  - Biliary system and gallbladder: □ normal □ gallstones
  - Spleen: □ normal □ cyst
  - Stomach: □ normal □ hiatal hernia
  - Small intestine and large intestine: □ normal □ malposition
  - Adrenal glands: □ normal □ cystic mass
  - Kidneys and female reproductive system: □ normal □ nephrectomy
  - Vascular system: □ normal □ extravasation at injection site

28.9.2 Solution

Additional Annotated Images

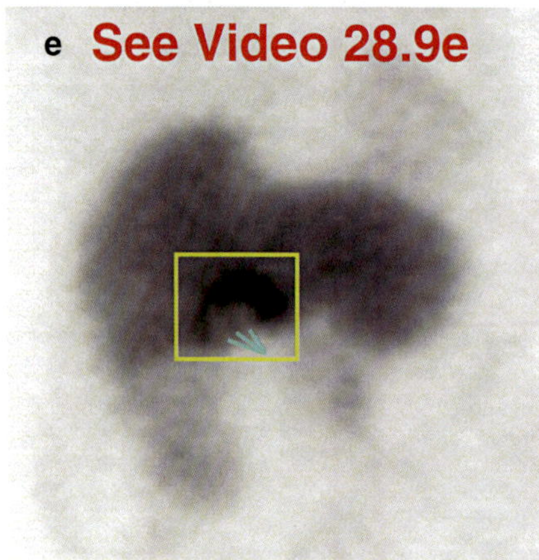

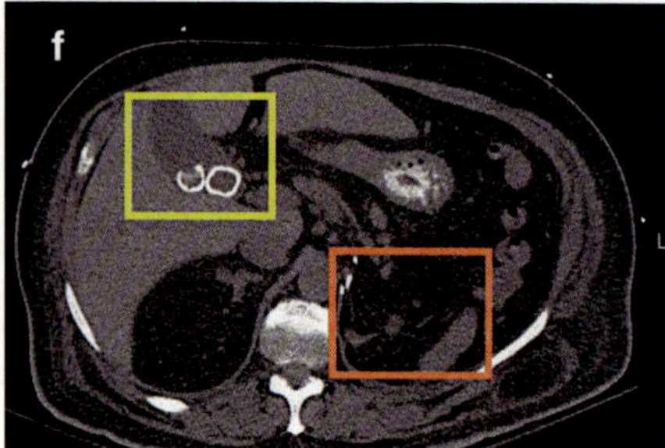

(**e**) Stress raw projection image (Video 28.9e, frame 6) adjusted to view liver and gallbladder, ^{99m}Tc sestamibi, gallbladder (*yellow box*), and gallstone (*blue lines*)

(**f**) CT scan through upper abdomen, gallbladder (*yellow box*), and left renal fossa (*orange box*)

The Pertinent Findings

- Chest
  - Not applicable
- Abdomen
  - Biliary system and gallbladder: □ hot ■ cold
  - Small intestine and large intestine: ■ hot □ cold
  - Kidneys and female reproductive system: □ hot ■ cold

The Relevant Diagnosis(es)

- Chest
  - Not applicable
- Abdomen
  - Biliary system and gallbladder: ■ gallstones
  - Small intestine and large intestine: ■ malposition
  - Kidneys and female reproductive system: ■ nephrectomy

Discussion

Chest

There are no abnormalities.

Abdomen

At rest, the gallbladder just begins to fill with radioactive bile (a), and at stress (c), it fills completely; there is a striking "cold" "filling defect" within its lumen (a, c, e). Correlative CT image (f) demonstrates large calcified gallstones as the cause.

The left kidney is surgically absent; it is not seen on the raw data (b, d). Note surgical clips and small bowel positioned in the posterior left upper quadrant (renal fossa) (f).

Relevant Chapter(s)

20, 23, and 25

28.10   Case Challenge #22

28.10.1   Problem

Clinical Highlights

A 64-year-old male presents with dyspnea and an abnormal ECG (low voltage).

Images for Review

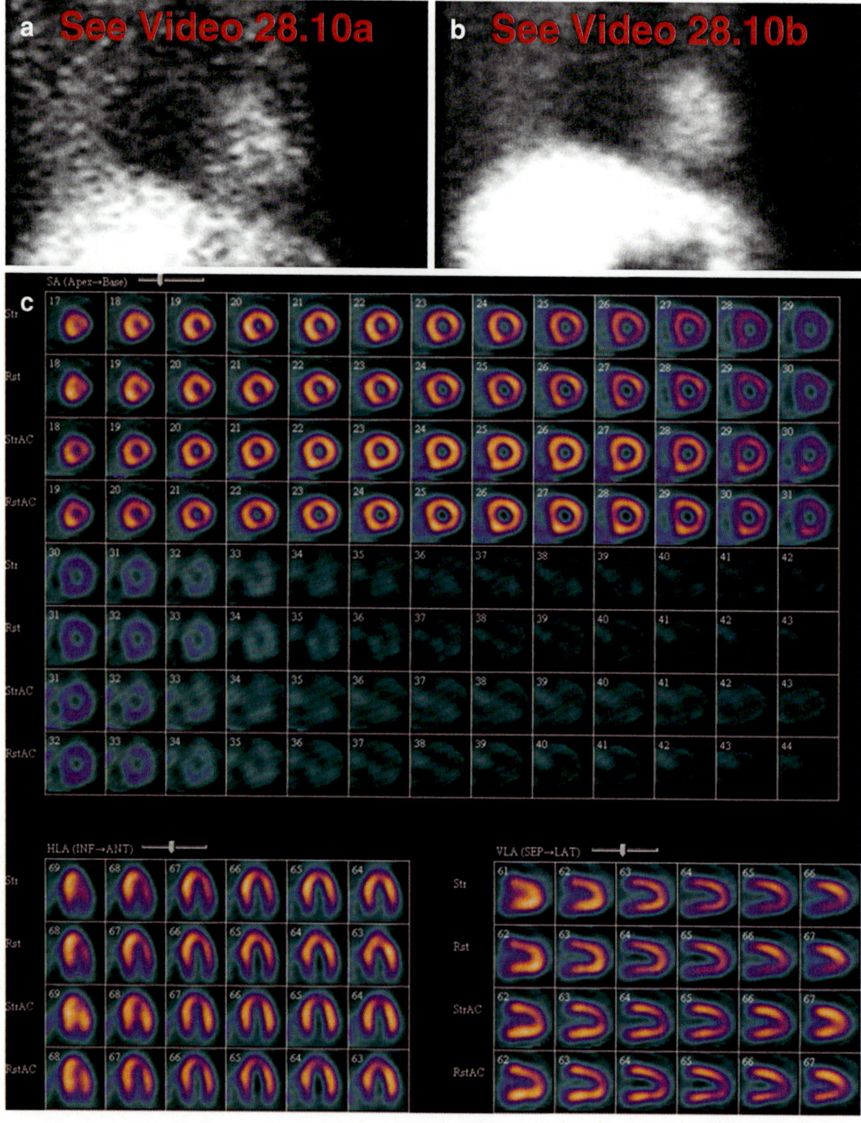

Fig. 28.10

(**a**) Rest "white-on-black" raw projection images contrast adjusted for chest (Video 28.10a, frame 1), ^{99m}Tc sestamibi

(**b**) Stress "white-on-black" raw projection images contrast adjusted for chest (Video 28.10b, frame 1), ^{99m}Tc sestamibi

(**c**) Stress/rest processed SPECT images (SA, HLA, VLA) (without and with AC)

Characterize the Pertinent Finding(s)

- Chest
    - Breasts: ☐ hot ☐ cold
    - Chest wall: ☐ hot ☐ cold
    - Skeleton: ☐ hot ☐ cold
    - Pleura: ☐ hot ☐ cold
    - Lungs: ☐ hot ☐ cold
    - Mediastinum: ☐ hot ☐ cold
    - Myocardium and pericardium: ☐ hot ☐ cold
    - Right atrium and right ventricle: ☐ hot ☐ cold
    - Diaphragm: ☐ hot ☐ cold
- Abdomen
    - Abdominal wall: ☐ hot ☐ cold
    - Peritoneum: ☐ hot ☐ cold
    - Liver: ☐ hot ☐ cold
    - Biliary system and gallbladder: ☐ hot ☐ cold
    - Stomach: ☐ hot ☐ cold
    - Small intestine and large intestine: ☐ hot ☐ cold
    - Adrenal glands: ☐ hot ☐ cold
    - Kidneys and female reproductive system: ☐ hot ☐ cold

State Your Relevant The Relevant Diagnosis(es)

- Chest
    - Breasts: ☐ normal ☐ malignancy
    - Chest wall: ☐ normal ☐ pacemaker
    - Skeleton: ☐ normal ☐ anemia
    - Pleura: ☐ normal ☐ bilateral effusions
    - Lungs: ☐ normal ☐ asymmetry due to transplant
    - Mediastinum: ☐ normal ☐ malignancy
    - Myocardium and pericardium: ☐ normal ☐ effusion
    - Right atrium and right ventricle: ☐ normal ☐ hypertrophy
    - Diaphragm: ☐ normal ☐ flattened
- Abdomen
    - Abdominal wall: ☐ normal ☐ external defibrillator device
    - Peritoneum: ☐ normal ☐ malignant ascites
    - Liver: ☐ normal ☐ pericholecystic rim sign of acute cholecystitis
    - Biliary system and gallbladder: ☐ normal ☐ acute cholecystitis
    - Stomach: ☐ normal ☐ gastroparesis
    - Small intestine and large intestine: ☐ normal ☐ primary neoplasm
    - Adrenal glands: ☐ normal ☐ primary neoplasm
    - Kidneys and female reproductive system: ☐ normal ☐ primary malignant neoplasm (renal cell carcinoma)

28.10.2 Solution

Additional Annotated Images

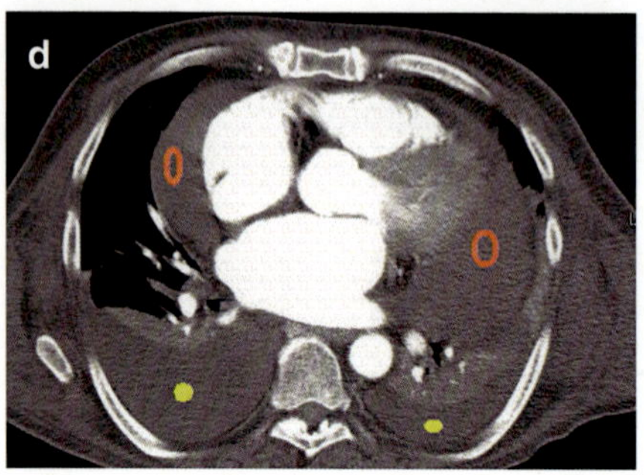

(**d**) Axial CT image of lower chest, pericardial fluid (*open orange ovals*), and pleural effusions (*closed yellow ovals*)

The Pertinent Findings
- Chest
    - Pleura: ☐ hot ■ cold
    - Myocardium and pericardium: ☐ hot ■ cold
- Abdomen
    - Not applicable

The Relevant Diagnosis(es)
- Chest
    - Pleura: ■ bilateral effusions
    - Myocardium and pericardium: ■ effusion
- Abdomen
    - Not applicable

Discussion
Chest

There is a striking large circumferential "cold" region around the heart (a, b). Note the photopenic ("cold") lower lungs, left much more apparent than right (a, b). On the processed non-AC images (c), there is a medium-sized, mildly severe, fixed defect involving the inferior lateral wall; this normalizes on the AC images (best noted on the VLA and HLA orientation) and is likely caused by attenuation artifact from the large pericardial and/or left pleural effusion. The CT scan (d) confirms fluid around the heart and at the lung bases.

Abdomen

There are no abnormalities.

Relevant Chapter(s)
9, and 12

28.11   Case Challenge #23

28.11.1   Problem

Clinical Highlights

A 56-year-old male presents with epigastric pain and suspicion of coronary artery disease.

Images for Review

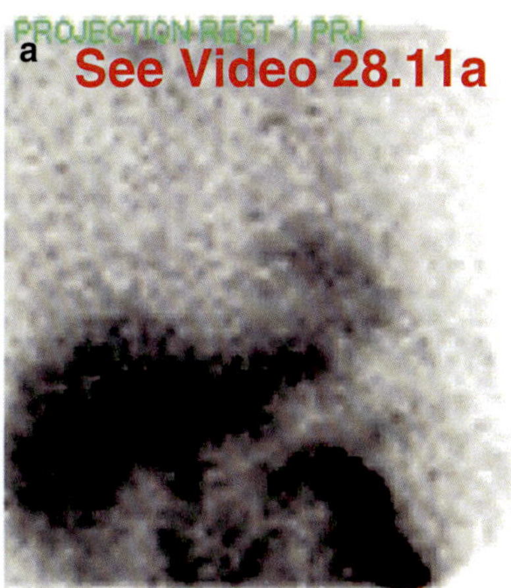

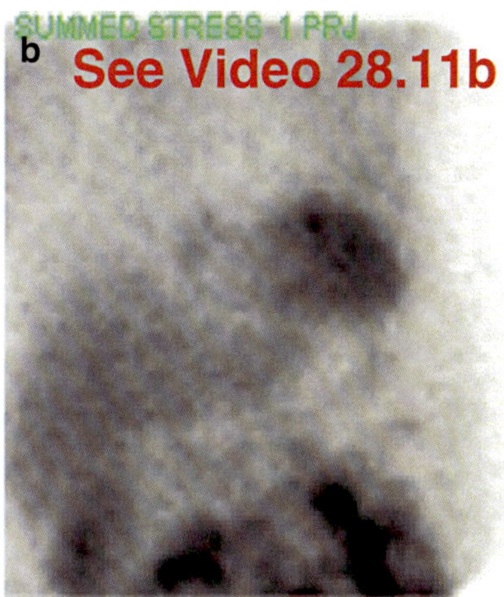

Fig. 28.11

(**a**) Rest raw projection images contrast adjusted for extracardiac structures (Video 28.11a, frame 1), ^{99m}Tc sestamibi

(**b**) Stress raw projection images at usual contrast settings for heart (Video 28.11b, frame 1), ^{99m}Tc sestamibi

Characterize the Pertinent Finding(s)
- Chest
    - Parathyroid glands: ☐ hot ☐ cold
    - Chest wall: ☐ hot ☐ cold
    - Skeleton: ☐ hot ☐ cold
    - Pleura: ☐ hot ☐ cold
    - Lungs: ☐ hot ☐ cold
    - Mediastinum: ☐ hot ☐ cold
    - Right atrium and right ventricle: ☐ hot ☐ cold
    - Vascular system: ☐ hot ☐ cold
    - Diaphragm: ☐ hot ☐ cold

- Abdomen
  - Abdominal wall: □ hot □ cold
  - Peritoneum: □ hot □ cold
  - Liver: □ hot □ cold
  - Biliary system and gallbladder: □ hot □ cold
  - Spleen: □ hot □ cold
  - Stomach: □ hot □ cold
  - Small intestine and large intestine: □ hot □ cold
  - Kidneys and female reproductive system: □ hot □ cold

State Your Relevant Diagnosis(es)

- Chest
  - Parathyroid glands: □ normal □ mediastinal adenoma
  - Chest wall: □ normal □ external artifact
  - Skeleton: □ normal □ metastases
  - Pleura: □ normal □ effusion
  - Lungs: □ normal □ malignancy
  - Mediastinum: □ normal □ esophageal reflux
  - Right atrium and right ventricle: □ normal □ right auricular appendage
  - Vascular system: □ normal □ extravasation
  - Diaphragm: □ normal □ flattening
- Abdomen
  - Abdominal wall: □ normal □ metallic object
  - Peritoneum: □ normal □ ascites
  - Liver: □ normal □ postoperative resection
  - Biliary system and gallbladder: □ normal □ cholecystectomy
  - Spleen: □ normal □ enlargement
  - Stomach: □ normal □ duodenogastric reflux
  - Small intestine and large intestine: □ normal □ stasis (slow peristalsis)
  - Kidneys and female reproductive system: □ normal □ left nephrectomy

28.11.2 Solution

Additional Images

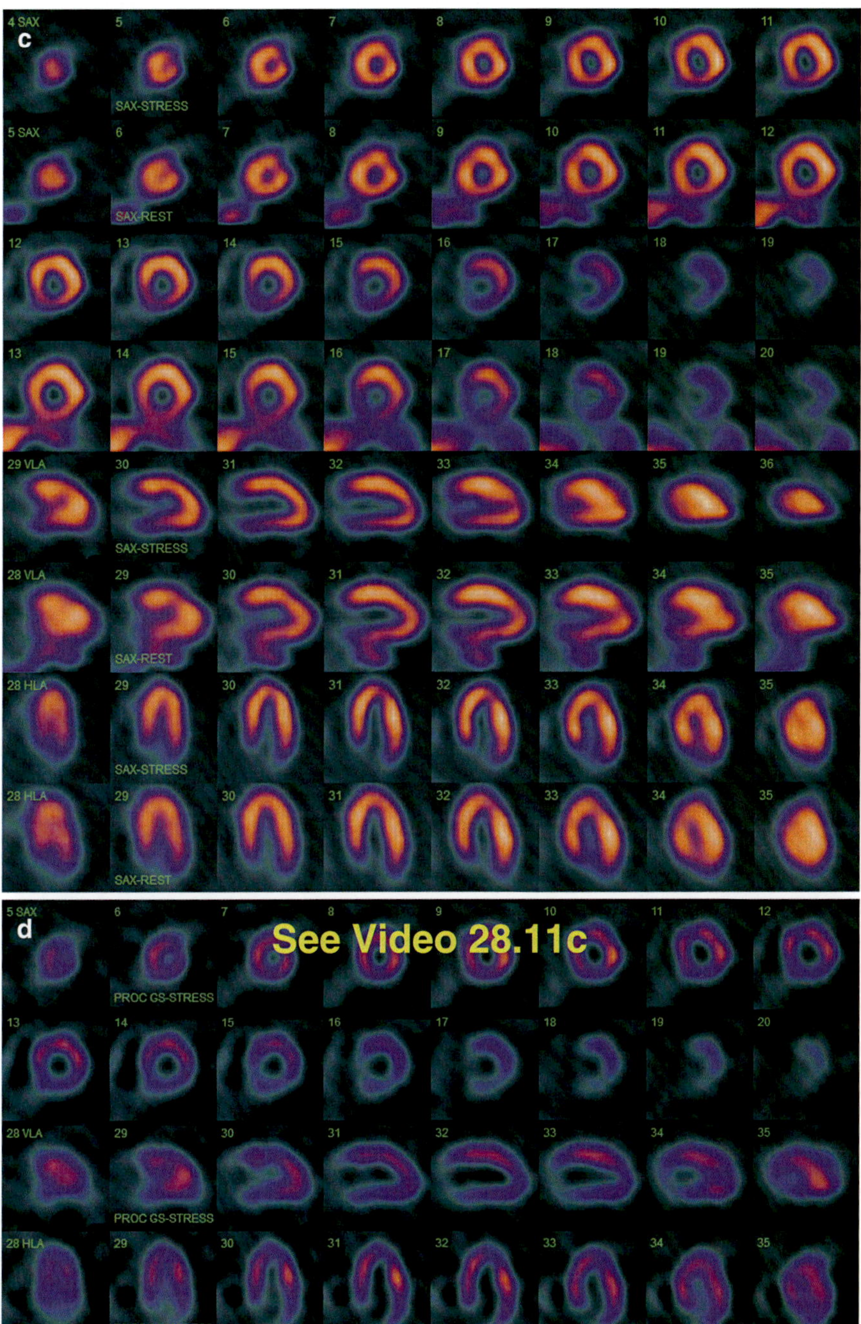

(**c**) Stress/rest processed SPECT images (SA, VLA, HLA)
(**d**) Stress gated SPECT (Video 28.11c, frame 1) (SA, VLA, HLA)

The Pertinent Findings
- Chest
  - Chest wall: ■ hot □ cold
- Abdomen
  - Biliary system and gallbladder: □ hot ■ cold
  - Stomach: ■ hot ■ cold
  - Small intestine and large intestine: ■ hot □ cold

The Relevant Diagnosis(es)
- Chest
  - Chest wall: ■ external artifact
- Abdomen
  - Biliary system and gallbladder: ■ cholecystectomy
  - Stomach: ■ duodenogastric reflux
  - Small intestine and large intestine: ■ normal

Discussion
Chest
On close inspection, one can detect the appearance of diffuse activity external to the patient's right side on frames 46–47 of the rest raw images (a); the explanation for this finding is that another radioactive patient walked past the gamma camera when it was positioned at just the right angle to register photons emanating from the "other human source."

The MPI is normal. An inferobasal wall fixed defect is likely diaphragmatic attenuation artifact in this male (c). Note the hepatic and gastric activity below the heart on the rest images. LVEF is 65 % and there is normal wall motion and wall thickening (d). The right ventricle is normal.

Abdomen
Absence of gallbladder on both rest raw (a) and stress raw (b) images is confirmed by history of cholecystectomy. Duodenogastric reflux is identified on raw rest images (a) and is cleared by water ingestion on stress raw images (b). Note the clue of a distended, "cold" stomach. The small intestine demonstrates physiologic peristalsis (a, b).

Relevant Chapter(s)
7, 20, 22, and 23

28.12 Case Challenge #24

28.12.1 Problem

Clinical Highlights

A 73-year-old man presents with a complicated medical history including dilated cardiomyopathy, coronary artery disease with right coronary artery stenting, congestive heart failure, hypertension, chronic renal failure, diabetes mellitus, and cirrhosis with elevated bilirubin level (1.3 mg/dL).

Images for Review

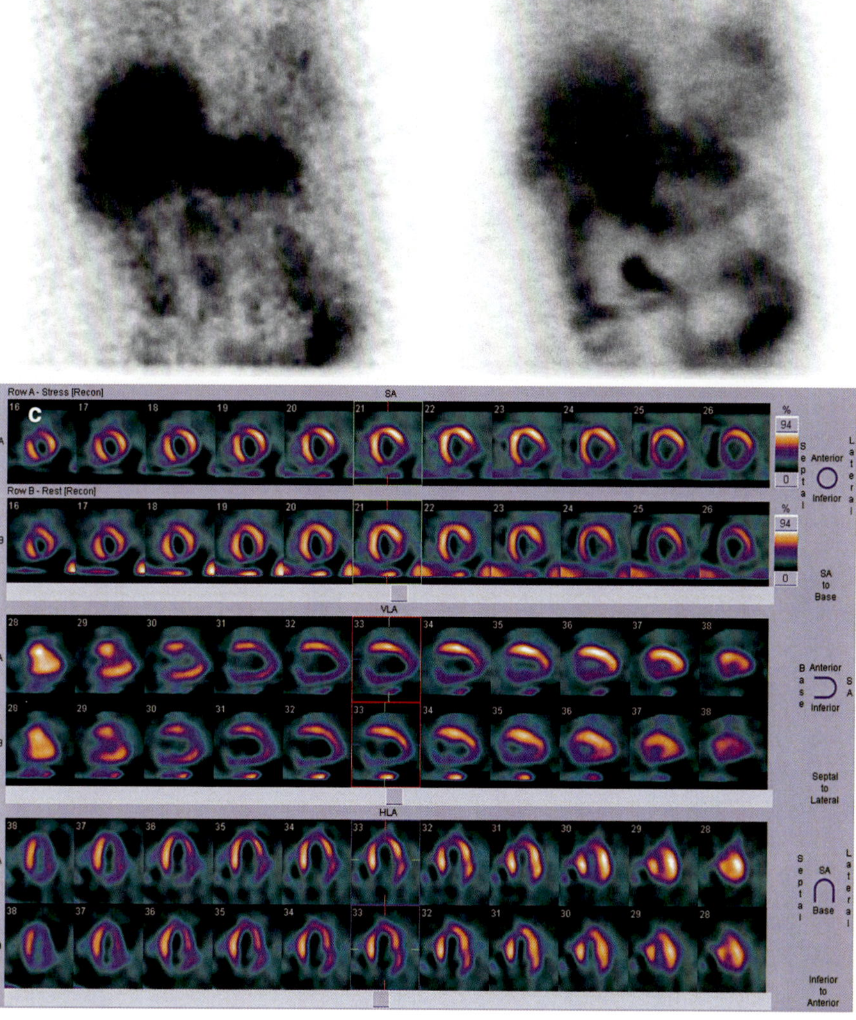

Fig. 28.12

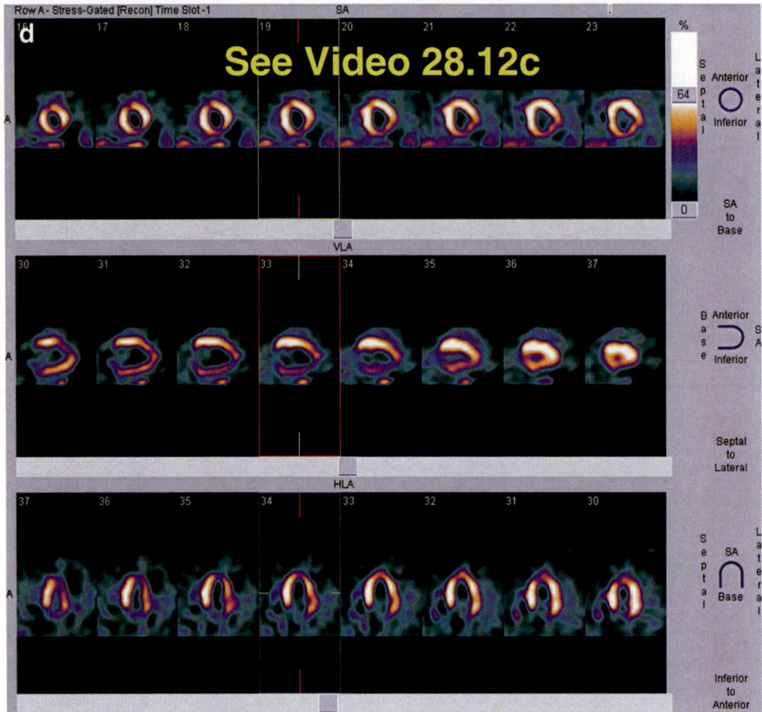

Fig. 28.12 (continued)

(**a**) Rest raw projection images (Video 28.12a, frame 1), ^{99m}Tc sestamibi
(**b**) Stress raw projection images (Video 28.12b, frame 1), ^{99m}Tc sestamibi
(**c**) Stress/rest processed SPECT images (SA, VLA, HLA)
(**d**) Stress gated SPECT images (Video 28.12c, frame 1) (SA, HLA, VLA)

Characterize the Pertinent Finding(s)

- Chest
  - Thyroid gland: ☐ hot ☐ cold
  - Breasts: ☐ hot ☐ cold
  - Chest wall: ☐ hot ☐ cold
  - Lungs: ☐ hot ☐ cold
  - Mediastinum: ☐ hot ☐ cold
  - Right atrium and right ventricle: ☐ hot ☐ cold
  - Vascular system: ☐ hot ☐ cold
  - Lymphatic system: ☐ hot ☐ cold
  - Diaphragm: ☐ hot ☐ cold

- Abdomen
    - Abdominal wall: ☐ hot ☐ cold
    - Peritoneum: ☐ hot ☐ cold
    - Liver: ☐ hot ☐ cold
    - Biliary system and gallbladder: ☐ hot ☐ cold
    - Spleen: ☐ hot ☐ cold
    - Stomach: ☐ hot ☐ cold
    - Small intestine and large intestine: ☐ hot ☐ cold
    - Vascular system: ☐ hot ☐ cold

State Your Relevant Diagnosis(es)

- Chest
    - Thyroid gland: ☐ normal ☐ multinodular goiter
    - Breasts: ☐ normal ☐ prostheses
    - Chest wall: ☐ normal ☐ holter monitor
    - Lungs: ☐ normal ☐ emphysema
    - Mediastinum: ☐ normal ☐ left hilar mass
    - Right atrium and right ventricle: ☐ normal ☐ dilatation
    - Vascular system: ☐ normal ☐ contamination during injection
    - Lymphatic system: ☐ normal ☐ right axillary metastases
    - Diaphragm: ☐ normal ☐ elevated right hemidiaphragm
- Abdomen
    - Abdominal wall: ☐ normal ☐ contamination artifact during injection
    - Peritoneum: ☐ normal ☐ ascites
    - Liver: ☐ normal ☐ slow physiologic clearance
    - Biliary system and gallbladder: ☐ normal ☐ chronic gallbladder disease
    - Spleen: ☐ normal ☐ infarction
    - Stomach: ☐ normal ☐ duodenogastric reflux
    - Small intestine and large intestine: ☐ normal ☐ rapid transit into large intestine
    - Vascular system: ☐ normal ☐ injection site

28.12.2   Solution

Additional Images

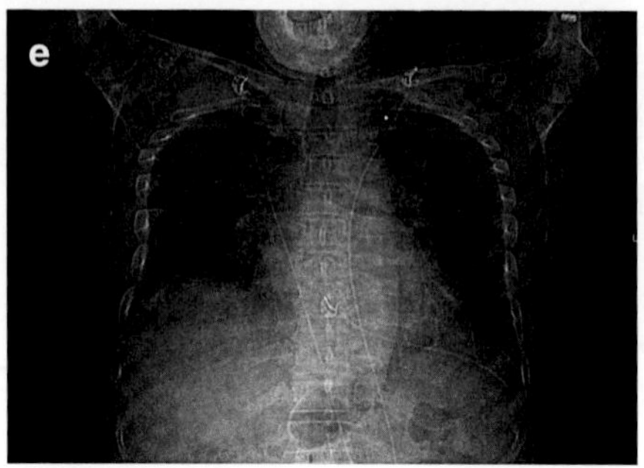

(**e**) Scout CT image of chest

The Pertinent Findings
- Chest
  - Right atrium and right ventricle: □ hot ■ cold
  - Diaphragm: ■ hot □ cold
- Abdomen
  - Liver: ■ hot □ cold
  - Biliary system and gallbladder: ■ hot ■ cold
  - Stomach: ■ hot □ cold
  - Small intestine and large intestine: ■ hot □ cold

The Relevant Diagnosis(es)
- Chest
  - Right atrium and right ventricle: ■ dilatation
  - Diaphragm: ■ elevated right hemidiaphragm
- Abdomen
  - Liver: ■ slow physiologic clearance
  - Biliary system and gallbladder: ■ chronic gallbladder disease
  - Stomach: ■ duodenogastric reflux
  - Small intestine and large intestine: ■ rapid transit into large intestine

Discussion
Chest

First take note of the elevated right hemidiaphragm and cardiomegaly (a, b), confirmed by scout chest CT (e). There is biventricular enlargement with "thinned" myocardial walls; the right atrium is dilated (a, b). The left ventricle demonstrates a medium-sized, moderately severe, fixed distal anterior wall defect and a large, moderately severe, fixed inferior/inferolateral wall defect consistent with scars (c). There is global hypokinesis with marked hypokinesis/akinesis of the anterior and inferior/inferolateral walls; the LVEF is markedly reduced at 20 % (d). The right ventricular function appears reduced as well (d).

Abdomen

The liver activity is prominent on both raw data sets (a, b) and suggests impaired hepatic excretion of the radiopharmaceutical. While the gallbladder is well visualized on the stress raw images (a), it is not seen on the earlier rest raw images (b); this pattern is abnormal and suggests chronic gallbladder disease with resistance in the cystic duct.

On the rest images only, there is clearly a "hot" stomach, indicating duodeno-gastric reflux, and it mostly clears with fluid on the stress raw images ("cold" stomach). The gastric activity, as well as the left hepatic lobe activity, can be seen on the rest SA processed images; it is inferior to and separate from the inferior myocardial wall. On the stress images, the gastrointestinal activity has reached the ascending and transverse portions of the large intestine; anatomically, the transverse colon overlies the region of the stomach, and it can be difficult to distinguish between the two.

Relevant Chapter(s)
13, 16, 19, 20, 22, and 23

Electronic supplementary material The online version of this chapter (doi:10.1007/978-3-319-25436-4_29) contains supplementary material, which is available to authorized users.

© Springer International Publishing Switzerland 2017
M.E. Oates, V.L. Sorrell, *Myocardial Perfusion Imaging - Beyond the Left Ventricle: Pathology, Artifacts and Pitfalls in the Chest and Abdomen,*
DOI 10.1007/978-3-319-25436-4_29

29.1   Case Challenge #25

29.1.1 Problem

Clinical Highlights
A 35-year-old female presents with "yellow eyes."

Images for Review

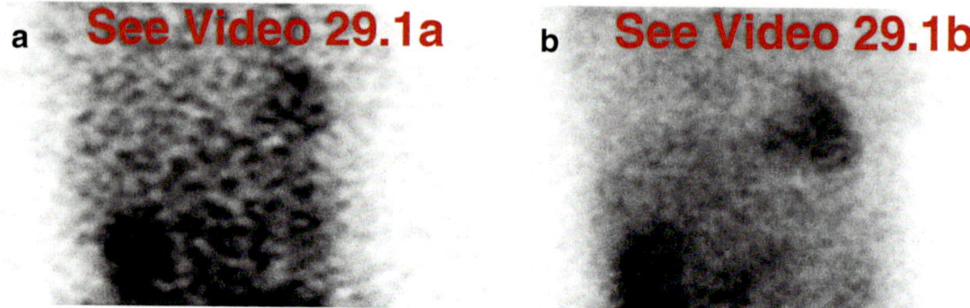

Fig. 29.1

(**a**) Rest raw projection images (Video 29.1a, frame 1), ^{99m}Tc sestamibi
(**b**) Stress raw projection images (Video 29.1b, frame 1), ^{99m}Tc sestamibi

Characterize the Pertinent Finding(s)
- Chest
    - Thyroid gland: □ hot □ cold
    - Parathyroid glands: □ hot □ cold
    - Breasts: □ hot □ cold
    - Chest wall: □ hot □ cold
    - Skeleton: □ hot □ cold
    - Pleura: □ hot □ cold
    - Lungs: □ hot □ cold
    - Mediastinum: □ hot □ cold
    - Myocardium and pericardium: □ hot □ cold
    - Right atrium and right ventricle: □ hot □ cold
    - Vascular system: □ hot □ cold
    - Lymphatic system: □ hot □ cold
    - Diaphragm: □ hot □ cold

- Abdomen
  - Abdominal wall: □ hot □ cold
  - Peritoneum: □ hot □ cold
  - Liver: □ hot □ cold
  - Biliary system and gallbladder: □ hot □ cold
  - Spleen: □ hot □ cold
  - Stomach: □ hot □ cold
  - Small intestine and large intestine: □ hot □ cold
  - Adrenal glands: □ hot □ cold
  - Kidneys and female reproductive system: □ hot □ cold
  - Vascular system: □ hot □ cold

State Your Relevant Diagnosis(es)

- Chest
  - Thyroid gland: □ normal □ diffuse toxic goiter
  - Parathyroid glands: □ normal □ adenoma, substernal location
  - Breasts: □ normal □ lactation
  - Chest wall: □ normal □ cross talk from another radioactive source
  - Skeleton: □ normal □ Gaucher disease
  - Pleura: □ normal □ neoplasm, metastatic
  - Lungs: □ normal □ postoperative change
  - Mediastinum: □ normal □ thymoma
  - Myocardium and pericardium: □ normal □ pericardial mass
  - Right atrium and right ventricle: □ normal □ prominent right auricular appendage
  - Vascular system: □ normal □ retention in central port
  - Lymphatic system: □ normal □ lymphoma
  - Diaphragm: □ normal □ eventration, left hemidiaphragm
- Abdomen
  - Abdominal wall: □ normal □ urinary contamination
  - Peritoneum: □ normal □ malignant metastatic implants
  - Liver: □ normal □ cirrhosis
  - Biliary system and gallbladder: □ normal □ cholecystectomy
  - Spleen: □ normal □ splenomegaly
  - Stomach: □ normal □ gastropathy with fluid distension
  - Small intestine and large intestine: □ normal □ diminished bile flow
  - Adrenal glands: □ normal □ hemorrhagic mass
  - Kidneys and female reproductive system: □ normal □ hyperfunctioning state (hepatic failure)
  - Vascular system: □ normal □ abdominal aortic aneurysm

29.1.2 Solution

Additional Annotated Images
None.

The Pertinent Findings
- Chest
  - Not applicable
- Abdomen
  - Liver: ☐ hot ■ cold
  - Biliary system and gallbladder: ☐ hot ■ cold
  - Spleen: ■ hot ☐ cold
  - Stomach: ■ hot ■ cold
  - Small intestine and large intestine: ☐ hot ■ cold
  - Kidneys and female reproductive system: ■ hot ☐ cold

The Relevant Diagnosis(es)
- Chest
  - Not applicable
- Abdomen
  - Liver: ■ cirrhosis
  - Biliary system and gallbladder: ■ cholecystectomy
  - Spleen: ■ splenomegaly
  - Stomach: ■ gastropathy with fluid distension
  - Small intestine and large intestine: ■ diminished bile flow
  - Kidneys and female reproductive system: ■ hyperfunctioning state

Discussion
Chest
There are no significant findings.

Abdomen
The liver and the small intestine are poorly visualized, suggesting severe liver dysfunction and reduced biliary clearance of the radiopharmaceutical (a, b). The patient has known autoimmune hepatitis, awaiting transplant. The gallbladder is surgically absent; however, in patients with such impaired bile flow, differential diagnosis of gallbladder non-visualization would include underlying liver dysfunction and not necessarily acute or chronic cholecystitis. The stomach appears collapsed on rest raw images (a) but appears distended and "cold" on stress raw images (b) after water ingestion. This pattern is characteristic of cirrhosis-related gastropathy. There is markedly greater visualization of the kidneys, the alternate route of biological clearance of the radiopharmaceutical (a, b); renal clearance compensates for liver dysfunction.

Relevant Chapter(s)
Chapters 19, 20, 21, 22, 23, and 25

29.2   Case Challenge #26

29.2.1 Problem

Clinical Highlights

A 66-year-old female provides a history of diabetes mellitus, coronary artery disease, and previous "heart attack."

Images for Review

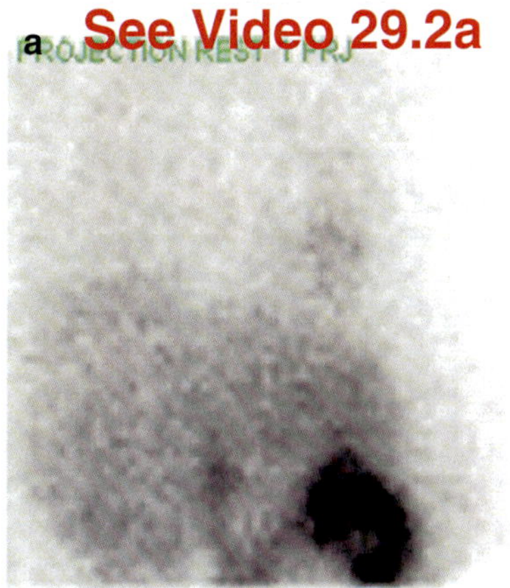

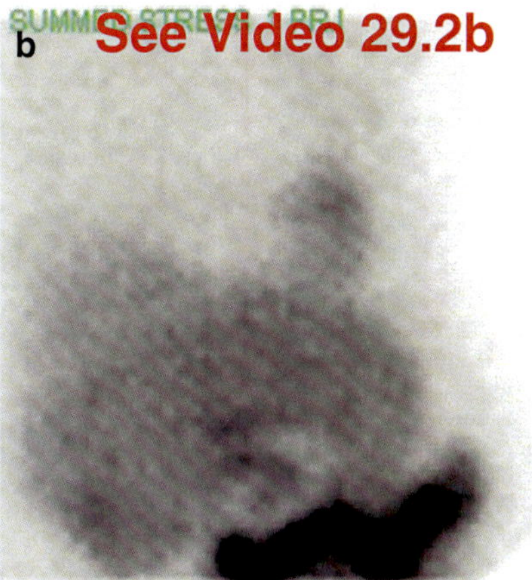

Fig. 29.2

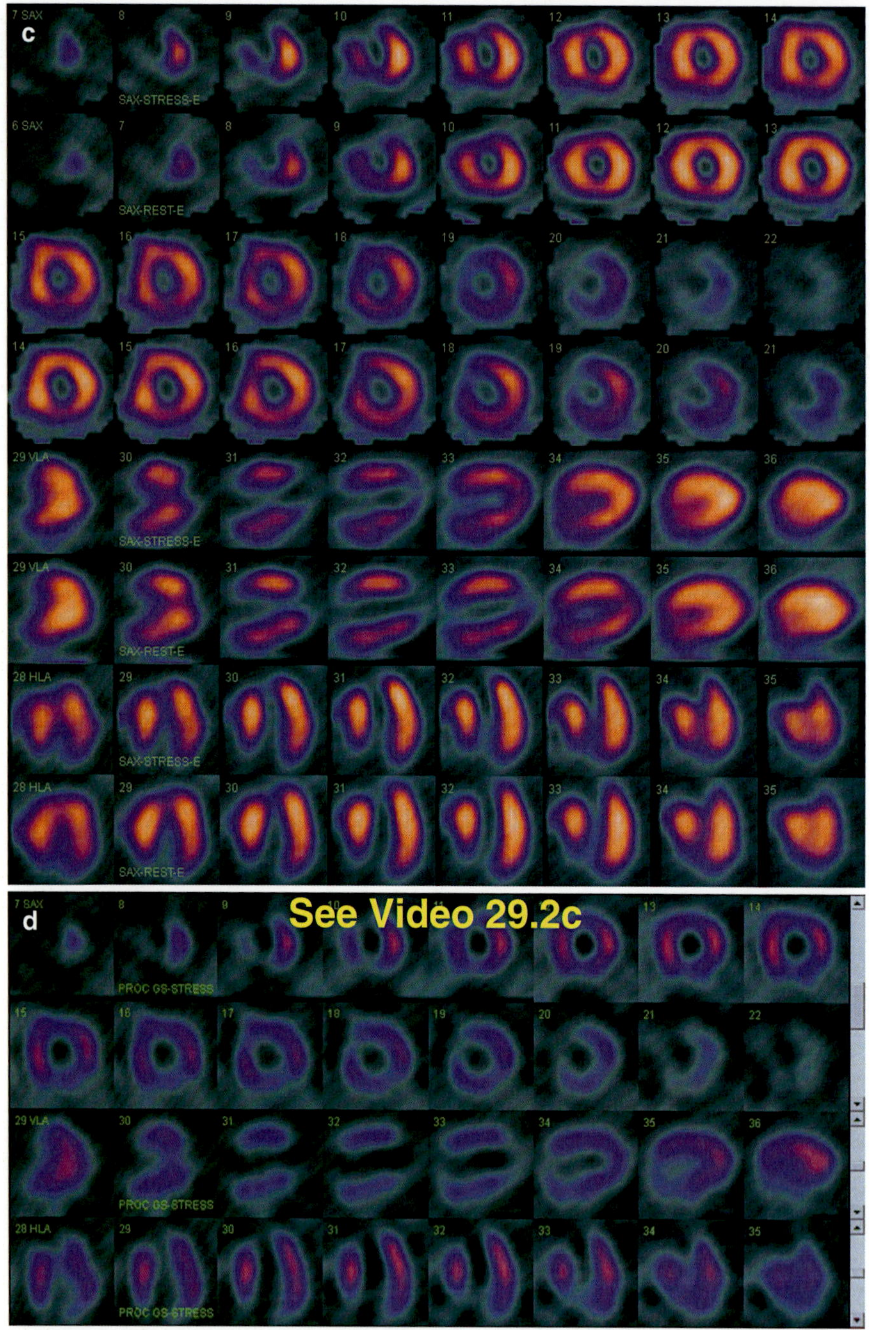

Fig. 29.2 (continued)

(**a**) Rest raw projection images (Video 29.2a, frame 1), ^{99m}Tc sestamibi
(**b**) Stress raw projection images (Video 29.2b, frame 1), ^{99m}Tc sestamibi
(**c**) Stress/rest processed SPECT images (SA, VLA, HLA)
(**d**) Stress gated SPECT images (Video 29.2c, frame 1) (SA, VLA, HLA)

Characterize the Pertinent Finding(s)

- Chest
    - Thyroid gland: □ hot □ cold
    - Parathyroid glands: □ hot □ cold
    - Breasts: □ hot □ cold
    - Chest wall: □ hot □ cold
    - Skeleton: □ hot □ cold
    - Pleura: □ hot □ cold
    - Lungs: □ hot □ cold
    - Mediastinum: □ hot □ cold
    - Myocardium and pericardium: □ hot □ cold
    - Right atrium and right ventricle: □ hot □ cold
    - Vascular system: □ hot □ cold
    - Lymphatic system: □ hot □ cold
    - Diaphragm: □ hot □ cold
- Abdomen
    - Abdominal wall: □ hot □ cold
    - Peritoneum: □ hot □ cold
    - Liver: □ hot □ cold
    - Biliary system and gallbladder: □ hot □ cold
    - Spleen: □ hot □ cold
    - Stomach: □ hot □ cold
    - Small intestine and large intestine: □ hot □ cold
    - Adrenal glands: □ hot □ cold
    - Kidneys and female reproductive system: □ hot □ cold
    - Vascular system: □ hot □ cold

State Your Relevant Diagnosis(es)

- Chest
    - Thyroid gland: □ normal □ lymphoma
    - Parathyroid glands: □ normal □ ectopic hyperplasia
    - Breasts: □ normal □ soft-tissue attenuation artifact
    - Chest wall: □ normal □ Holter monitor
    - Skeleton: □ normal □ multiple metastases
    - Pleura: □ normal □ mesothelioma
    - Lungs: □ normal □ posttransplant asymmetry
    - Mediastinum: □ normal □ lymphoma
    - Myocardium and pericardium: □ normal □ "hot" mass
    - Right atrium and right ventricle: □ normal □ dilatation
    - Vascular system: □ normal □ chest port injection site
    - Lymphatic system: □ normal □ necrotic axillary lymph nodes, malignant
    - Diaphragm: □ normal □ muscular (soft-tissue attenuation)

- Abdomen
    - Abdominal wall: ☐ normal ☐ overlying patient's arms and hands
    - Peritoneum: ☐ normal ☐ ascites
    - Liver: ☐ normal ☐ hepatitis
    - Biliary system and gallbladder: ☐ normal ☐ cholecystectomy
    - Spleen: ☐ normal ☐ infarct
    - Stomach: ☐ normal ☐ duodenogastric reflux and fluid
    - Small intestine and large intestine: ☐ normal ☐ visualization of large intestine
    - Adrenal glands: ☐ normal ☐ cystic neoplasm
    - Kidneys and female reproductive system: ☐ normal ☐ left nephrectomy
    - Vascular system: ☐ normal ☐ extravasation

29.2.2 Solution

Additional Annotated Images

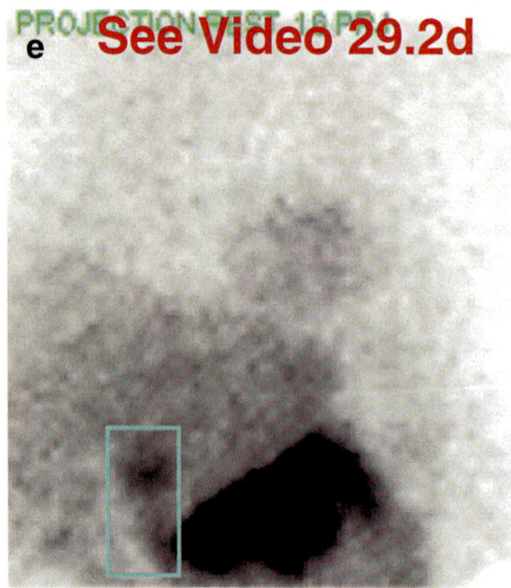

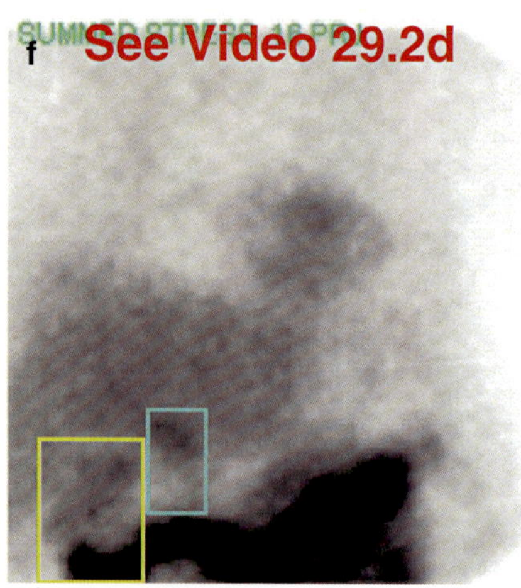

(**e**) Rest raw projection image (Video 29.2d, frame 16), ^{99m}Tc sestamibi, duodenum (*blue box*)

(**f**) Stress raw projection image (Video 29.2e, frame 16), ^{99m}Tc sestamibi, hepatic flexure of large intestine (*yellow box*), duodenum (*blue box*)

The Pertinent Findings

- Chest
  - Breasts: ☐ hot ■ cold
- Abdomen
  - Biliary system and gallbladder: ☐ hot ■ cold
  - Stomach: ■ hot ■ cold
  - Small intestine and large intestine: ■ hot ☐ cold

The Relevant Diagnosis(es)

- Chest
  - Breasts: ■ soft-tissue attenuation artifact
- Abdomen
  - Biliary system and gallbladder: ■ cholecystectomy
  - Stomach: ■ duodenogastric reflux and fluid
  - Small intestine and large intestine: ■ visualization of large intestine

Discussion

Chest

The breast tissue creates an attenuation artifact on the heart (a, b, c, d). On processed images (c), there is a medium-size, severe, fixed anteroseptal-apical perfusion defect that represents myocardial scar (her "heart attack"?); there is no ischemia. There is anteroseptal-apical akinesis, but preserved global function with LVEF greater than 60 % (d). Thus, despite the potential for breast attenuation artifact, this perfusion defect is "real" and correlates with "true" coronary artery disease.

Abdomen

The gallbladder is absent (a, b). The rest raw images (a, e) demonstrate duodenal ("C-loop") activity that could be mistaken for the gallbladder. The first portion of the duodenum is posterior and gravity dependent in the supine position used for imaging. The gallbladder is usually anteriorly situated, whereas the duodenum is posteriorly situated, and should appear focally intense and constant during the acquisition. On later same-day stress raw (b, f) images, large intestinal activity is seen in the right upper quadrant. As is the case for the early duodenal activity, activity in the hepatic flexure of the large intestine could be misconstrued as gallbladder.

On stress raw images (b), the stomach appears "cold" due to water ingestion, but there is no artifactual attenuation effect on the processed images (c).

Relevant Chapter(s)

Chapters 6, 20, 22, and 23

29.3   Case Challenge #27

29.3.1 Problem

Clinical Highlights

A 62-year-old male presents with chronic disease.

Images for Review

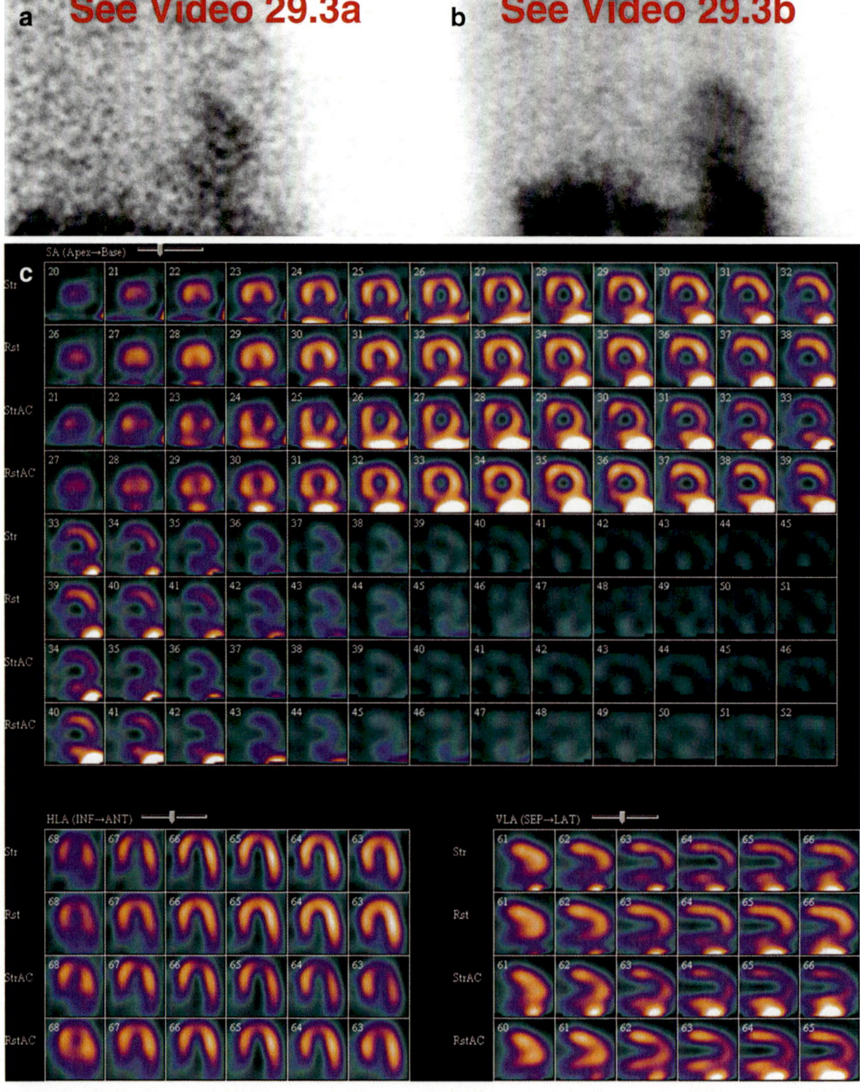

Fig. 29.3

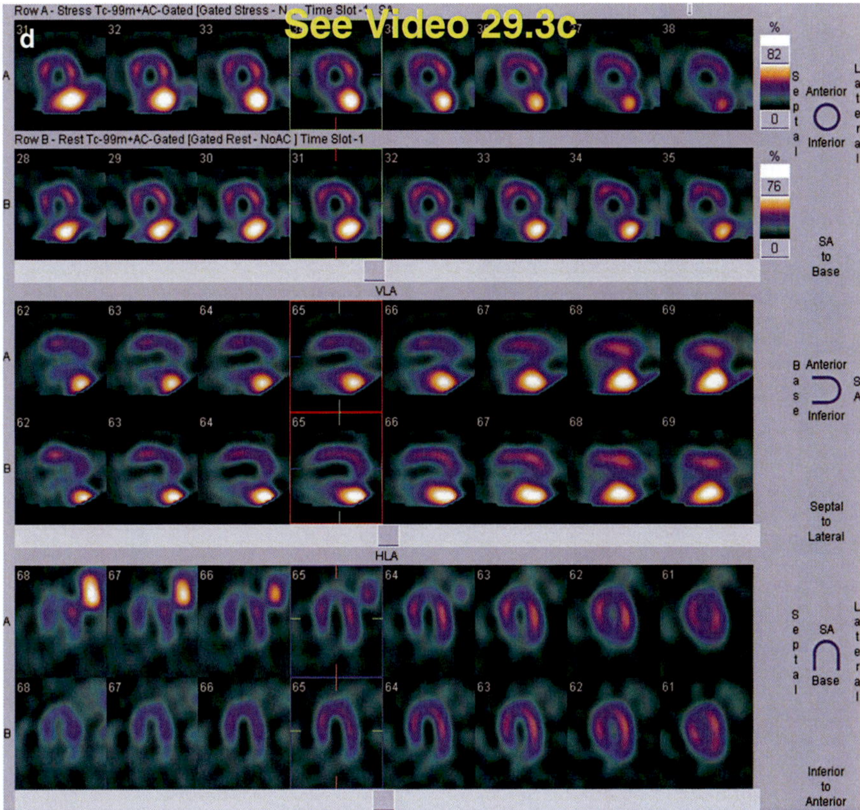

Fig. 29.3   (continued)

(**a**) Rest raw projection images (Video 29.3a, frame 1), ^{99m}Tc sestamibi
(**b**) Stress raw projection images (Video 29.3b, frame 1), ^{99m}Tc sestamibi
(**c**) Stress/rest processed SPECT images (SA, HLA, VLA) (without and with AC)
(**d**) Stress and rest gated SPECT images (Video 29.3c, frame 1) (SA, VLA, HLA)

Characterize the Pertinent Finding(s)

- Chest
    - Thyroid gland: ☐ hot ☐ cold
    - Parathyroid glands: ☐ hot ☐ cold
    - Breasts: ☐ hot ☐ cold
    - Chest wall: ☐ hot ☐ cold
    - Skeleton: ☐ hot ☐ cold
    - Pleura: ☐ hot ☐ cold
    - Lungs: ☐ hot ☐ cold
    - Mediastinum: ☐ hot ☐ cold
    - Myocardium and pericardium: ☐ hot ☐ cold
    - Right atrium and right ventricle: ☐ hot ☐ cold
    - Vascular system: ☐ hot ☐ cold
    - Lymphatic system: ☐ hot ☐ cold
    - Diaphragm: ☐ hot ☐ cold

- Abdomen
  - Abdominal wall: ☐ hot ☐ cold
  - Peritoneum: ☐ hot ☐ cold
  - Liver: ☐ hot ☐ cold
  - Biliary system and gallbladder: ☐ hot ☐ cold
  - Spleen: ☐ hot ☐ cold
  - Stomach: ☐ hot ☐ cold
  - Small intestine and large intestine: ☐ hot ☐ cold
  - Adrenal glands: ☐ hot ☐ cold
  - Kidneys and female reproductive system: ☐ hot ☐ cold
  - Vascular system: ☐ hot ☐ cold

State Your Relevant Diagnosis(es)

- Chest
  - Thyroid gland: ☐ normal ☐ multinodular goiter
  - Parathyroid glands: ☐ normal ☐ multiple adenomas
  - Breasts: ☐ normal ☐ gynecomastia
  - Chest wall: ☐ normal ☐ jewelry
  - Skeleton: ☐ normal ☐ myelofibrosis
  - Pleura: ☐ normal ☐ bilateral effusions
  - Lungs: ☐ normal ☐ hyperinflation
  - Mediastinum: ☐ normal ☐ esophageal malignancy
  - Myocardium and pericardium: ☐ normal ☐ effusion
  - Right atrium and right ventricle: ☐ normal ☐ enlargement
  - Vascular system: ☐ normal ☐ extravasation around chest port during injection
  - Lymphatic system: ☐ normal ☐ metastatic neoplasm
  - Diaphragm: ☐ normal ☐ hiccups
- Abdomen
  - Abdominal wall: ☐ normal ☐ umbilical hernia
  - Peritoneum: ☐ normal ☐ ascites
  - Liver: ☐ normal ☐ cirrhosis
  - Biliary system and gallbladder: ☐ normal ☐ calculous cholecystitis, chronic
  - Spleen: ☐ normal ☐ splenomegaly
  - Stomach: ☐ normal ☐ gastropathy
  - Small intestine and large intestine: ☐ normal ☐ visualization of large intestine
  - Adrenal glands: ☐ normal ☐ metastasis
  - Kidneys and female reproductive system: ☐ normal ☐ atrophic left kidney
  - Vascular system: ☐ normal ☐ chest port for injection

29.3.2 Solution

Additional Annotated Images

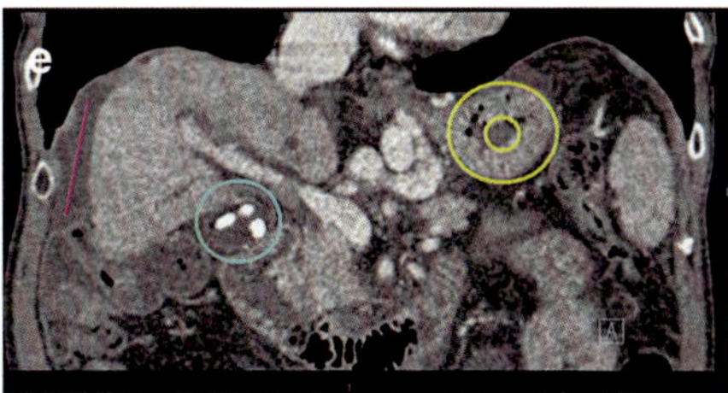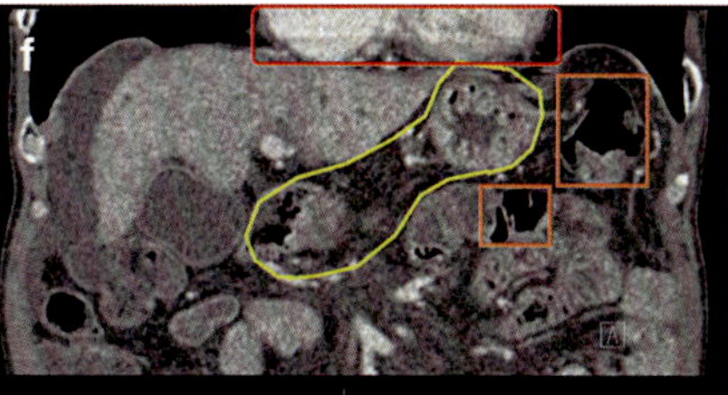

(**e**) Coronal CT most anterior through the liver, gallbladder with gallstones (*blue circle*), and stomach (*yellow circles*, outer wall and inner lumen), perihepatic ascites (*pink line*)

(**f**) Coronal CT most posterior through the stomach (*yellow outline*) and splenic flexure (*orange boxes*), heart for reference (*red box*)

The Pertinent Findings
- Chest
  - Not applicable
- Abdomen
  - Peritoneum: ☐ hot ■ cold
  - Liver: ☐ hot ■ cold
  - Biliary system and gallbladder: ☐ hot ■ cold
  - Stomach: ■ hot ☐ cold
  - Small intestine and large intestine: ■ hot ☐ cold

The Relevant Diagnosis(es)
- Chest
  - Not applicable
- Abdomen
  - Peritoneum: ■ ascites
  - Liver: ■ cirrhosis
  - Biliary system and gallbladder: ■ calculous cholecystitis, chronic
  - Stomach: ■ gastropathy
  - Small intestine and large intestine: ■ visualization of large intestine

Discussion

Chest

There are no abnormal findings.

Abdomen

There is ascites and poor visualization of the liver (a, b, e), consistent with cirrhosis. There might be visualization of the gallbladder on stress raw images (b), but it is difficult to separate from the "hot" large intestine. On the rest raw images (a), the gallbladder is out of the field-of-view and cannot be evaluated. There are multiple large calcified gallstones (e).

Marked gastric activity appears on the rest raw images (a). On the stress raw images (b), the gastric activity is even more marked; this likely represents gastropathy. There is also marked activity in the large intestine (splenic flexure) that overlaps the stomach on the raw images (a, b); their anatomic relationships are correlated on CT images (f). The gastric activity and large intestinal activity are problematic because they create a significant processing artifact affecting the adjacent inferior myocardial wall where there is a fixed perfusion defect (c). This is almost certainly an artifactual defect because the gated SPECT images demonstrate normal wall motion and thickening (d).

Relevant Chapter(s)

Chapters 18, 19, 20, 22, and 23

29.4   Case Challenge #28

29.4.1 Problem

Clinical Highlights

A 56-year-female presents with three-vessel coronary calcifications on chest CT and a long history of hypertension.

Images for Review

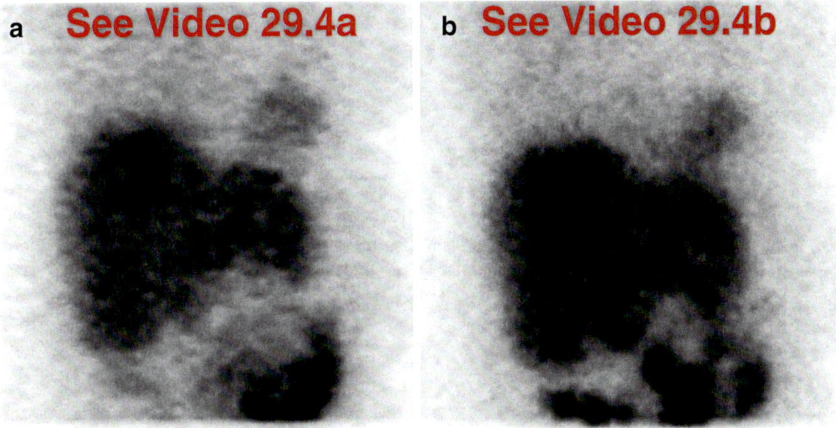

Fig. 29.4

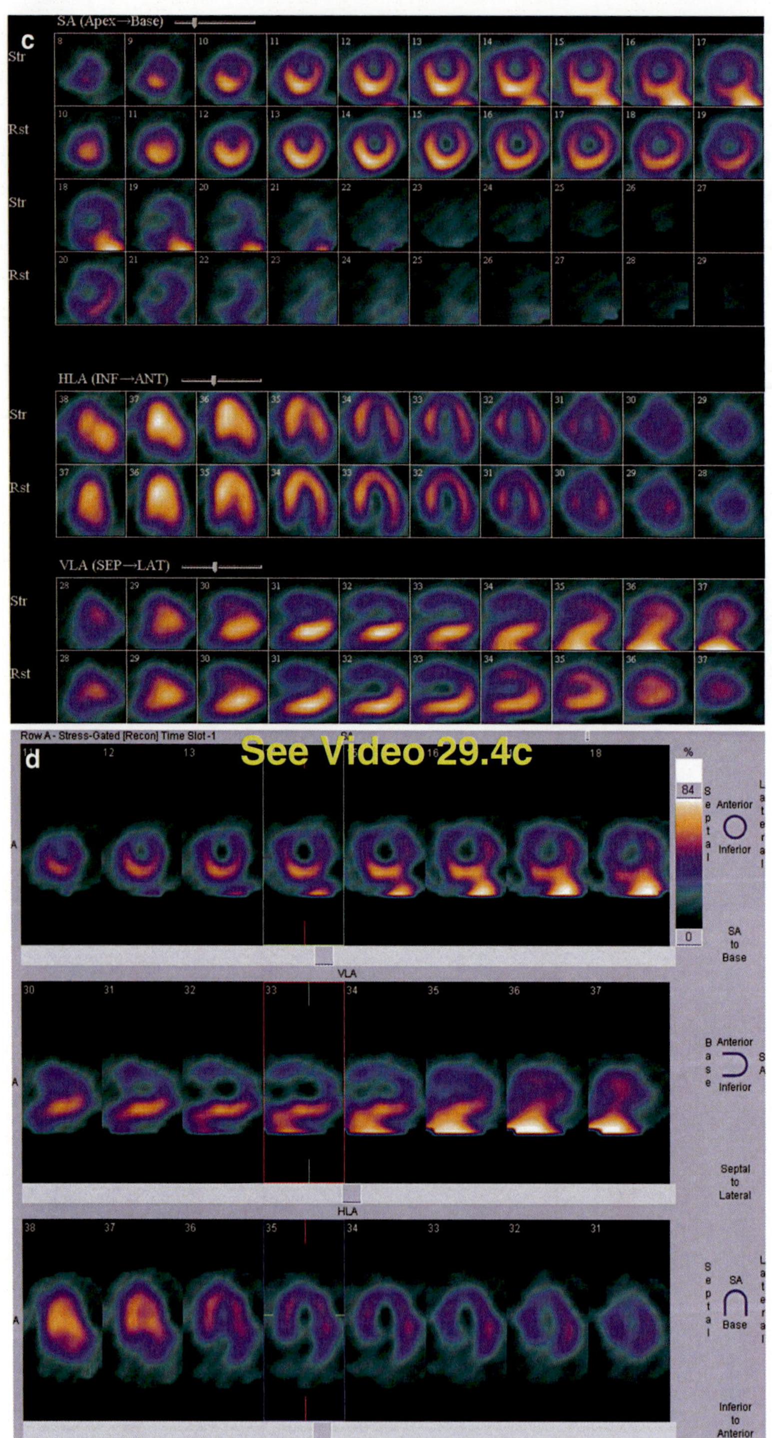

Fig. 29.4 (continued)

(**a**) Rest raw projection images (Video 29.4a, frame 1), ^{99m}Tc sestamibi
(**b**) Stress raw projection images (Video 29.4b, frame 1), ^{99m}Tc sestamibi
(**c**) Stress/rest processed SPECT images (SA, HLA, VLA)
(**d**) Stress gated SPECT images (Video 29.4c, frame 1) (SA, VLA, HLA)

Characterize the Pertinent Finding(s)

- Chest
    - Thyroid gland: □ hot □ cold
    - Parathyroid glands: □ hot □ cold
    - Breasts: □ hot □ cold
    - Chest wall: □ hot □ cold
    - Skeleton: □ hot □ cold
    - Pleura: □ hot □ cold
    - Lungs: □ hot □ cold
    - Mediastinum: □ hot □ cold
    - Myocardium and pericardium: □ hot □ cold
    - Right atrium and right ventricle: □ hot □ cold
    - Vascular system: □ hot □ cold
    - Lymphatic system: □ hot □ cold
    - Diaphragm: □ hot □ cold
- Abdomen
    - Abdominal wall: □ hot □ cold
    - Peritoneum: □ hot □ cold
    - Liver: □ hot □ cold
    - Biliary system and gallbladder: □ hot □ cold
    - Spleen: □ hot □ cold
    - Stomach: □ hot □ cold
    - Small intestine and large intestine: □ hot □ cold
    - Adrenal glands: □ hot □ cold
    - Kidneys and female reproductive system: □ hot □ cold
    - Vascular system: □ hot □ cold

State Your Relevant Diagnosis(es)

- Chest
    - Thyroid gland: □ normal □ free ^{99m}Tc pertechnetate
    - Parathyroid glands: □ normal □ ectopic adenoma
    - Breasts: □ normal □ soft-tissue attenuation artifact
    - Chest wall: □ normal □ photomultiplier tube malfunction
    - Skeleton: □ normal □ anemia
    - Pleura: □ normal □ effusion
    - Lungs: □ normal □ congestive heart failure
    - Mediastinum: □ normal □ solid mass
    - Myocardium and pericardium: □ normal □ effusion
    - Right atrium and right ventricle: □ normal □ hypertrophy
    - Vascular system: □ normal □ extravasation
    - Lymphatic system: □ normal □ lymphoma, multifocal
    - Diaphragm: □ normal □ flattening

- Abdomen
  - Abdominal wall: ☐ normal ☐ metallic object
  - Peritoneum: ☐ normal ☐ ascites
  - Liver: ☐ normal ☐ postoperative effect
  - Biliary system and gallbladder: ☐ normal ☐ cholecystectomy
  - Spleen: ☐ normal ☐ enlargement
  - Stomach: ☐ normal ☐ duodenogastric reflux
  - Small intestine and large intestine: ☐ normal ☐ duodenal stasis
  - Adrenal glands: ☐ normal ☐ neoplasm
  - Kidneys and female reproductive system: ☐ normal ☐ large left renal cyst
  - Vascular system: ☐ normal ☐ extravasation

29.4.2 Solution

Additional Images

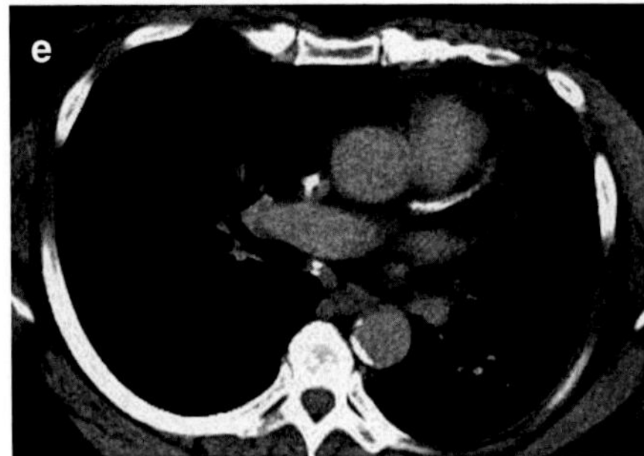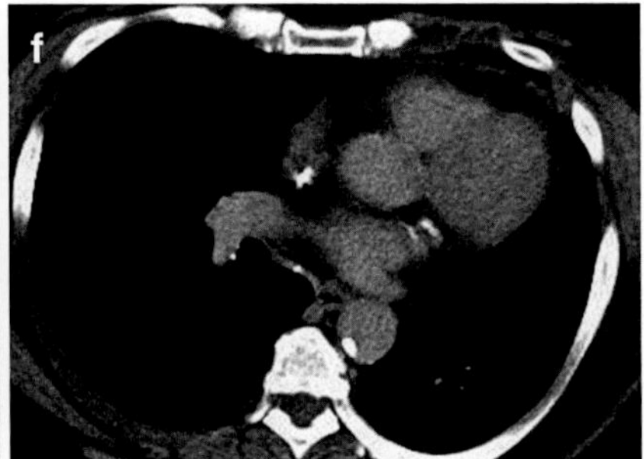

(**e**) Axial image from chest CT at level of LAD coronary artery
(**f**) Axial image from chest CT at level of left circumflex coronary artery

The Pertinent Findings

- Chest
  - Breasts: ☐ hot ■ cold
- Abdomen
  - Biliary system and gallbladder: ☐ hot ■ cold
  - Stomach: ■ hot ☐ cold
  - Small intestine and large intestine: ■ hot ☐ cold

The Relevant Diagnosis(es)

- Chest
  - Breasts: ■ soft-tissue attenuation artifact
- Abdomen
  - Biliary system and gallbladder: ■ cholecystectomy
  - Stomach: ■ duodenogastric reflux
  - Small intestine and large intestine: ■ duodenal stasis

Discussion
Chest
Breast attenuation artifact is evident on review of the raw data (a, b). Take note of how the curvilinear edge of the breast overlies most of the heart but spares the inferior wall. This observation permits one to predict (correctly) that there will be an attenuation effect on the anterior wall and that the inferior wall will not be subject to that same effect, thus creating relative differences in the processed perfusion pattern. As predicted, there is a characteristic large, moderately severe, fixed anterior myocardial wall perfusion defect (c). Normal wall thickening and wall motion (d, especially on the VLA images) favor attenuation artifact rather than myocardial scar.

Normal myocardial perfusion in the setting of extensive coronary artery and vascular calcifications, as seen on routine chest CT (e, f), is an important and relatively common clinical situation that confirms that there is coronary atherosclerosis in the absence of significant stenosis.

Abdomen
There is non-visualization of the gallbladder (a, b) (history of cholecystectomy). Prominent duodenal activity (note: posterior location) and marked gastric activity due to duodenogastric reflux are more apparent on stress raw images (b) compared to rest raw images (a). The gastric activity creates a "bleeding in" artifact involving the adjacent inferolateral myocardial wall on the stress processed images (c). There is normal function on gated SPECT images (d).

Relevant Chapter(s)
Chapters 6, 20, 22, and 23

29.5   Case Challenge #29

29.5.1 Problem

Clinical Highlights
A 66-year-old male has a recent abdominal surgical history.

Images for Review

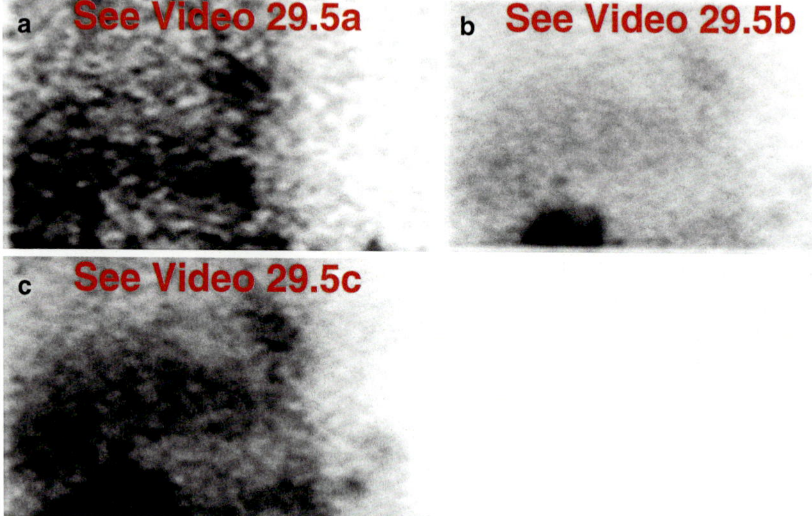

Fig. 29.5

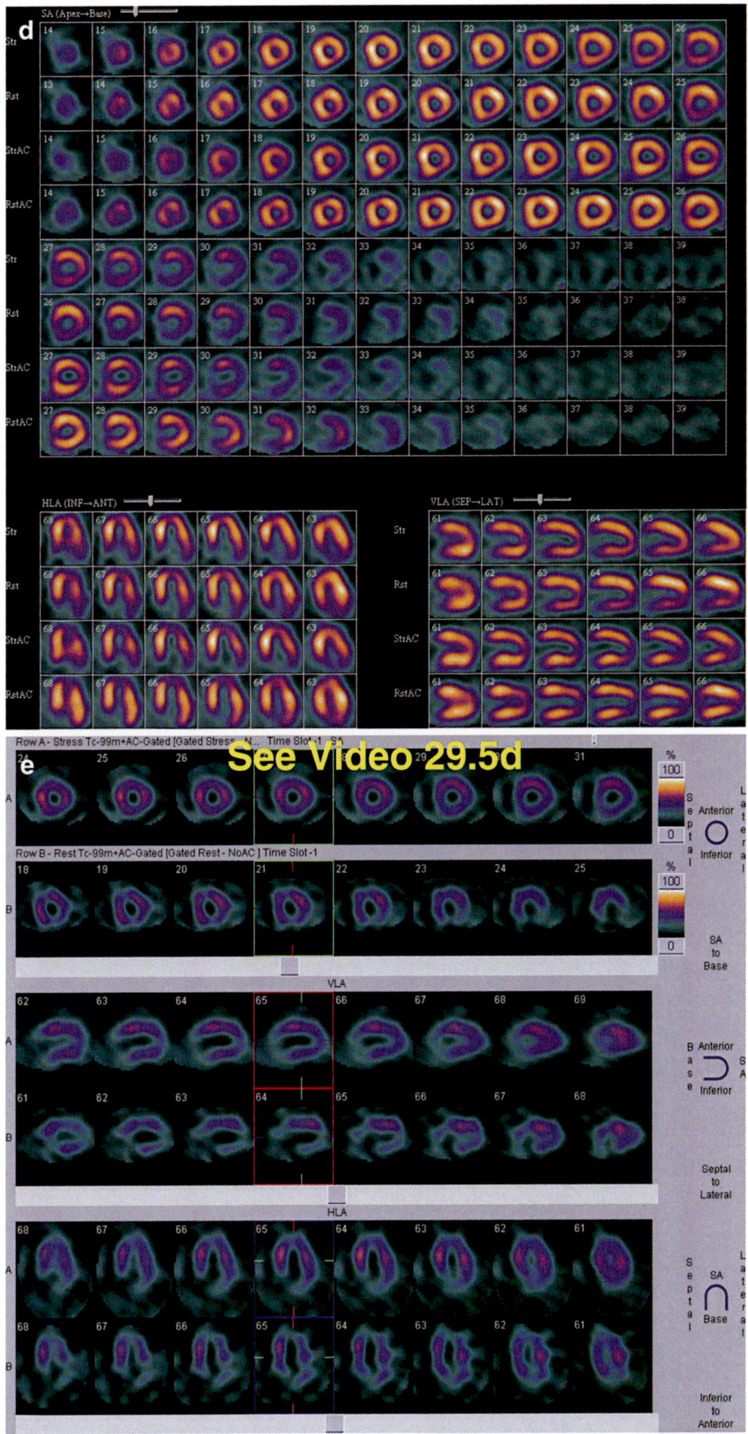

Fig. 29.5 (continued)

(a) Rest raw projection images (Video 29.5a, frame 1), ^{99m}Tc sestamibi
(b) Stress raw projection images contrast adjusted for the heart (Video 29.5b, frame 1), ^{99m}Tc sestamibi
(c) Stress raw projection images contrast adjusted for extracardiac structures (Video 29.5c, frame 1), ^{99m}Tc sestamibi
(d) Stress/rest processed SPECT images (SA, HLA, VLA) (without and with AC)
(e) Stress and rest gated SPECT images (Video 29.5d, frame 1) (SA, VLA, HLA)

Characterize the Pertinent Finding(s)

- Chest
    - Thyroid gland: ☐ hot ☐ cold
    - Parathyroid glands: ☐ hot ☐ cold
    - Breasts: ☐ hot ☐ cold
    - Chest wall: ☐ hot ☐ cold
    - Skeleton: ☐ hot ☐ cold
    - Pleura: ☐ hot ☐ cold
    - Lungs: ☐ hot ☐ cold
    - Mediastinum: ☐ hot ☐ cold
    - Myocardium and pericardium: ☐ hot ☐ cold
    - Right atrium and right ventricle: ☐ hot ☐ cold
    - Vascular system: ☐ hot ☐ cold
    - Lymphatic system: ☐ hot ☐ cold
    - Diaphragm: ☐ hot ☐ cold
- Abdomen
    - Abdominal wall: ☐ hot ☐ cold
    - Peritoneum: ☐ hot ☐ cold
    - Liver: ☐ hot ☐ cold
    - Biliary system and gallbladder: ☐ hot ☐ cold
    - Spleen: ☐ hot ☐ cold
    - Stomach: ☐ hot ☐ cold
    - Small intestine and large intestine: ☐ hot ☐ cold
    - Adrenal glands: ☐ hot ☐ cold
    - Kidneys and female reproductive system: ☐ hot ☐ cold
    - Vascular system: ☐ hot ☐ cold

State Your Relevant Diagnosis(es)

- Chest
  - Thyroid gland: ☐ normal ☐ substernal goiter
  - Parathyroid glands: ☐ normal ☐ carcinoma
  - Breasts: ☐ normal ☐ gynecomastia
  - Chest wall: ☐ normal ☐ metallic object
  - Skeleton: ☐ normal ☐ sternal fracture
  - Pleura: ☐ normal ☐ effusion
  - Lungs: ☐ normal ☐ lobectomy
  - Mediastinum: ☐ normal ☐ hiatal hernia
  - Myocardium and pericardium: ☐ normal ☐ effusion
  - Right atrium and right ventricle: ☐ normal ☐ hypertrophy and pulmonary hypertension
  - Vascular system: ☐ normal ☐ extravasation
  - Lymphatic system: ☐ normal ☐ axillary nodes related to extravasation
  - Diaphragm: ☐ normal ☐ talking and laughing throughout acquisition
- Abdomen
  - Abdominal wall: ☐ normal ☐ metallic object
  - Peritoneum: ☐ normal ☐ ascites
  - Liver: ☐ normal ☐ non-alcoholic steatohepatitis (NASH)
  - Biliary system and gallbladder: ☐ normal ☐ cholecystostomy
  - Spleen: ☐ normal ☐ splenomegaly
  - Stomach: ☐ normal ☐ gastropathy and duodenogastric reflux
  - Small intestine and large intestine: ☐ normal ☐ prominent duodenum
  - Adrenal glands: ☐ normal ☐ bilateral malignant masses
  - Kidneys and female reproductive system: ☐ normal ☐ polycystic disease
  - Vascular system: ☐ normal ☐ extravasation

29.5.2 Solution

Additional Annotated Images

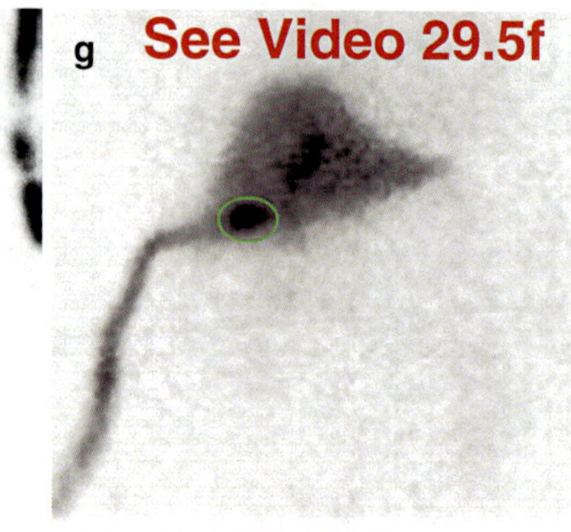

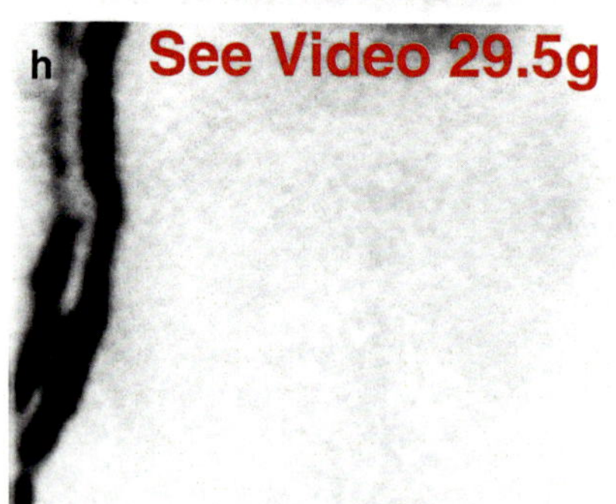

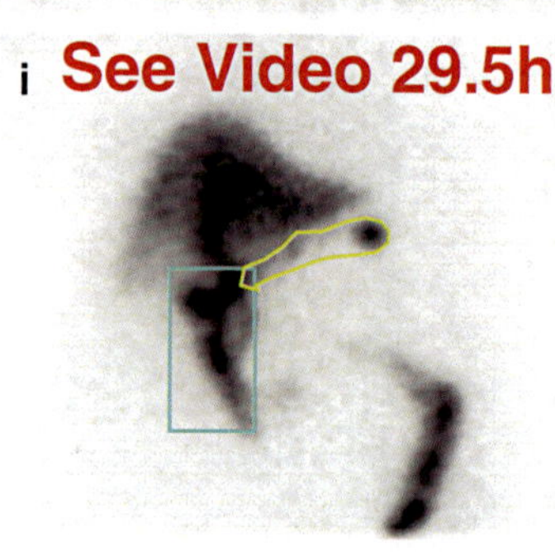

(**f**) Follow up hepatobiliary images (Video 29.5e, frame 1), ^{99m}Tc iminodiacetic acid (IDA)

(**g**) Follow up hepatobiliary image (Video 29.5f, frame 55), ^{99m}Tc iminodiacetic acid (IDA), gallbladder (*green oval*)

(**h**) Original hepatobiliary images (Video 29.5g, frame 1), ^{99m}Tc iminodiacetic acid (IDA)

(**i**) Original hepatobiliary image (Video 29.5h, frame 48), ^{99m}Tc iminodiacetic acid (IDA), duodenum (*blue box*), stomach (*yellow outline*)

The Pertinent Findings
- Chest
    - Breasts: ■ hot □ cold
    - Chest wall: □ hot ■ cold
- Abdomen
    - Abdominal wall: □ hot ■ cold
    - Liver: □ hot ■ cold
    - Biliary system and gallbladder: ■ hot ■ cold
    - Spleen: ■ hot □ cold
    - Stomach: ■ hot ■ cold
    - Small intestine and large intestine: ■ hot □ cold

The Relevant Diagnosis(es)

- Chest
  - Breasts: ■ gynecomastia
  - Chest wall: ■ metallic object
- Abdomen
  - Abdominal wall: ■ metallic object
  - Liver: ■ non-alcoholic steatohepatitis (NASH)
  - Biliary system and gallbladder: ■ cholecystostomy
  - Spleen: ■ splenomegaly
  - Stomach: ■ gastropathy and duodenogastric reflux
  - Small intestine and large intestine: ■ prominent duodenum

Discussion

Chest

There is gynecomastia (a, b, c) with large breast tissue and slight periareolar uptake. Incidental note is made of a subtle "cold" metallic object overlying the lower chest/upper abdominal wall in the midline and projecting over the left hepatic lobe (a, b, c). The heart is normal (d, e).

Abdomen

The liver is small, consistent with known history of non-alcoholic steatohepatitis (NASH). There is non-visualization of the externally decompressed gallbladder (a, b, c). However, external tubing containing radioactive bile courses across the superficial upper abdomen (a, b, c). Its presence is affirmed by correlative hepatobiliary scintigraphy (f) showing bile drainage into external cholecystostomy tubing (g). Interestingly, on the original hepatobiliary scan (h), the gallbladder failed to visualize due to cystic duct obstruction and acute cholecystitis; note how this scan demonstrates the normal duodenal location (i) that can be used for anatomic reference when interpreting MPI in order to avoid the interpretative pitfall.

On rest images, there is duodenogastric reflux and/or gastropathy (a), while the stomach appears "cold" at stress, likely related to fluid ingestion. Interestingly, duodenogastric reflux is demonstrated on hepatobiliary scan (i), which again can be used for reference. Splenomegaly is quite apparent (a, b, c); it can be appreciated on the hepatobiliary scan during the early blood pool phase (f, h). No ascites was present on same-day ultrasonography.

Relevant Chapter(s)

Chapters 6, 7, 17, 19, 20, 21, 22, and 23

29.6   Case Challenge #30

29.6.1 Problem

Clinical Highlights

A 60-year-old male has very weak arms. He has hypertension and hyperlipidemia but no known coronary artery disease.

Images for Review

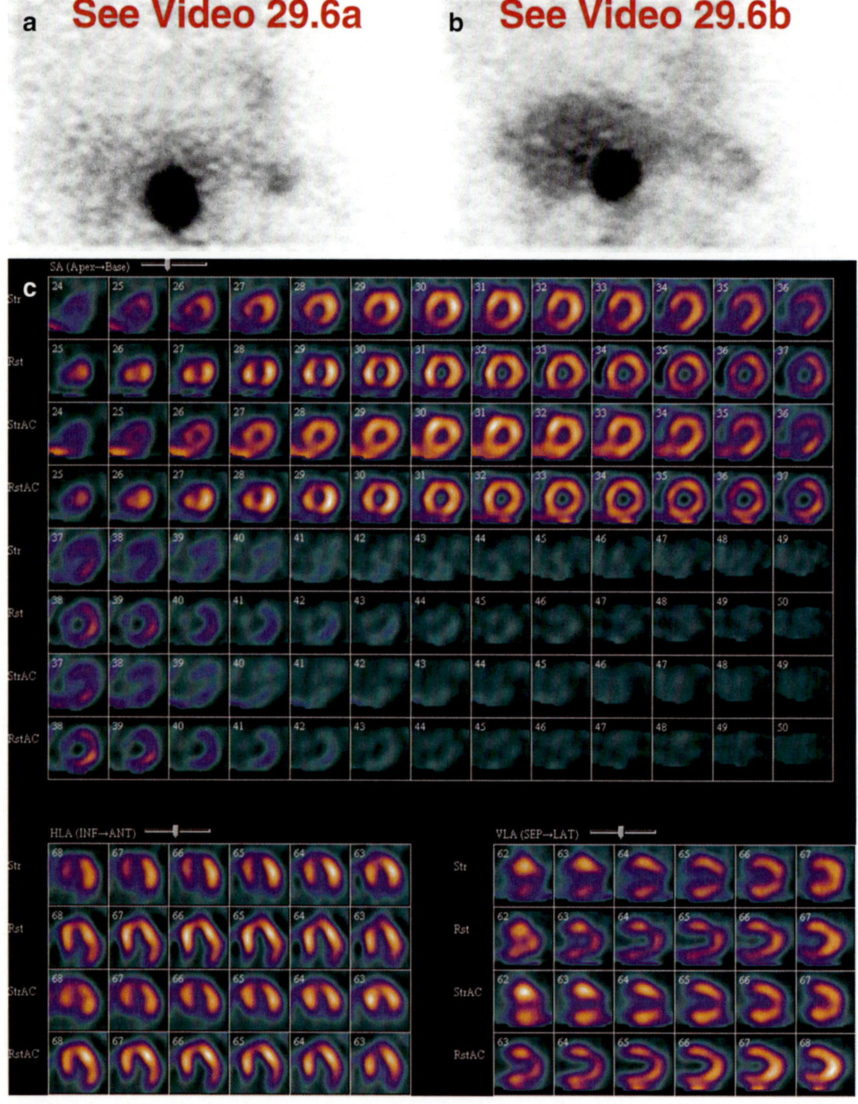

Fig. 29.6

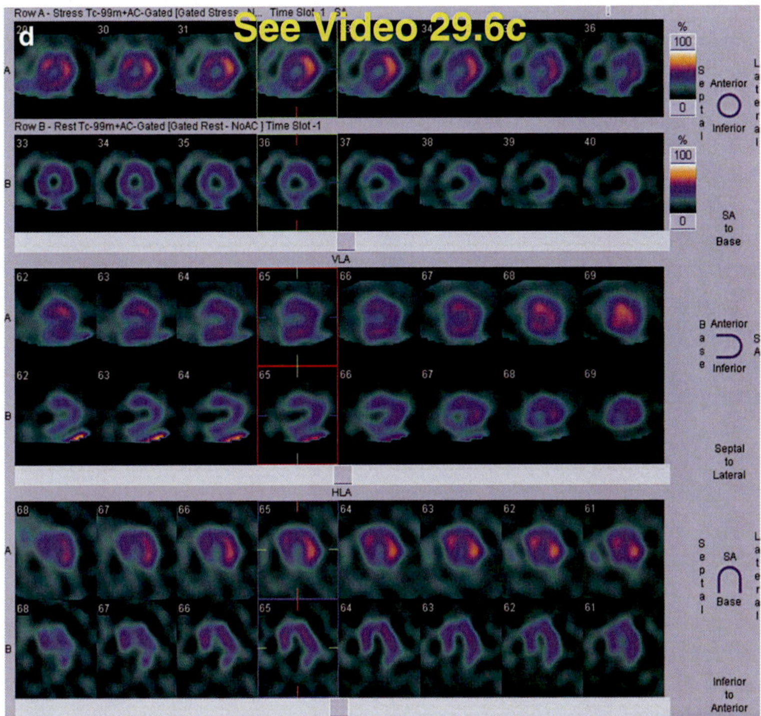

Fig. 29.5   (continued)

(**a**) Rest raw projection images (Video 29.6a, frame 1), ^{99m}Tc sestamibi

(**b**) Stress raw projection images (Video 29.6b, frame 1), ^{99m}Tc sestamibi

(**c**) Stress/rest SPECT images (SA, HLA, VLA) (without and with AC)

(**d**) Stress and rest gated SPECT images (Video 29.6c, frame 1) (SA, VLA, HLA)

Characterize the Pertinent Finding(s)

- Chest
    - Thyroid gland: ☐ hot ☐ cold
    - Parathyroid glands: ☐ hot ☐ cold
    - Breasts: ☐ hot ☐ cold
    - Chest wall: ☐ hot ☐ cold
    - Skeleton: ☐ hot ☐ cold
    - Pleura: ☐ hot ☐ cold
    - Lungs: ☐ hot ☐ cold
    - Mediastinum: ☐ hot ☐ cold
    - Myocardium and pericardium: ☐ hot ☐ cold
    - Right atrium and right ventricle: ☐ hot ☐ cold
    - Vascular system: ☐ hot ☐ cold
    - Lymphatic system: ☐ hot ☐ cold
    - Diaphragm: ☐ hot ☐ cold

- Abdomen
    - Abdominal wall: ☐ hot ☐ cold
    - Peritoneum: ☐ hot ☐ cold
    - Liver: ☐ hot ☐ cold
    - Biliary system and gallbladder: ☐ hot ☐ cold
    - Spleen: ☐ hot ☐ cold
    - Stomach: ☐ hot ☐ cold
    - Small intestine and large intestine: ☐ hot ☐ cold
    - Adrenal glands: ☐ hot ☐ cold
    - Kidneys and female reproductive system: ☐ hot ☐ cold
    - Vascular system: ☐ hot ☐ cold

State Your Relevant Diagnosis(es)

- Chest
    - Thyroid gland: ☐ normal ☐ multinodular goiter
    - Parathyroid glands: ☐ normal ☐ adenoma
    - Breasts: ☐ normal ☐ hematoma
    - Chest wall: ☐ normal ☐ injection site artifact
    - Skeleton: ☐ normal ☐ anemia
    - Pleura: ☐ normal ☐ effusion
    - Lungs: ☐ normal ☐ malignancy
    - Mediastinum: ☐ normal ☐ malignancy
    - Myocardium and pericardium: ☐ normal ☐ effusion
    - Right atrium and right ventricle: ☐ normal ☐ hypertrophy
    - Vascular system: ☐ normal ☐ injection site
    - Lymphatic system: ☐ normal ☐ axillary lymph nodes
    - Diaphragm: ☐ normal ☐ eventration, right hemidiaphragm
- Abdomen
    - Abdominal wall: ☐ normal ☐ metallic object
    - Peritoneum: ☐ normal ☐ ascites
    - Liver: ☐ normal ☐ hydatid cyst
    - Biliary system and gallbladder: ☐ normal ☐ obstructed common bile duct
    - Spleen: ☐ normal ☐ splenectomy
    - Stomach: ☐ normal ☐ duodenogastric reflux
    - Small intestine and large intestine: ☐ normal ☐ visualization of large intestine
    - Adrenal glands: ☐ normal ☐ cystic enlargement
    - Kidneys and female reproductive system: ☐ normal ☐ left nephrectomy
    - Vascular system: ☐ normal ☐ extravasation, left arm

29.6.2 Solution

Additional Annotated Images
None

The Pertinent Findings
- Chest
  - Chest wall: ■ hot □ cold
  - Vascular system: ■ hot □ cold
- Abdomen
  - Stomach: ■ hot ■ cold

The Relevant Diagnosis(es)
- Chest
  - Chest wall: ■ injection site artifact
  - Vascular system: ■ injection site
- Abdomen
  - Stomach: ■ duodenogastric reflux

Discussion
Chest

There is intense, ill-defined, and variable activity across the top of the field-of-view during the stress acquisition (b); this is not seen on the rest acquisition (a). The patient was too weak to keep his arms above his head, and the technologist held them in place throughout the acquisition (a, b). The activity is related to extravasation at the injection site which periodically slipped into the field-of-view as his arms moved (b). There was no significant detrimental effect from this "hot" artifact on the processed images (c, d).

However, motion affected the quality of the examination and the confidence in the interpretation. Both sets of images are compromised by motion artifact (a, b, c, d). There is minimal motion on the rest data (a) but marked motion on the stress data (b). Both original and motion-corrected stress data sets were reviewed with the rest images; there was no significant change in the appearance of the apparent small, severe, reversible apical defect. During a follow-up examination one year later, the patient was able to cooperate, and the examination was normal.

Abdomen

There is a "beating gallbladder" due to motion on the stress images (b). There is a "hot" stomach at rest (a) and a "cold" stomach at stress (b), consistent with variable duodenogastric reflux.

Relevant Chapter(s)
Chapters 7, 14, and 22

29.7 Case Challenge #31

29.7.1 Problem

Clinical Highlights

A 44-year-old male with NASH cirrhosis presents for routine preoperative risk stratification. Unable to exercise, he underwent regadenoson stress.

Images for Review

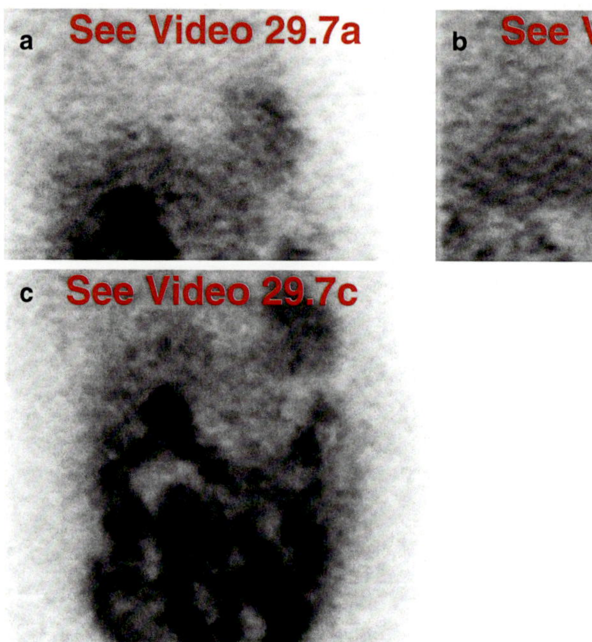

Fig. 29.7

(**a**) Current: stress raw projection images (Video 29.7a, frame 1), ^{99m}Tc sestamibi
(**b**) Previous: stress raw projection images (Video 29.7b, frame 1), ^{99m}Tc sestamibi
(**c**) Original: stress raw projection images (Video 29.7c, frame 1), ^{99m}Tc sestamibi

Characterize the Pertinent Finding(s)

- Chest
  - Thyroid gland: □ hot □ cold
  - Parathyroid glands: □ hot □ cold
  - Breasts: □ hot □ cold
  - Chest wall: □ hot □ cold
  - Skeleton: □ hot □ cold
  - Pleura: □ hot □ cold
  - Lungs: □ hot □ cold
  - Mediastinum: □ hot □ cold
  - Myocardium and pericardium: □ hot □ cold
  - Right atrium and right ventricle: □ hot □ cold
  - Vascular system: □ hot □ cold
  - Lymphatic system: □ hot □ cold
  - Diaphragm: □ hot □ cold
- Abdomen
  - Abdominal wall: □ hot □ cold
  - Peritoneum: □ hot □ cold
  - Liver: □ hot □ cold
  - Biliary system and gallbladder: □ hot □ cold
  - Spleen: □ hot □ cold
  - Stomach: □ hot □ cold
  - Small intestine and large intestine: □ hot □ cold
  - Adrenal glands: □ hot □ cold
  - Kidneys and female reproductive system: □ hot □ cold
  - Vascular system: □ hot □ cold

State Your Relevant Diagnosis(es)

- Chest
  - Thyroid gland: □ normal □ benign neoplasm
  - Parathyroid glands: □ normal □ adenoma
  - Breasts: □ normal □ gynecomastia
  - Chest wall: □ normal □ cracked crystal
  - Skeleton: □ normal □ sarcoma
  - Pleura: □ normal □ effusion
  - Lungs: □ normal □ pneumonectomy
  - Mediastinum: □ normal □ thymoma
  - Myocardium and pericardium: □ normal □ effusion
  - Right atrium and right ventricle: □ normal □ dilatation due to valvular heart disease
  - Vascular system: □ normal □ retention in central veins
  - Lymphatic system: □ normal □ axillary lymph nodes, malignant
  - Diaphragm: □ normal □ herniation of small intestine

- Abdomen
  - Abdominal wall: ☐ normal ☐ metallic object
  - Peritoneum: ☐ normal ☐ ascites
  - Liver: ☐ normal ☐ cirrhosis
  - Biliary system and gallbladder: ☐ normal ☐ chronic cholecystitis
  - Spleen: ☐ normal ☐ splenomegaly
  - Stomach: ☐ normal ☐ gastropathy
  - Small intestine and large intestine: ☐ normal ☐ malposition
  - Adrenal glands: ☐ normal ☐ cystic neoplasm
  - Kidneys and female reproductive system: ☐ normal ☐ partial left nephrectomy
  - Vascular system: ☐ normal ☐ extravasation

29.7.2 Solution

Additional Images

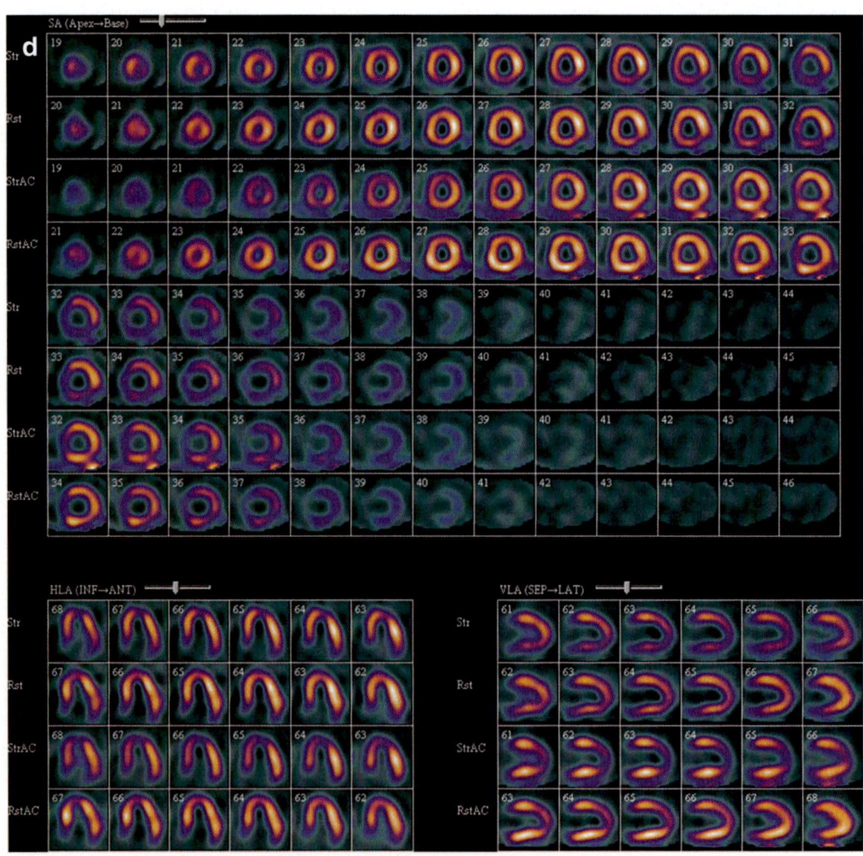

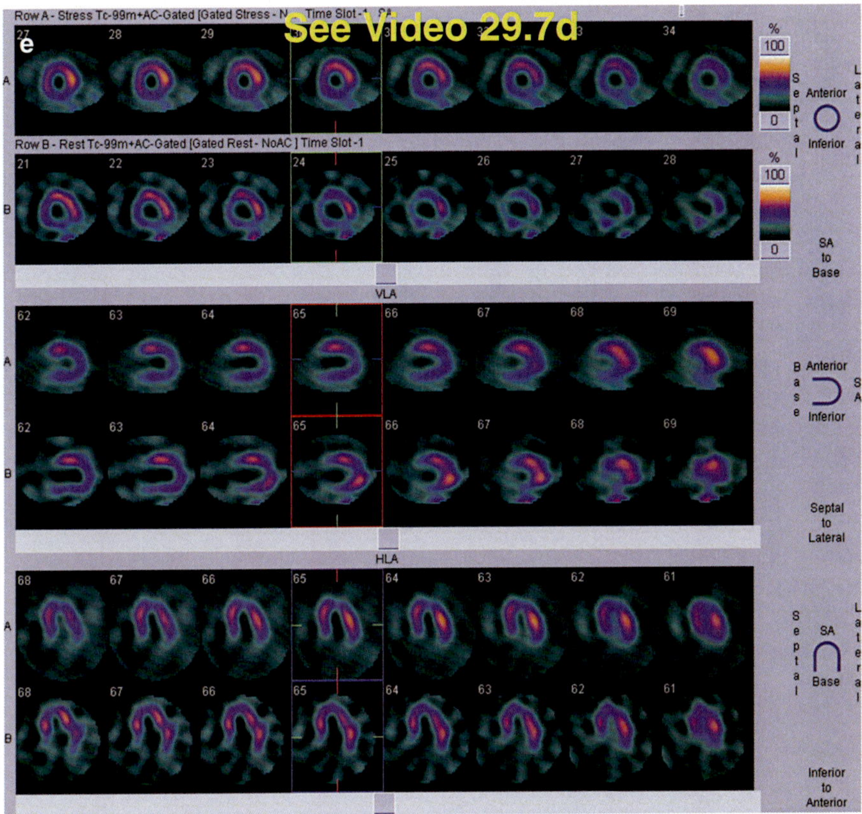

(**d**) Current: stress/rest processed SPECT images (SA, HLA, VLA) (without and with AC)

(**e**) Current: stress and rest gated SPECT images (Video 29.7d, frame 1) (SA, VLA, HLA)

The Pertinent Findings

- Chest
  - Not applicable
- Abdomen
  - Liver: □ hot ■ cold
  - Biliary system and gallbladder: ■ hot ■ cold
  - Spleen: ■ hot □ cold
  - Stomach: ■ hot □ cold

The Relevant Diagnosis(es)

- Chest
  - Not applicable

- Abdomen
    - Liver: ■ cirrhosis
    - Biliary system and gallbladder: ■ chronic cholecystitis
    - Spleen: ■ splenomegaly
    - Stomach: ■ gastropathy

Discussion
Chest
The chest is normal. Heart size is at the upper level of normal for a male; there is no change during over serial examinations. His vasodilator nuclear stress tests have been normal, with LVEF ranging from 62 to 68 %. The current processed images and gated images are shown in Fig. 29.9d, e.

Abdomen
Minimal to no ascites is apparent on serial contemporaneous CT scans (not shown). Note a small liver (a, b, c). A "small" gallbladder is intermittently visualized: it is seen on the current (a) and original (c) serial examinations, but is not identified on the one in-between (b). This pattern is suggestive of chronic gallbladder disease. Review of previous examinations is an important step in interpretation.

Note an enlarged spleen (a, b, c), consistent with underlying cirrhosis. On the current examination, there is faint gastric activity which might signal gastropathy.

Relevant Chapter(s)
Chapters 19, 20, 21, and 22

29.8 Case Challenge #32

29.8.1 Problem

Clinical Highlights

An 87-year-old female with left bundle branch block and heart failure.

Images for Review

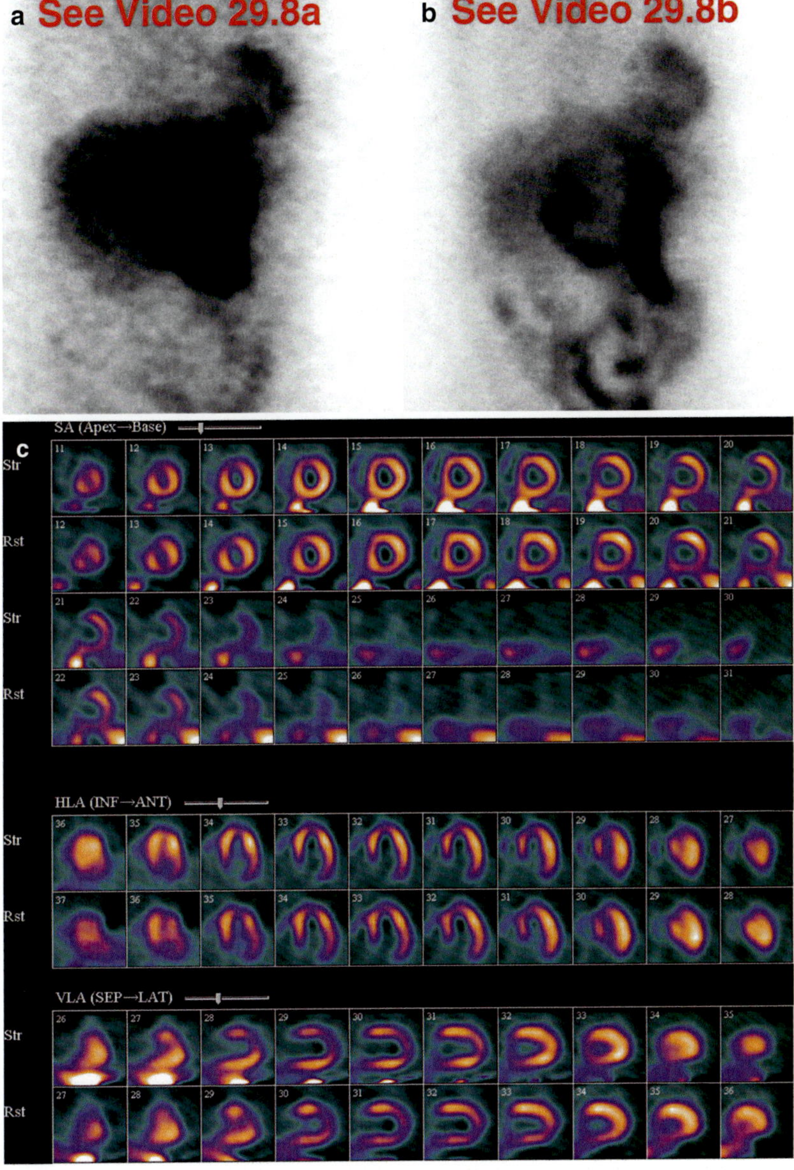

Fig. 29.8

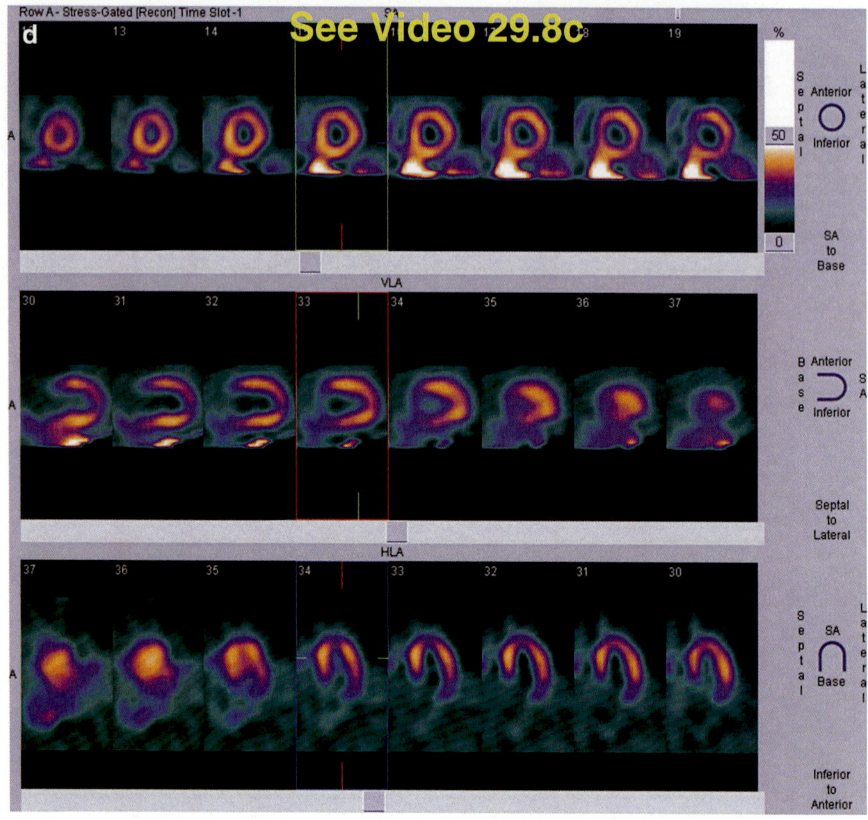

Fig. 29.8 (continued)

(**a**) Rest raw projection images (Video 29.8a, frame 1), ^{99m}Tc sestamibi
(**b**) Stress raw projection images (Video 29.8b, frame 1), ^{99m}Tc sestamibi
(**c**) Stress processed SPECT images (SA, HLA, VLA)
(**d**) Stress gated SPECT (Video 29.8c, frame 1) (SA, VLA, HLA)

Characterize the Pertinent Finding(s)

- Chest
    - Thyroid gland: ☐ hot ☐ cold
    - Parathyroid glands: ☐ hot ☐ cold
    - Breasts: ☐ hot ☐ cold
    - Chest wall: ☐ hot ☐ cold
    - Skeleton: ☐ hot ☐ cold
    - Pleura: ☐ hot ☐ cold
    - Lungs: ☐ hot ☐ cold
    - Mediastinum: ☐ hot ☐ cold
    - Myocardium and pericardium: ☐ hot ☐ cold
    - Right atrium and right ventricle: ☐ hot ☐ cold
    - Vascular system: ☐ hot ☐ cold
    - Lymphatic system: ☐ hot ☐ cold
    - Diaphragm: ☐ hot ☐ cold

- Abdomen
  - Abdominal wall: ☐ hot ☐ cold
  - Peritoneum: ☐ hot ☐ cold
  - Liver: ☐ hot ☐ cold
  - Biliary system and gallbladder: ☐ hot ☐ cold
  - Spleen: ☐ hot ☐ cold
  - Stomach: ☐ hot ☐ cold
  - Small intestine and large intestine: ☐ hot ☐ cold
  - Adrenal glands: ☐ hot ☐ cold
  - Kidneys and female reproductive system: ☐ hot ☐ cold
  - Vascular system: ☐ hot ☐ cold

State Your Relevant Diagnosis(es)

- Chest
  - Thyroid gland: ☐ normal ☐ benign neoplasm
  - Parathyroid glands: ☐ normal ☐ carcinoma
  - Breasts: ☐ normal ☐ large, with periareolar uptake
  - Chest wall: ☐ normal ☐ metallic artifact
  - Skeleton: ☐ normal ☐ osteosarcoma
  - Pleura: ☐ normal ☐ effusion
  - Lungs: ☐ normal ☐ pneumothorax
  - Mediastinum: ☐ normal ☐ esophageal reflux
  - Myocardium and pericardium: ☐ normal ☐ effusion
  - Right atrium and right ventricle: ☐ normal ☐ dilatation and hypertrophy
  - Vascular system: ☐ normal ☐ retention in central veins
  - Lymphatic system: ☐ normal ☐ axillary lymph nodes, malignant
  - Diaphragm: ☐ normal ☐ herniation of large intestine
- Abdomen
  - Abdominal wall: ☐ normal ☐ metallic object
  - Peritoneum: ☐ normal ☐ ascites
  - Liver: ☐ normal ☐ hepatomegaly
  - Biliary system and gallbladder: ☐ normal ☐ cholecystectomy
  - Spleen: ☐ normal ☐ cystic mass
  - Stomach: ☐ normal ☐ hiatal hernia
  - Small intestine and large intestine: ☐ normal ☐ prominent duodenum with duodenogastric reflux
  - Adrenal glands: ☐ normal ☐ cyst
  - Kidneys and female reproductive system: ☐ normal ☐ congenitally absent left kidney
  - Vascular system: ☐ normal ☐ extravasation

29.8.2 Solution

Additional Annotated Images

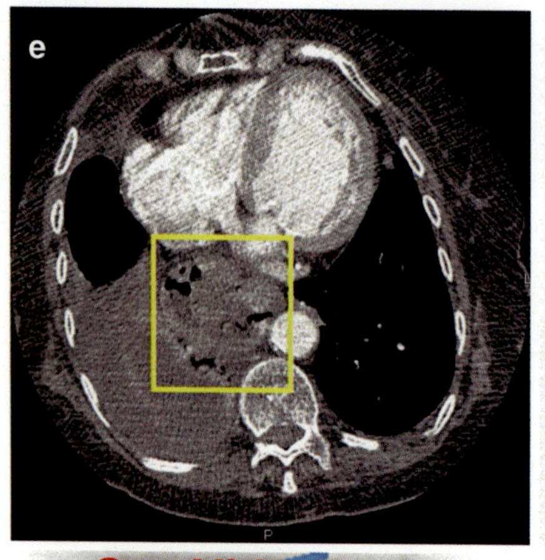

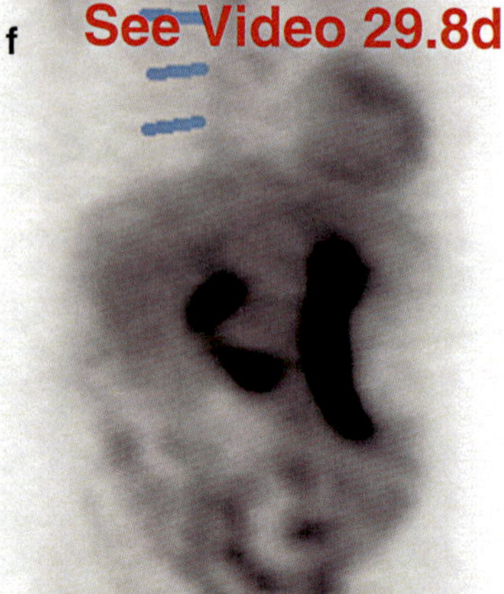

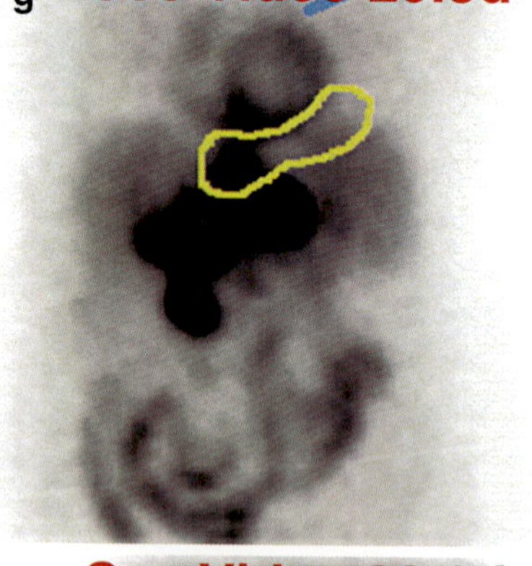

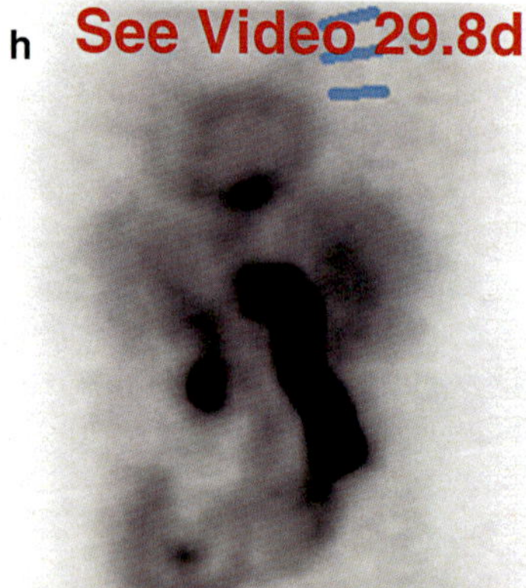

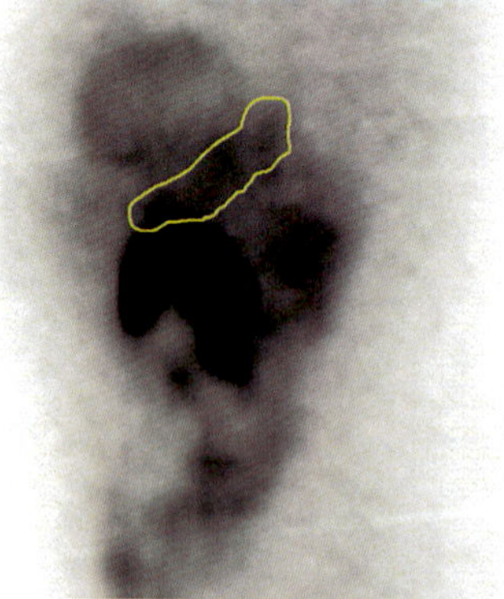

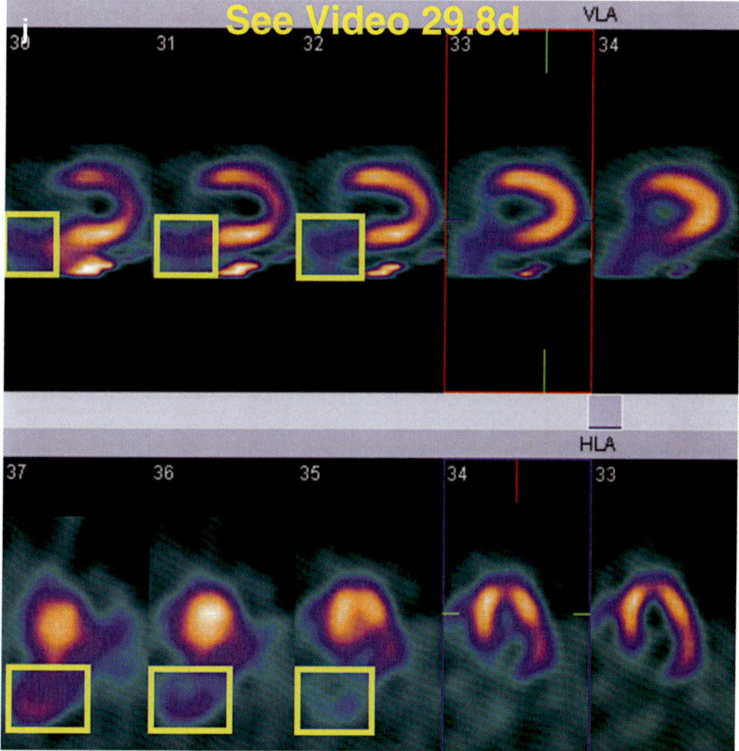

(**e**) Axial contrast-enhanced CT through lower chest at level of hiatal hernia containing gas (*yellow box*)

(**f**) Stress raw projection image (Video 29.8c, frame 2), ^{99m}Tc sestamibi, esophageal activity (*blue lines*)

(**g**) Stress raw projection image (Video 29.8c, frame 24), ^{99m}Tc sestamibi, esophageal activity (*blue lines*), stomach (*yellow outline*)

(**h**) Stress raw projection image (Video 29.8c, frame 34), ^{99m}Tc sestamibi, esophageal activity (*blue lines*)

(**i**) Stress raw projection image (Video 29.8c, frame 44), ^{99m}Tc sestamibi, stomach (*yellow outline*)

(**j**) Stress gated SPECT (Video 29.8d, frame 2), selected VLA and HLA images, stomach (*yellow boxes*)

The Pertinent Findings

- Chest
    - Chest wall: ☐ hot ☒ cold
    - Pleura: ☐ hot ☒ cold
    - Mediastinum: ☒ hot ☐ cold

- Abdomen
    - Abdominal wall: ☐ hot ■ cold
    - Biliary system and gallbladder: ☐ hot ■ cold
    - Stomach: ■ hot ☐ cold
    - Small intestine and large intestine: ■ hot ☐ cold

The Relevant Diagnosis(es)

- Chest
    - Chest wall: ■ metallic artifact
    - Pleura: ■ effusion
    - Mediastinum: ■ esophageal reflux
- Abdomen
    - Abdominal wall: ■ metallic artifact
    - Biliary system and gallbladder: ■ cholecystectomy
    - Stomach: ■ hiatal hernia
    - Small intestine and large intestine: ■ prominent duodenum with duodenogastric reflux

Discussion

Chest

On the raw data (a, b), there is a small round "cold" defect (metallic object on clothing or a cardiac lead) that overlies the left lower chest wall and left upper abdominal wall; it can be discerned when it is contrasted against the "hot" spleen, particularly on the stress data (b). It is of no consequence, but it is useful to notice such artifacts because they could potentially affect the processed images and could lead to misinterpretation.

The right hemithorax is "cold," consistent with a significant right pleural effusion (a, b, e). There are multiple episodes of transient linear (tubular) activity appearing in the midline chest, behind and superior to the heart, particularly striking on the stress acquisition (b, f, g, h). This activity is located within the esophagus and is contiguous with the stomach. The stomach appears "hot," and the fundus is located posteriorly and to the right of the heart (b, e, g, i, j), suggesting a hiatal hernia, which is confirmed by the CT scan (e). The "hot" anterior antral portion of the stomach is immediately adjacent to the inferior right heart, while the fundus and hiatal hernia are more posterior on the processed images (c, j). Careful review of the raw data demonstrates the relative position of the hiatal hernia to the right heart (a, b).

The left ventricle is enlarged, with severe dysfunction (LVEF of 15 %) (c, d). Note the dyskinetic septal rocking motion on the gated SPECT images (d); this is consistent with underlying left bundle branch block conduction abnormality.

Abdomen

The duodenal activity appears prominent and should not be misconstrued as the gallbladder, which has been surgically removed. As discussed above, the entire stomach is "hot" on both acquisitions, consistent with duodenogastric reflux into the stomach and the hiatal hernia, and with reflux into the esophagus.

Relevant Chapter(s)

Chapters 7, 9, 11, 17, 20, 22, and 23

29.9   Case Challenge #33

29.9.1 Problem

Clinical Highlights
A 70-year-old female previously treated for ventricular arrhythmia.

Images for Review

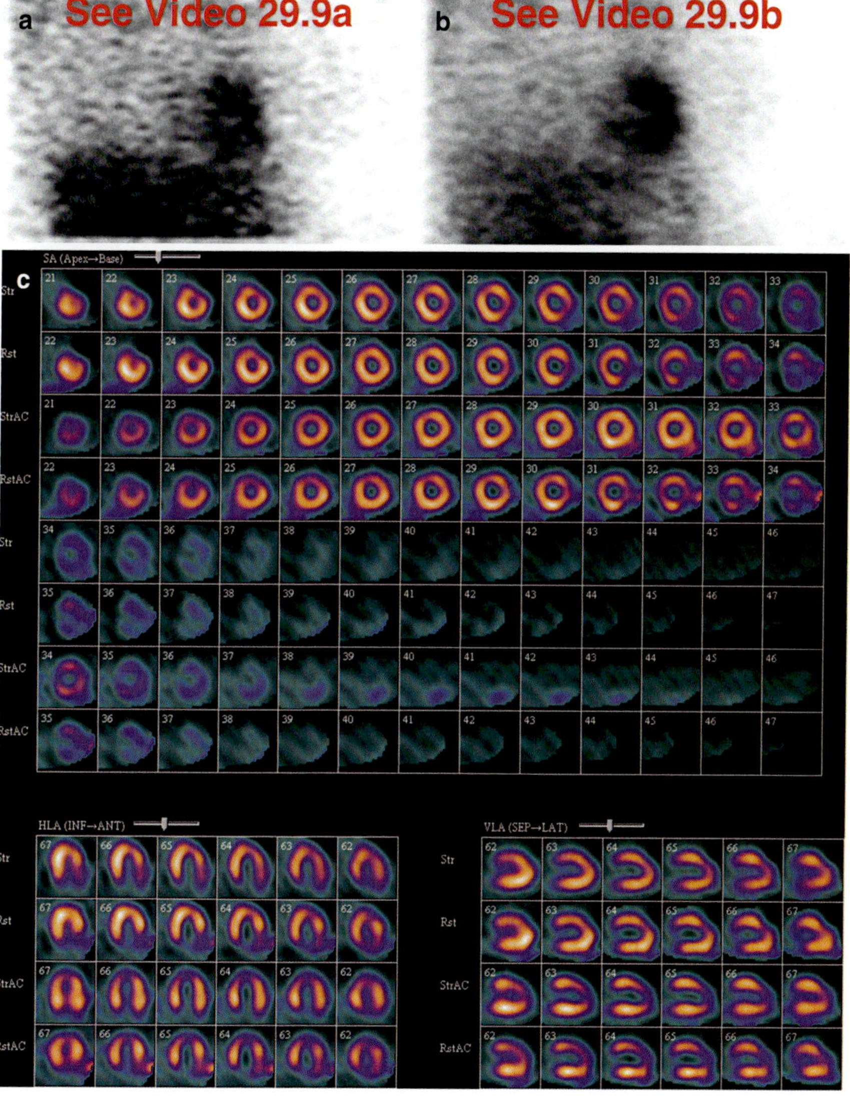

Fig. 29.9

(**a**) Rest raw projection images (Video 29.9a, frame 1), ^{99m}Tc sestamibi
(**b**) Stress raw projection images (Video 29.9b, frame 1), ^{99m}Tc sestamibi
(**c**) Stress/rest processed SPECT images (SA, HLA, VLA) (without and with AC)

Characterize the Pertinent Finding(s)

- Chest
    - Thyroid gland: ☐ hot ☐ cold
    - Parathyroid glands: ☐ hot ☐ cold
    - Breasts: ☐ hot ☐ cold
    - Chest wall: ☐ hot ☐ cold
    - Skeleton: ☐ hot ☐ cold
    - Pleura: ☐ hot ☐ cold
    - Lungs: ☐ hot ☐ cold
    - Mediastinum: ☐ hot ☐ cold
    - Myocardium and pericardium: ☐ hot ☐ cold
    - Right atrium and right ventricle: ☐ hot ☐ cold
    - Vascular system: ☐ hot ☐ cold
    - Lymphatic system: ☐ hot ☐ cold
    - Diaphragm: ☐ hot ☐ cold
- Abdomen
    - Abdominal wall: ☐ hot ☐ cold
    - Peritoneum: ☐ hot ☐ cold
    - Liver: ☐ hot ☐ cold
    - Biliary system and gallbladder: ☐ hot ☐ cold
    - Spleen: ☐ hot ☐ cold
    - Stomach: ☐ hot ☐ cold
    - Small intestine and large intestine: ☐ hot ☐ cold
    - Adrenal glands: ☐ hot ☐ cold
    - Kidneys and female reproductive system: ☐ hot ☐ cold
    - Vascular system: ☐ hot ☐ cold

State Your Relevant Diagnosis(es)

- Chest
    - Thyroid gland: ☐ normal ☐ malignant neoplasm, metastatic
    - Parathyroid glands: ☐ normal ☐ cystic adenoma
    - Breasts: ☐ normal ☐ implants
    - Chest wall: ☐ normal ☐ defibrillator device
    - Skeleton: ☐ normal ☐ sternotomy
    - Pleura: ☐ normal ☐ effusion
    - Lungs: ☐ normal ☐ emphysema
    - Mediastinum: ☐ normal ☐ hiatal hernia
    - Myocardium and pericardium: ☐ normal ☐ effusion
    - Right atrium and right ventricle: ☐ normal ☐ dilatation and hypertrophy
    - Vascular system: ☐ normal ☐ chest port injection site
    - Lymphatic system: ☐ normal ☐ axillary lymph nodes, benign
    - Diaphragm: ☐ normal ☐ elevated right hemidiaphragm

- Abdomen
  - Abdominal wall: ☐ normal ☐ contamination
  - Peritoneum: ☐ normal ☐ peritoneal dialysate
  - Liver: ☐ normal ☐ rapid clearance
  - Biliary system and gallbladder: ☐ normal ☐ contracted gallbladder
  - Spleen: ☐ normal ☐ splenomegaly
  - Stomach: ☐ normal ☐ duodenogastric reflux into hiatal hernia
  - Small intestine and large intestine: ☐ normal ☐ stasis
  - Adrenal glands: ☐ normal ☐ benign cystic mass
  - Kidneys and female reproductive system: ☐ normal ☐ transplant
  - Vascular system: ☐ normal ☐ extravasation

29.9.2 Solution

Additional Annotated Images

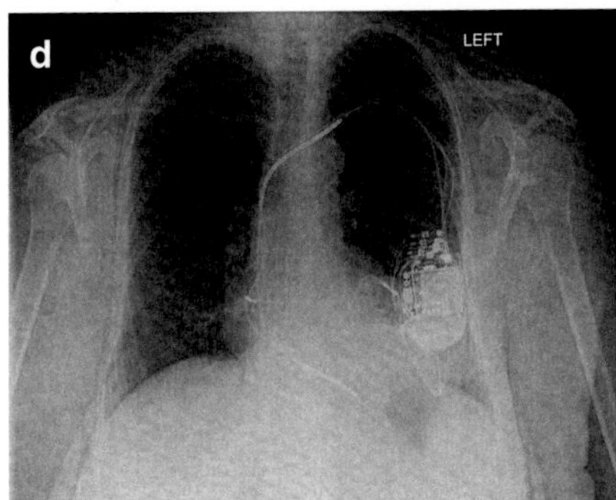

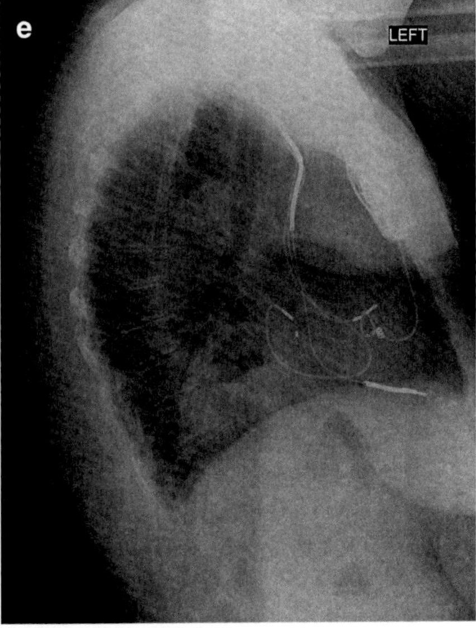

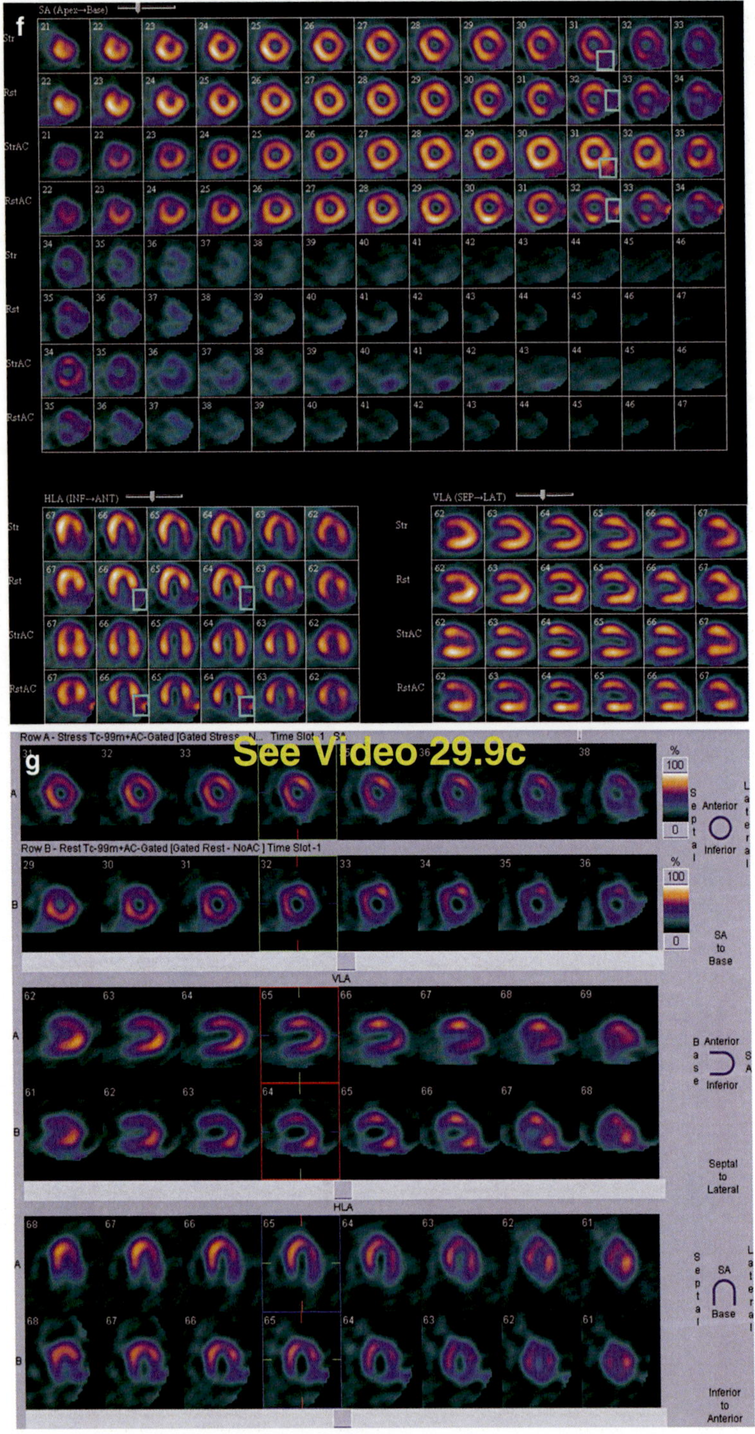
f
SA (Apex→Base)
Str
Rst
StrAC
RstAC
Str
Rst
StrAC
RstAC
HLA (INF→ANT)
VLA (SEP→LAT)
Str
Rst
StrAC
RstAC
Row A - Stress Tc-99m+AC-Gated [Gated Stress - N... Time Slot -1
g
%
100
0
Septal
Lateral
Anterior
Inferior
Row B - Rest Tc-99m+AC-Gated [Gated Rest - NoAC] Time Slot -1
%
100
0
SA
to
Base
VLA
Base
Anterior
Inferior
SA
A
Septal
to
Lateral
HLA
Septal
Lateral
SA
Base
Inferior
to
Anterior
See Video 29.9c

(**d**) PA chest radiograph
(**e**) Lateral chest radiograph
(**f**) Stress/rest processed SPECT images (SA, HLA, VLA) (without and with AC), stomach proper/hiatal hernia (*blue boxes*)
(**g**) Stress and rest gated SPECT images (Video 29.9c, frame 1) (SA, VLA, HLA)

The Pertinent Findings
- Chest
  - Chest wall: □ hot ■ cold
  - Mediastinum: ■ hot □ cold
- Abdomen
  - Stomach: ■ hot □ cold

The Relevant Diagnosis(es)
- Chest
  - Chest wall: ■ defibrillator device
  - Mediastinum: ■ hiatal hernia
- Abdomen
  - Stomach: ■ duodenogastric reflux into hiatal hernia

Discussion
Chest
There is an implanted defibrillator device that produces a subtle "cold" defect in the superior left chest wall (a, b) and is confirmed by radiography (d, e). Note that such implanted devices often project more cephalad on nuclear images (with arms up) as compared to the chest radiographs which may be taken with the arms down, as in this patient.

There is focal activity projecting lateral and posterior to the heart on the rest raw images (a); this activity is likely related to duodenogastric bile reflux into a hiatal hernia as correlated with chest radiographs which demonstrates the retrocardiac air-fluid level (d, e). The activity becomes less apparent on the stress raw images (b). It can be identified on the processed rest SPECT images (c, f). Intense activity in a hiatal hernia can potentially create a significant processing artifact in the adjacent myocardium. As seen on these images, the basal/mid-inferolateral defect corrects with AC (best seen on the HLA displays) and demonstrates normal wall motion and wall thickening (g). Interesting, there is normal regional septal wall motion. This may reflect normal conduction rather than pacing or this may be due to a biventricular pacemaker setting that creates a more coordinated regional septal contraction pattern.

Abdomen
There is variable duodenogastric reflux into a large hiatal hernia (a, b, c, d, f).

Relevant Chapter(s)
Chapters 7, 11, and 22

29.10 Case Challenge #34

29.10.1 Problem

Clinical Highlights

A 57-year-old male presents with epigastric pain suspected to be an angina equivalent.

Images for Review

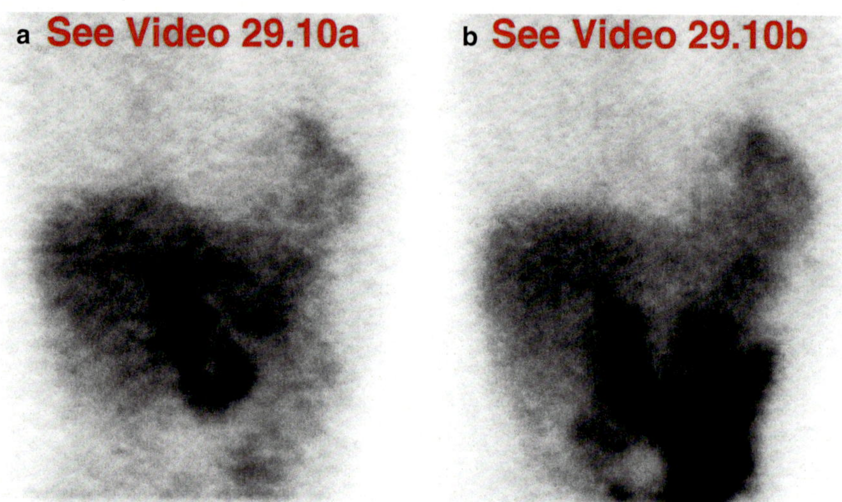

Fig. 29.10

(**a**) Rest raw projection images (Video 29.10a, frame 1), ^{99m}Tc sestamibi
(**b**) Stress raw projection images (Video 29.10b, frame 1), ^{99m}Tc sestamibi

Characterize the Pertinent Finding(s)
- Chest
    - Thyroid gland: ☐ hot ☐ cold
    - Parathyroid glands: ☐ hot ☐ cold
    - Breasts: ☐ hot ☐ cold
    - Chest wall: ☐ hot ☐ cold
    - Skeleton: ☐ hot ☐ cold
    - Pleura: ☐ hot ☐ cold
    - Lungs: ☐ hot ☐ cold
    - Mediastinum: ☐ hot ☐ cold
    - Myocardium and pericardium: ☐ hot ☐ cold
    - Right atrium and right ventricle: ☐ hot ☐ cold
    - Vascular system: ☐ hot ☐ cold
    - Lymphatic system: ☐ hot ☐ cold
    - Diaphragm: ☐ hot ☐ cold

- Abdomen
  - Abdominal wall: ☐ hot ☐ cold
  - Peritoneum: ☐ hot ☐ cold
  - Liver: ☐ hot ☐ cold
  - Biliary system and gallbladder: ☐ hot ☐ cold
  - Spleen: ☐ hot ☐ cold
  - Stomach: ☐ hot ☐ cold
  - Small intestine and large intestine: ☐ hot ☐ cold
  - Adrenal glands: ☐ hot ☐ cold
  - Kidneys and female reproductive system: ☐ hot ☐ cold
  - Vascular system: ☐ hot ☐ cold

State Your Relevant Diagnosis(es)

- Chest
  - Thyroid gland: ☐ normal ☐ goitrous right lobe
  - Parathyroid glands: ☐ normal ☐ ectopic adenoma
  - Breasts: ☐ normal ☐ prostheses
  - Chest wall: ☐ normal ☐ metallic object
  - Skeleton: ☐ normal ☐ multiple myeloma
  - Pleura: ☐ normal ☐ effusion
  - Lungs: ☐ normal ☐ hyperinflation/chronic obstructive pulmonary disease (COPD)
  - Mediastinum: ☐ normal ☐ hiatal hernia
  - Myocardium and pericardium: ☐ normal ☐ effusion
  - Right atrium and right ventricle: ☐ normal ☐ right auricular appendage
  - Vascular system: ☐ normal ☐ injection site
  - Lymphatic system: ☐ normal ☐ lymphoma
  - Diaphragm: ☐ normal ☐ flattening
- Abdomen
  - Abdominal wall: ☐ normal ☐ metallic object
  - Peritoneum: ☐ normal ☐ ascites
  - Liver: ☐ normal ☐ cysts
  - Biliary system and gallbladder: ☐ normal ☐ chronic calculous cholecystitis
  - Spleen: ☐ normal ☐ enlargement
  - Stomach: ☐ normal ☐ duodenogastric reflux
  - Small intestine and large intestine: ☐ normal ☐ stasis in jejunum
  - Adrenal glands: ☐ normal ☐ mass, left side
  - Kidneys and female reproductive system: ☐ normal ☐ chronic/end-stage renal disease
  - Vascular system: ☐ normal ☐ extravasation

29.10.2   Solution

Additional Annotated Images

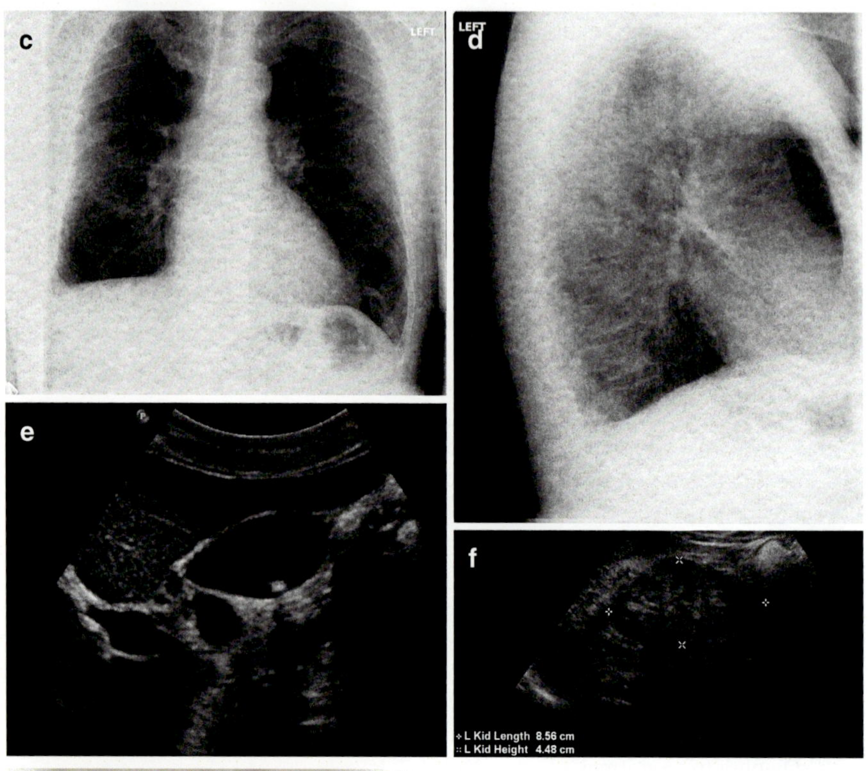

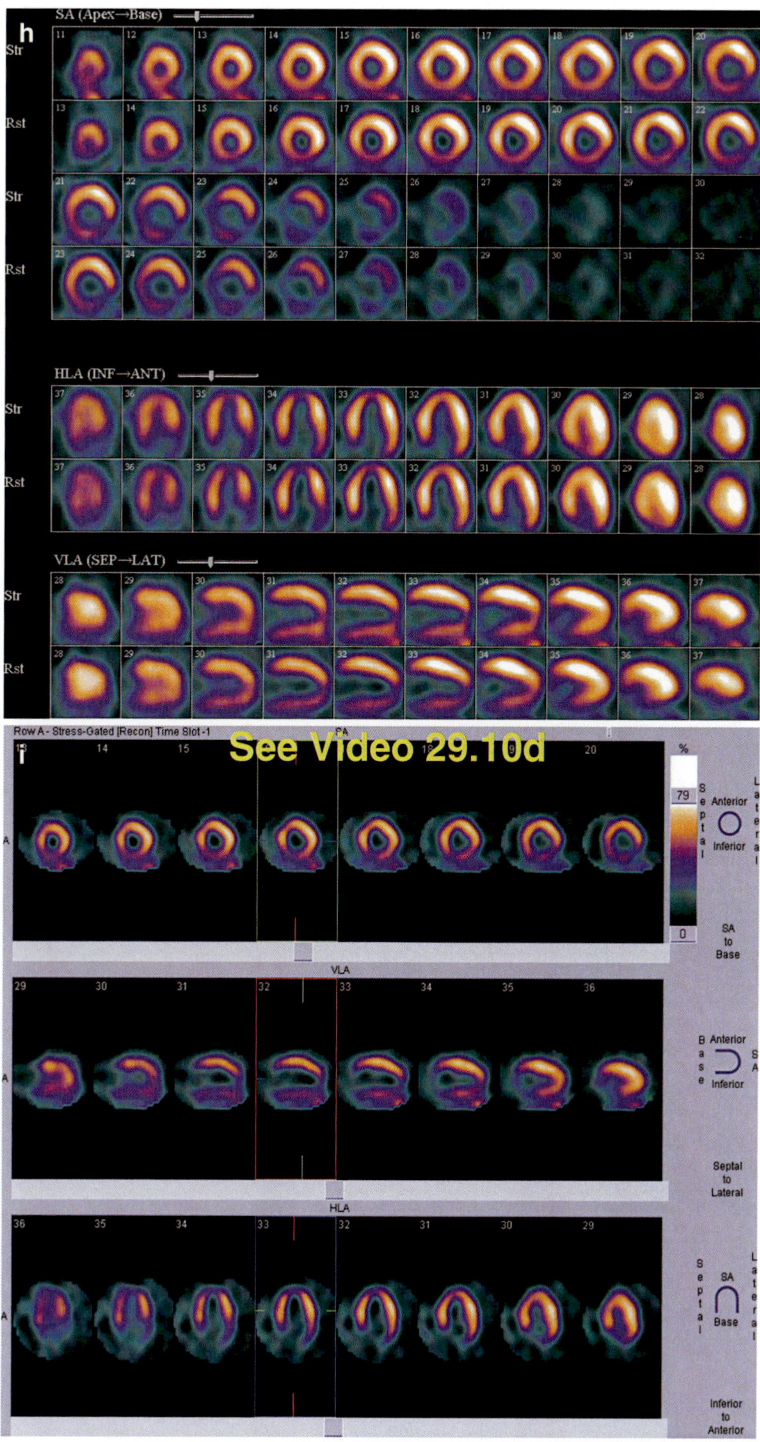

SA (Apex→Base)
Str
Rst
Str
Rst
HLA (INF→ANT)
Str
Rst
VLA (SEP→LAT)
Str
Rst
h
Row A - Stress-Gated [Recon] Time Slot -1
See Video 29.10d
i
SA
%
79
0
Septal
Anterior
Inferior
Lateral
SA to Base
VLA
Base
Anterior
Inferior
SA
Septal to Lateral
HLA
Septal
SA Base
Lateral
Inferior to Anterior

(**c**) PA chest radiograph
(**d**) Lateral chest radiograph
(**e**) Ultrasound of gallbladder
(**f**) Ultrasound of left kidney
(**g**) Stress raw projection image (Video 29.10c, frame 56), ^{99m}Tc sestamibi, metallic object (*pink circle*), left kidney (*yellow box*)
(**h**) Stress/rest processed SPECT images (SA, HLA, VLA)
(**i**) Stress gated SPECT (Video 29.10d, frame 1) (SA, VLA, HLA)

The Pertinent Findings

- Chest
    - Breasts: ☐ hot ■ cold
    - Chest wall: ☐ hot ■ cold
    - Pleura: ☐ hot ■ cold
    - Lungs: ☐ hot ■ cold
    - Right atrium and right ventricle: ■ hot ☐ cold
    - Diaphragm: ☐ hot ■ cold
- Abdomen
    - Abdominal wall: ☐ hot ■ cold
    - Biliary system and gallbladder: ■ hot ■ cold
    - Stomach: ■ hot ☐ cold
    - Small intestine and large intestine: ■ hot ☐ cold
    - Kidneys and female reproductive system: ☐ hot ■ cold

The Relevant Diagnosis(es)

- Chest
    - Breasts: ■ prostheses
    - Chest wall: ■ metallic object
    - Skeleton: ■ normal
    - Pleura: ■ effusion
    - Lungs: ■ hyperinflation/hyperinflation/chronic obstructive pulmonary disease (COPD)
    - Right atrium and right ventricle: ■ right auricular appendage
    - Diaphragm: ■ flattening
- Abdomen
    - Abdominal wall: ■ metallic object
    - Biliary system and gallbladder: ■ chronic calculous cholecystitis
    - Stomach: ■ duodenogastric reflux
    - Small intestine and large intestine: ■ stasis in jejunum
    - Kidneys and female reproductive system: ■ chronic/end-stage renal disease

Discussion

Chest

A "cold" defect is present in a superficial location on the left lateral chest wall/upper abdominal wall; on some projections, it overlies the spleen and on others, the left ventricular apex (b, g). There is a subtle photopenia at the right lung base (b), correlating with pleural effusion radiographically (c, d); right pleural effusions may be difficult to appreciate due to the axis of rotation from the right anterior oblique projection to the left posterior oblique. The radiographic left pleural effusion (in the upright position) is too small to detect by MPI (in the supine position). The lungs appear hyperinflated with flattened diaphragms (a, b, c, d), characteristic of chronic obstructive pulmonary disease.

The right auricular appendage is faintly seen (a, b). There is cardiomegaly and the left ventricular cavity is enlarged (a, b, h, i). Processed SPECT (h) and gated SPECT (i) show a medium-size, mild, fixed inferolateral wall defect with associated hypokinesis. LV end-diastolic volume is 189 mL and LVEF is 49 %.

Abdomen

There is duodenogastric reflux accounting for the "hot" stomach (a, b). Note how the jejunum appears quite "hot" and localized in the left upper quadrant on the rest images, but the activity moves along with peristalsis by the time of the stress imaging. The stone-filled gallbladder (e) is not visualized on rest raw images (a) but visualizes on later same-day stress raw images (b). There are gallstones (e). The diagnosis is chronic calculous cholecystitis. The left kidney is small (a, b, f, g), consistent with chronic renal disease.

Relevant Chapter(s)

Chapters 6, 7, 9, 10, 13, 16, 17, 20, 22, 23, and 25

29.11 Case Challenge #35

29.11.1 Problem

Clinical Highlights

A 43-year-old female awaits organ transplant. She exercised 6 minutes on a treadmill achieving 7 METS, without chest pain nor ECG changes.

Images for Review

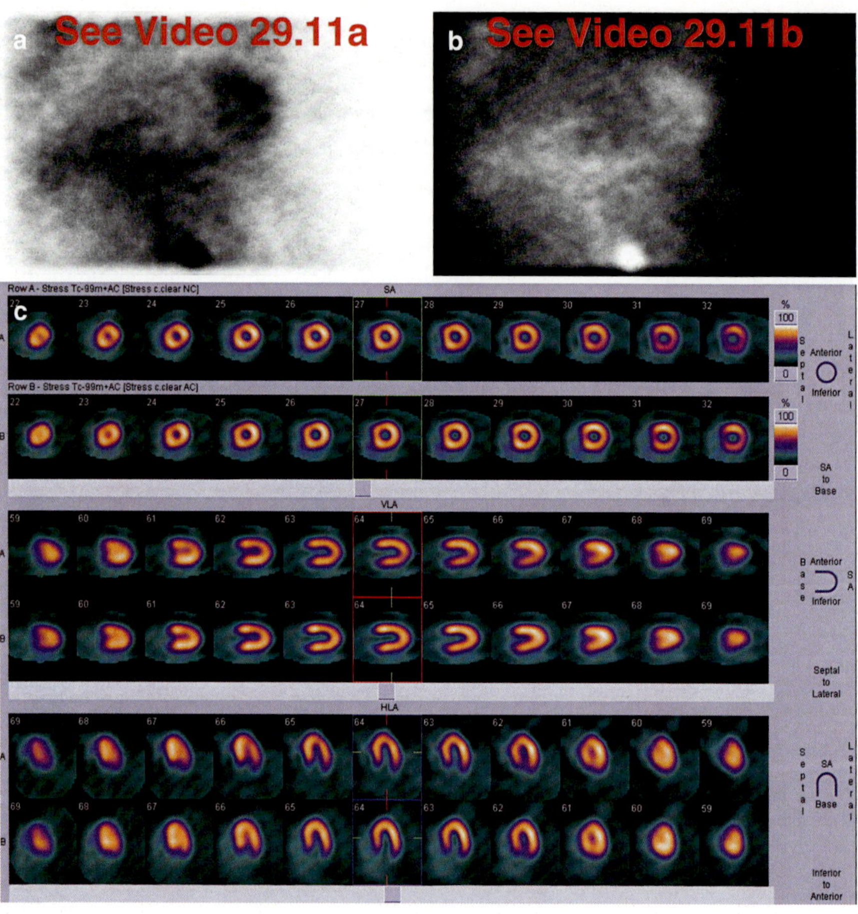

Fig. 29.11

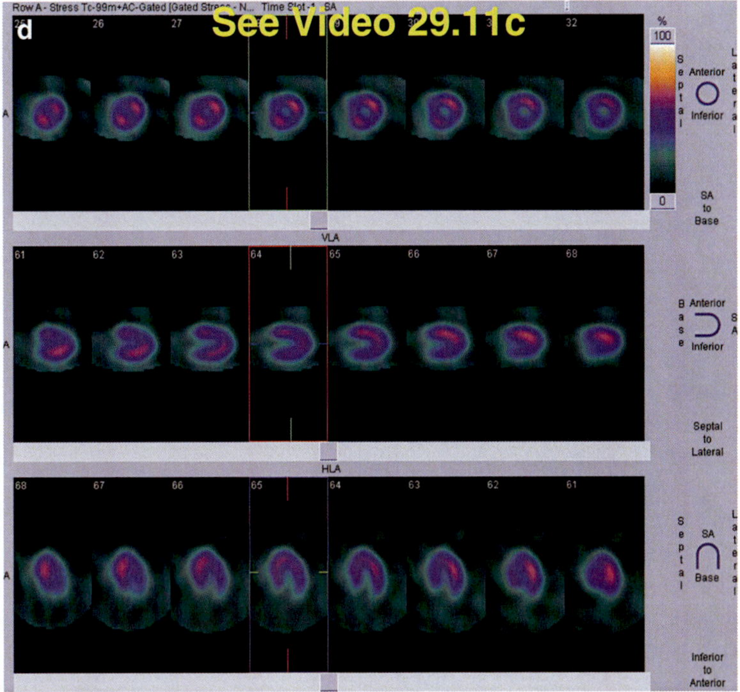

Fig. 29.11   (continued)

(**a**) Stress "black-on-white" raw projection images (Video 29.11a, frame 1), ^{99m}Tc sestamibi

(**b**) Stress "white-on-black" raw projection images (Video 29.11b, frame 1), ^{99m}Tc sestamibi

(**c**) Stress processed SPECT images (SA, VLA, HLA) without and with AC [*top row*: non-AC; *bottom row*: AC]

(**d**) Stress gated SPECT (Video 29.11c, frame 1) (SA, VLA, HLA)

Characterize the Pertinent Finding(s)

- Chest
    - Thyroid gland: ☐ hot ☐ cold
    - Parathyroid glands: ☐ hot ☐ cold
    - Breasts: ☐ hot ☐ cold
    - Chest wall: ☐ hot ☐ cold
    - Skeleton: ☐ hot ☐ cold
    - Pleura: ☐ hot ☐ cold
    - Lungs: ☐ hot ☐ cold
    - Mediastinum: ☐ hot ☐ cold
    - Myocardium and pericardium: ☐ hot ☐ cold
    - Right atrium and right ventricle: ☐ hot ☐ cold
    - Vascular system: ☐ hot ☐ cold
    - Lymphatic system: ☐ hot ☐ cold
    - Diaphragm: ☐ hot ☐ cold

- Abdomen
    - Abdominal wall: □ hot □ cold
    - Peritoneum: □ hot □ cold
    - Liver: □ hot □ cold
    - Biliary system and gallbladder: □ hot □ cold
    - Spleen: □ hot □ cold
    - Stomach: □ hot □ cold
    - Small intestine and large intestine: □ hot □ cold
    - Adrenal glands: □ hot □ cold
    - Kidneys and female reproductive system: □ hot □ cold
    - Vascular system: □ hot □ cold

State Your Relevant Diagnosis(es)

- Chest
    - Thyroid gland: □ normal □ primary malignancy
    - Parathyroid glands: □ normal □ multigland hyperplasia
    - Breasts: □ normal □ large, with periareolar uptake
    - Chest wall: □ normal □ multifocal melanoma
    - Skeleton: □ normal □ sternotomy
    - Pleura: □ normal □ effusion
    - Lungs: □ normal □ pneumothorax
    - Mediastinum: □ normal □ esophageal tumor
    - Myocardium and pericardium: □ normal □ effusion
    - Right atrium and right ventricle: □ normal □ dilatation
    - Vascular system: □ normal □ injection site
    - Lymphatic system: □ normal □ lymphoma
    - Diaphragm: □ normal □ paralysis
- Abdomen
    - Abdominal wall: □ normal □ multifocal melanoma
    - Peritoneum: □ normal □ ascites
    - Liver: □ normal □ metastases, colon carcinoma
    - Biliary system and gallbladder: □ normal □ cholecystectomy
    - Spleen: □ normal □ splenomegaly
    - Stomach: □ normal □ gastropathy
    - Small intestine and large intestine: □ normal □ stasis
    - Adrenal glands: □ normal □ cystic mass
    - Kidneys and female reproductive system: □ normal □ polycystic disease
    - Vascular system: □ normal □ extravasation

29.11.2 Solution

Additional Annotated Images

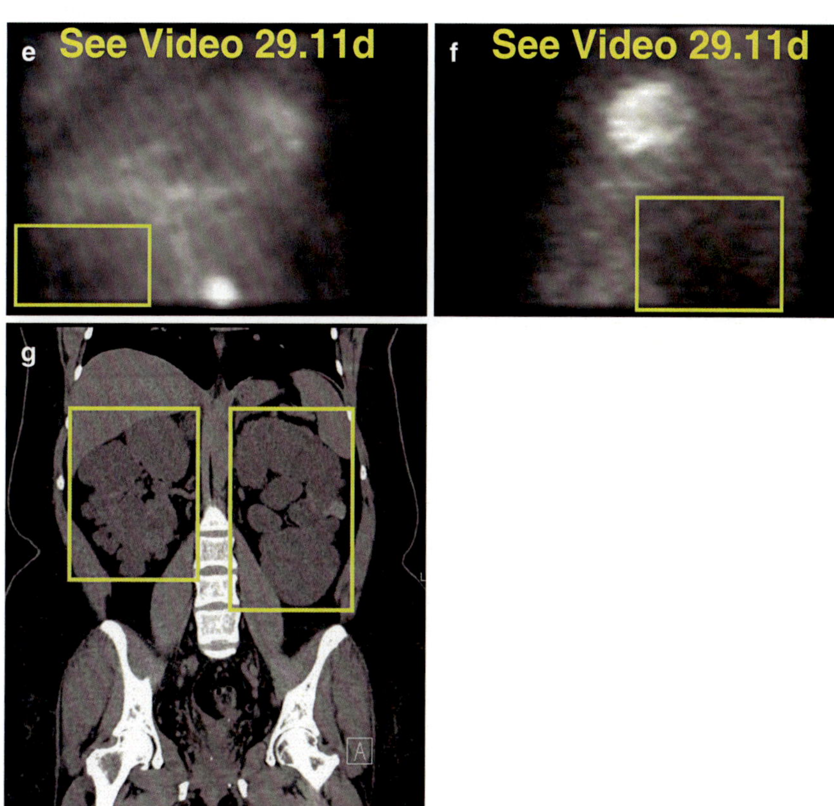

(**e**) Stress "white-on-black" raw projection image (Video 29.11d, frame 1), [99mTc] sestamibi, right kidney (*yellow box*)

(**f**) Stress "white-on-black" raw projection image (Video 29.11d, frame 46), [99mTc] sestamibi, left kidney (*yellow box*)

(**g**) Coronal CT of posterior abdomen at level of kidneys (*yellow boxes*)

The Pertinent Findings

- Chest
  - Breasts: ■ hot ■ cold
- Abdomen
  - Kidneys and female reproductive system: ☐ hot ■ cold

The Relevant Diagnosis(es)

- Chest
  - Breasts: ■ large, with periareolar uptake
- Abdomen
  - Kidneys and female reproductive system: ■ polycystic disease

Discussion

Chest

There are prominent "cold" breasts with symmetric slight increased ("hot") peri-areolar uptake. This is a normal appearance. Note that the breasts are large and create "photopenia" that extends to the lateral chest wall. There is also curvilinear increased uptake along the underside of the lower breasts where they overlie the chest wall; this is due to low-angle scatter artifact at the skinfold interface.

The stress-only processed images (c) are normal, with a very small left ventricular cavity (end-diastolic volume of 45 mL) and a calculated LVEF of 87 % (d) (note: high LVEFs are often seen in such patients with low EDVs).

Abdomen

There are striking large "cold" regions in the abdomen (a), better appreciated on "white-on-black" (b, e, f) rendering of the images. The left-sided abnormality is better seen due to the axis of rotation for imaging. These "cold" regions are located within markedly enlarged "lumpy-bumpy" kidneys as shown on the CT image (g). Note that the "hot" gallbladder is slightly more medially positioned than usual; this may be related to some mass effect on the liver from the enlarged right kidney. A normal-size spleen is anatomically present but difficult to appreciate due to the large "cold" left kidney occupying the left upper quadrant (a, b). The final diagnosis is adult polycystic kidney disease.

Relevant Chapter(s)

Chapters 6 and 25

29.12 Case Challenge #36

29.12.1 Problem

Clinical Highlights
A 60-year-old female needs a preoperative assessment.

Images for Review

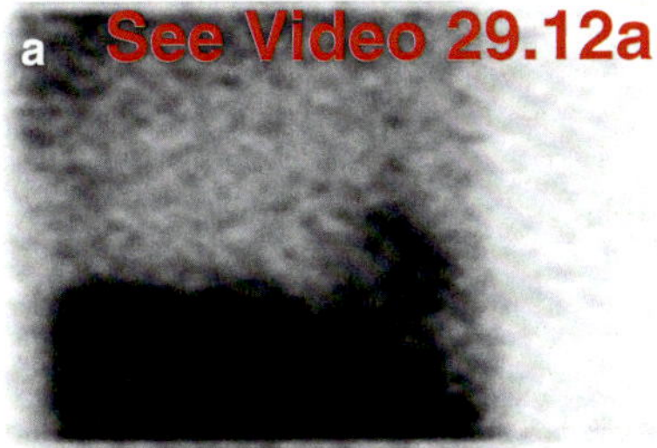

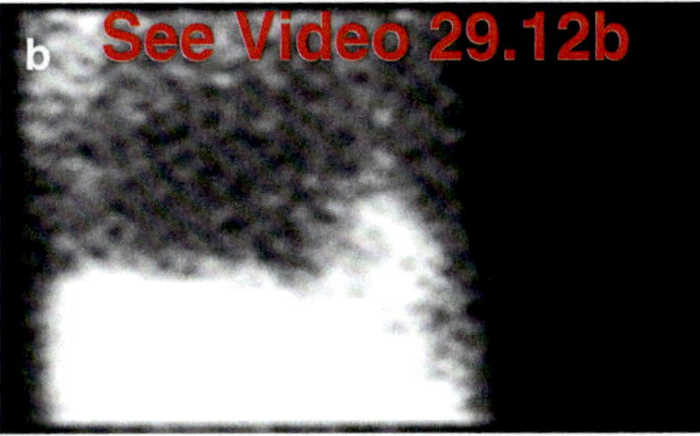

Fig. 29.12

(**a**) Stress "black-on-white" raw projection images contrast-adjusted for chest (Video 29.12a, frame 1), ^{99m}Tc sestamibi

(**b**) Stress "white-on-black" raw projection images contrast-adjusted for chest (Video 29.12b, frame 1), ^{99m}Tc sestamibi

Characterize the Pertinent Finding(s)
- Chest
    - Thyroid gland: ☐ hot ☐ cold
    - Parathyroid glands: ☐ hot ☐ cold
    - Breasts: ☐ hot ☐ cold
    - Chest wall: ☐ hot ☐ cold
    - Skeleton: ☐ hot ☐ cold
    - Pleura: ☐ hot ☐ cold
    - Lungs: ☐ hot ☐ cold
    - Mediastinum: ☐ hot ☐ cold
    - Myocardium and pericardium: ☐ hot ☐ cold
    - Right atrium and right ventricle: ☐ hot ☐ cold
    - Vascular system: ☐ hot ☐ cold
    - Lymphatic system: ☐ hot ☐ cold
    - Diaphragm: ☐ hot ☐ cold

- Abdomen
  - Abdominal wall: □ hot □ cold
  - Peritoneum: □ hot □ cold
  - Liver: □ hot □ cold
  - Biliary system and gallbladder: □ hot □ cold
  - Spleen: □ hot □ cold
  - Stomach: □ hot □ cold
  - Small intestine and large intestine: □ hot □ cold
  - Adrenal glands: □ hot □ cold
  - Kidneys and female reproductive system: □ hot □ cold
  - Vascular system: □ hot □ cold

State Your Relevant Diagnosis(es)

- Chest
  - Thyroid gland: □ normal □ cyst
  - Parathyroid glands: □ normal □ ectopic adenoma
  - Breasts: □ normal □ implants
  - Chest wall: □ normal □ contamination
  - Skeleton: □ normal □ anemia
  - Pleura: □ normal □ effusion
  - Lungs: □ normal □ malignant neoplasm
  - Mediastinum: □ normal □ hiatal hernia
  - Myocardium and pericardium: □ normal □ effusion
  - Right atrium and right ventricle: □ normal □ hypertrophy
  - Vascular system: □ normal □ chest port injection site
  - Lymphatic system: □ normal □ lymphatic channels
  - Diaphragm: □ normal □ flattening
- Abdomen
  - Abdominal wall: □ normal □ contamination
  - Peritoneum: □ normal □ ascites
  - Liver: □ normal □ rapid clearance
  - Biliary system and gallbladder: □ normal □ contracted gallbladder
  - Spleen: □ normal □ splenomegaly
  - Stomach: □ normal □ duodenogastric reflux into hiatal hernia
  - Small intestine and large intestine: □ normal □ previous radiopharmaceutical
  - Adrenal glands: □ normal □ benign cystic mass
  - Kidneys and female reproductive system: □ normal □ metastatic disease to left kidney
  - Vascular system: □ normal □ extravasation

29.12.2 Solution

Additional Annotated Images

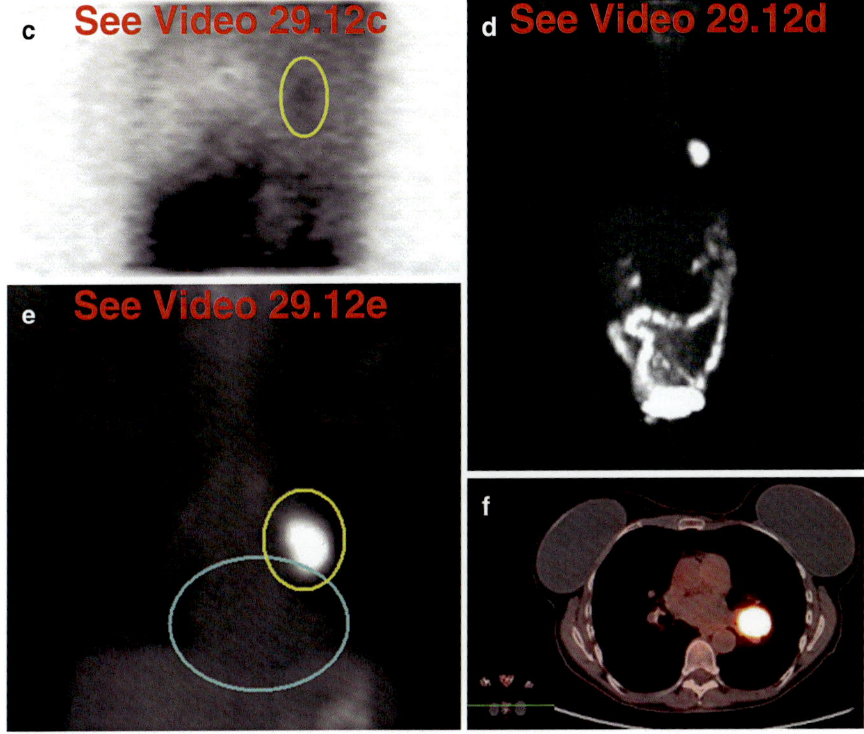

(**c**) Stress "black-on-white" raw projection images contrast-adjusted for chest (Video 29.12c, frame 1), ^{99m}Tc sestamibi, left hilar mass (*yellow oval*)

(**d**) Maximum intensity projection PET images (Video 29.12d, frame 1), ^{18}F FDG

(**e**) Maximum intensity projection PET image (Video 29.12e, frame 1), ^{18}F FDG, left hilar mass (*yellow oval*), heart blood pool for reference (*blue oval*)

(**f**) Axial fused ^{18}F FDG PET/CT image

The Pertinent Findings
- Chest
  - Breasts: ☐ hot ■ cold
  - Lungs: ■ hot ☐ cold
- Abdomen
  - Not applicable

The Relevant Diagnosis(es)
- Chest
  - Breasts: ■ implants
  - Lungs: ■ malignant neoplasm
- Abdomen
  - Not applicable

Discussion
Chest
Note the sharply photopenic ("cold") breasts (a); "cold" findings are often better appreciated using a "white-on-black" color scale (b).

There is focal radiopharmaceutical localization in the left mid-chest superior to the heart; it is partially obscured by marked attenuation artifact by the breast implants; on close scrutiny it can be glimpsed on some frames of the cinematic display of the raw data (a, b, c).

Correlative imaging with ^{18}F FDG PET/CT (d, e) depicts the breast implants as well-defined, low-attenuation "breasts" on the anterior chest wall. It also confirms the presence of a strikingly ^{18}F FDG-avid left pulmonary mass near the hilum corresponding to the sestamibi-avid mass. Left pneumonectomy revealed an invasive moderately differentiated adenosquamous cell carcinoma arising in the upper lobe.

Abdomen
The abdomen is normal.

Relevant Chapter(s)
Chapters 6 and 10

References

ACR–SNM–SPR practice guideline for the performance of cardiac scintigraphy (revised 2009). http://snmmi.files.cms-plus.com/docs/Cardiac_Scintigraphy_1382731812393_3.pdf. Accessed 4 June 2015.

Afzelius P, Henriksen JH. Extra cardiac activity detected on myocardial perfusion scintigraphy after intra-arterial injection of 99mTc-MIBI. Clin Physiol Funct Imaging. 2008;28(5):285–6. doi:10.1111/j.1475-097X.2008.00811.x. Epub 2008 Jun 5.

Aktolun C, Bayhan H. Tc-99m MIBI uptake in pulmonary sarcoidosis. Preliminary clinical results and comparison with Ga-67. Clin Nucl Med. 1994;19:1063–5.

Aktolun C, Bayhan H, Pabuccu Y, Bilgic H, Acar H, Koylu R. Assessment of tumour necrosis and detection of mediastinal lymph node metastasis in bronchial carcinoma with technetium-99m sestamibi imaging: comparison with CT scan. Eur J Nucl Med. 1994;21(9):973–9.

Aras T, Ergun EL, Bozkurt MF. Visualization of the pulmonary artery on 99m Tc-MIBI myocardial perfusion scintigraphy: a cause for focal uptake in the lung. Semin Nucl Med. 2003;33(4):338–41.

Arbab AS, Koizumi K, Arai T, Mera K, Miyazaki A, Otaka M. Incidental detection of breast cancer during T1-201 myocardial SPECT study. Ann Nucl Med. 1995;9(3):143–4.

Bhambhvani P, Dubovsky E, Nath H, Heo J, Iskandrian A. Unusual incidental findings by SPECT myocardial perfusion imaging and CT in the same patient. J Nucl Cardiol. 2010a;17(5):937–8. doi:10.1007/s12350-010-9219-1.

Bhambhvani P, Dubovsky E, Heo J, Iskandrian A. Incidental detection of hepatocellular carcinoma by SPECT myocardial perfusion imaging. J Nucl Cardiol. 2010b;17(6):1116–7. doi:10.1007/s12350-010-9267-6.

Bom H-S, Kim Y-C, Song H-C, Min J-J, Kim J-Y, Park K-O. Technetium-99m-MIBI uptake in small cell lung cancer. J Nucl Med. 1998;39:91–4.

Boz A, Gungor F, Karayalçin B, Yildiz A. The effects of solid food in prevention of intestinal activity in Tc-99m tetrofosmin myocardial perfusion scintigraphy. J Nucl Cardiol. 2003;10(2):161–7.

Burrell S, MacDonald A. Artifacts and pitfalls in myocardial perfusion imaging. J Nucl Med Technol. 2006;34:193–211.

Caner B, Kitapcl M, Unlu M, Erbengi G, Calikoglu T, Gogus T. Technetium-99m-MIBI uptake in benign and malignant bone lesions: a comparative study with technetium-99m-MDP. J Nucl Med. 1992;33:319–24.

Chadika S, Kokkirala AR, Giedd KN, Johnson LL, Giardina EG, Bokhari S. Focal uptake of radioactive tracer in the mediastinum during SPECT myocardial perfusion imaging. J Nucl Cardiol. 2005;12(3):359–61.

Chamarthy M, Travin MI. Altered biodistribution and incidental findings on myocardial perfusion imaging. Semin Nucl Med. 2010;40:257–70.

Chatziioannou SN, Alfaro-Franco C, Moore WH, Alanis-Williams L, Dhekne RD, Ford PV. The significance of incidental noncardiac findings in Tc-99m sestamibi myocardial perfusion imaging: illustrated by a case. Tex Heart Instit J. 1999;26:229–31.

© Springer International Publishing Switzerland 2017

M.E. Oates, V.L. Sorrell, *Myocardial Perfusion Imaging - Beyond the Left Ventricle: Pathology, Artifacts and Pitfalls in the Chest and Abdomen*, DOI 10.1007/978-3-319-25436-4

Cherng SC, Chen YH, Lee MS, Yang SP, Huang WS, Cheng CY. Acceleration of hepatobiliary excretion by lemon juice on 99mTc-tetrofosmin cardiac SPECT. Nucl Med Commun. 2006; 27(11):859–64.

Chin BB, Zukerberg BW, Buchpiguel C, Alavi A. Thallium-201 uptake in lung cancer. J Nucl Med. 1995;36:1514–9.

Coakley AJ, Kettle AG, Wells CP. 99m Tc sestamibi: a new agent for parathyroid imaging. Nucl Med Commun. 1989;10:791–4.

Cote C, Dumont M. The clinical meaning of gastric-wall hyperactivity observed on sestamibi cardiac single-photon emission computed tomography. Can Assoc Radiol J. 2004;55:178–83.

Eftekhari M, Gholamrezanezhad A. Incidental detection of malignant pleural effusion on sestamibi myocardial perfusion scan. Int J Cardiovasc Imaging. 2006;22:775–7.

Fisher C, Vehec A, Kashlan B, Longa G, Houpt L, Howe K, Stark L, Cavanaugh D. Incidental detection of skeletal uptake on sestamibi cardiac imaging in a patient with previously undiagnosed multiple myeloma. Clin Nucl Med. 2000;25:213–4.

Friedman J, Van Train K, Maddahi J, Rozanski A, Prigent F, Bietendorf J, Waxman A, Berman DS. "Upward creep" of the heart: a frequent source of false-positive reversible defects during thallium-201 stress-redistribution SPECT. J Nucl Med. 1989;30(10):1718–22.

Fukushima K, Kono M, Ishii K, Sakai E, Hirota S, Yuri H. Technetium-99m methoxyisobutylisonitrile single-photon emission tomography in hepatocellular carcinoma. Eur J Nucl Med. 1997;24(11):1426–8.

García-Talavera P, Olmos R, Sainz-Esteban A, Ruiz MÁ, González ML, Gamazo C. Evaluation by SPECT-CT of an incidental finding of a thymoma and breast cancer in a myocardial perfusion SPECT with 99mTc-MIBI. Rev Esp Med Nucl Imagen Mol. 2013;32(4):260–2. doi:10.1016/j. remn.2012.10.010. Epub 2012 Dec 23.

Garg J, Palaniswamy C, Huang T, Pradhan TS, Gerard P, Jain D. Large photopenic mass in abdomen on myocardial perfusion imaging. J Nucl Cardiol. 2013;20(4):644–7. doi:10.1007/ s12350-013-9733-z. Epub 2013 May 25.

Gedik GK, Ergun EL, Aslan M, Caner B. Unusual extracardiac findings detected on myocardial perfusion single photon emission computed tomography studies with Tc-99m sestamibi. Clin Nucl Med. 2007;32:920–6.

Gentili A, Miron SD, Adler LP. Review of some common artifacts in nuclear medicine. Clin Nucl Med. 1994;19:138–43.

Germano G, Chua T, Kiat H, Areeda JS, Berman DS. A quantitative phantom analysis of artifacts due to hepatic activity in technetium-99m myocardial perfusion SPECT studies. J Nucl Med. 1994;35:356–9.

Ghanbarinia A, Chandra S, Chhabra K, Jain D. Renal abnormalities as incidental findings on myocardial single photon emission computed tomography perfusion imaging. Nucl Med Commun. 2008;29(7):588–92. doi:10.1097/MNM.0b013e3282f8148b.

Gholamrezanezhad A, Mirpour S. An important but easily forgettable review: extracardiac activity in myocardial perfusion scans. Int J Cardiovasc Imaging. 2007;23(2):207–8. Epub 2006 Sep 14.

Gholamrezanezhad A, Moinian D, Eftekhari M, Mirpour S, Hajimohammadi H. The prevalence and significance of increased gastric wall radiotracer uptake in sestamibi myocardial perfusion SPECT. Int J Cardiovasc Imaging. 2006;22:435–41.

Goetze S, Lavely WC, Ziessman HA, Wahl RL. Visualization of brown adipose tissue with 99mTc-Methoxyisobutylisonitrile on SPECT/CT. J Nucl Med. 2008;49:752–6.

Gowda A, Peddinghaus L, Shandilya V, Gavriluke A, Jain D. Abnormal intense skeletal radiotracer uptake on myocardial perfusion imaging with Tc-99m sestamibi. J Nucl Cardiol. 2006;13:427–31.

Gupta V, Boyechko Y, Oates ME, Sorrell V. The railroad track sign: intense gastric wall uptake on Tc-99m sestamibi single photon emission computed tomography myocardial perfusion imaging in patients with end-stage liver disease. Presented as poster at the American College of Cardiology Annual Scientific Session, San Diego, CA, March 2015. J Am Coll Cardiol. 2015;65(10_S). doi:10.1016/S0735-1097(15)61283-9.

Hardebeck CJ, Herman C, Auseon A. Identification of incidental hepatic malignancy as photopenic defect on 99mTc-sestamibi myocardial perfusion imaging. Clin Nucl Med. 2013;38(10):821–2. doi:10.1097/RLU.0b013e31829af8f9.

Hassan IM, Mohammad MMJ, Constantinides C, Nair M, Belan N, Abdel-Dayem HH. Problems of duodeno-gastric reflux in Tc-99m HexaMIBI planar, tomographic and bull's eye display. Clin Nucl Med. 1991;14:286–9.

Hawkins M, Scarsbrook AF, Pavlitchouk S, Moore NR, Bradley KM. Detection of an occult thymoma on 99Tcm-tetrofosmin myocardial scintigraphy. Brit J Radiol. 2007;80:e72–4.

Hendel RC, Gibbons RJ, Bateman TM. Use of rotating (cine) planar projection images in the interpretation of a tomographic myocardial perfusion study. J Nucl Cardiol. 1999;6:234–40.

Henzlova MJ, Cerqueira MD, Hansen CL, Taillefer R, Yao S-S. ASNC Imaging Guidelines for Nuclear Cardiology Procedures. Stress protocols and tracers. 2009. http://www.asnc.org/imageuploads/ImagingGuidelinesStressProtocols021109.pdf. Accessed 4 June 2015.

Hesse B, Tägil K, Cuocolo A, Anagnostopoulos C, Bardiés M, Bax J, Bengel F, Busemann Sokole E, Davies G, Dondi M, Edenbrandt L, Franken P, Kjaerl A, Knuutil J, Lassmann M, Ljungberg M, Marcassa C, Marie PY, McKiddie F, OConnor M, Prvulovich E, Underwood R, van Eck-Smit B. EANM/ESC procedural guidelines for myocardial perfusion imaging in nuclear cardiology. Eur J Nucl Med Mol Imaging. 2005;32:855–97. Epub 21 May 2005. http://www.eanm.org/publications/guidelines/gl_cardio_myocard_perf.pdf. Accessed June 8, 2015.

Hofman M, McKay J, Nandurkar D. Efficacy of milk versus water to reduce interfering infracardiac activity in 99mTc-sestamibi myocardial perfusion scintigraphy. Nucl Med Commun. 2006;27(11):837–42.

Holbrook A, Newel MS. Alternative screening for women with dense breasts: breast-specific gamma imaging (molecular breast imaging). AJR Am J Roentgenol. 2015;204(2):252–6. doi:10.2214/AJR.14.13525.

Holly TA, Abbott BG, Al-Mallah M, Calnon DA, Cohen MC, DiFilippo FP, Ficaro EP, Freeman M, Hendel RC, Jain D, Leonard SM, Nichols KJ, Polk DM, Soman P. ASNC Imaging Guidelines for Nuclear Cardiology Procedures. (2010) Single photon-emission computed tomography. J Nucl Cardiol. Epub 15 June 2010. http://asnc.org/imageuploads/ImagingGuidelineSPECTJune2010.pdf. Accessed 8 June 2015.

Howarth DM, Forstrom LA, O'Connor MK, Thomas PA, Cardew AP. Patient-related pitfalls and artifacts in nuclear medicine imaging. Semin Nucl Med. 1996;26:295–307.

Hurwitz GA, Clark EM, Slomka PJ, Siddiq KS. Investigation of measures to reduce interfering abdominal activity on rest myocardial images with Tc-99m sestamibi. Clin Nucl Med. 1993;18:735–41.

Joy PS, Chhabra A, Ghanbarinia A, Jain D. Extracardiac abnormalities on myocardial perfusion imaging in a patient undergoing liver transplantation. J Nucl Cardiol. 2007;14:126–8.

Kasi VS, Ahsanuddin AN, Gilbert C, Orr L, Moran J, Sorrell VL. Isolated metastatic myocardial carcinoid tumor in a 48-year-old man. Mayo Clinic Proc. 2002;77(6):591–4.

Khary W, Nance RW, Stevens JS, Wilson RA. Gastric activity on dipyridamole 201Tl myocardial perfusion imaging: a clinically useful finding. Nucl Med Commun. 1995;16:477–82.

Lamont AE, Joyce JM, Grossman SJ. Acute cholecystitis detected on a Tc-99m sestamibi myocardial imaging. Clin Nucl Med. 1996;21:879.

Lazar HL, Oates E, Beazley RM. Excision of a mediastinal parathyroid adenoma after coronary artery bypass surgery. Ann Thorac Surg. 2005;80:1105–6.

Malhotra G, Upadhye TS, Nabar A, Asopa RV, Nayak UN, Rajan MG. Can carbonated lime drink intake prior to myocardial perfusion imaging with Tc-99m MIBI reduce the extracardiac activity that degrades the image quality and leads to fallacies in interpretation? Clin Nucl Med. 2010;35(3):160–4. doi:10.1097/RLU.0b013e3181cc63a1.

Mariani G, Filocamo M, Giona F, Villa G, Amendola A, Erba P, Buffoni F, Copello F, Pierini A, Minichilli F, Gatti R, Brady RO. Severity of bone marrow involvement in patients with Gaucher's disease evaluated by scintigraphy with ^{99m}Tc-sestamibi. J Nucl Med. 2003;44:1253–62.

Maurea S, Klain M, Lastoria S, Cuocolo A, Colao A, Salvatore M. Technetium-99m-tetrofosmin imaging of differentiated mixed thyroid cancer. J Nucl Med. 1995;36:2248–51.

Meesala M, Raza M, Chhabra A, Mehta N, Jain D. Hepatobiliary abnormalities on nuclear perfusion imaging. J Nucl Cardiol. 2006;13:297–9.

Middleton GW, Williams JH. Significant gastric reflux of technetium-99m-MIBI in SPECT myocardial imaging. J Nucl Med. 1994;35:619–20.

Middleton GW, Williams JH. Interference from duodeno-gastric reflux of 99Tcm radiopharmaceuticals in SPET myocardial perfusion imaging. Nucl Med Commun. 1996;17:114–8.

Mlikotic A, Mishkin FS. Visualization of the right atrial appendage during sestamibi scintigraphy. Clin Nucl Med. 2000;25:848–9.

Mohr WM, Gibson DL, Pang W. Extra-cardiac update of technetium-99m-MIBI: normal and abnormal variants. J Nucl Med Technol. 1996;24:104–11.

Niederkohr RD, Chiu E, Nielsen KRK, Maclean M. Extramedullary hematopoiesis within paravertebral masses demonstrating prominent sestamibi and thallium uptake. Clin Nucl Med. 2009;34:506–7.

Nishiyama Y, Kawasaki Y, Yamamoto Y, Fukunaga K, Satoh K, Takashima H, Ohkawa M, Tanabe M. Technetium-99m-MIBI and thallium-201 scintigraphy of primary lung cancer. J Nucl Med. 1997;38:1358–61.

O'Doherty MJ, Kettle AG, Wells P, Collins REC, Coakley AJ. Parathyroid imaging with technetium-99m-sestamibi: preoperative localization and tissue uptake studies. J Nucl Med. 1992;33:313–8.

Onsel C, Sonmezoglu K, Camsari G, Atay S, Cetin S, Erdil YT, Uslu I, Uzun A, Kanmaz B, Sayman HB. Technetium-99m-MIBI scintigraphy in pulmonary tuberculosis. J Nucl Med. 1996;37:233–8.

Panjrath GS, Narra K, Jain D. Myocardial perfusion imaging in a patient with chest pain. J Nucl Cardiol. 2004;11(4):515–7.

Pitman AG, Kalff V, Van Every B, Risa B, Barnden LR, Kelly MJ. Contributions of subdiaphragmatic activity, attenuation, and diaphragmatic motion to inferior wall artifact in attenuation-corrected Tc-99m myocardial perfusion SPECT. J Nucl Cardiol. 2005;12(4):401–9.

Ramakrishna G, Miller TD. Significant breast uptake of Tc-99m sestamibi in an actively lactating woman during SPECT myocardial perfusion imaging. J Nucl Cardiol. 2004;11(2):222–3.

Raza M, Meesala M, Jain D. Unusual radiotracer uptake in the lower mediastinum on sestamibi perfusion images. J Nucl Cardiol. 2005a;12:740–1.

Raza M, Meesala M, Panjrath GS, Ghanbarinia A, Jain D. Abnormal photopenic area on nuclear perfusion imaging. J Nucl Cardiol. 2005b;12:607–9.

Raza M, Panjrath GS, Haider A, Jain D. Extracardiac abnormalities on myocardial perfusion imaging. J Nucl Cardiol. 2005c;12(Suppl):S36 (abstr).

Raza M, Panjrath GS, Meesala M, Jain D. Prevalence of incidental non-cardiac findings on SPECT perfusion studies. J Nucl Cardiol. 2005d;12:S121–2 (abstr).

Rehm PK, Atkins FB, Ziessman HA, Green SE, Fox LM, Hixson DJ. Frequency of extra-cardiac activity and its effect on 99mTc-MIBI cardiac SPET interpretation. Nucl Med Commun. 1996;17:851–6.

Reyhan M, Aydin M, Yapar AF, Bolat FA, Tercan F. Atypical carcinoid tumor detected incidentally on Tc-99m sestamibi myocardial perfusion scintigraphy. Clin Nucl Med. 2004;29:129–31.

Seabold JE, Gurll N, Schurrer ME, Aktay R, Kirchner PT. Comparison of 99mTc-methoxyisobutylisonitrile and 201Tl scintigraphy for detection of residual thyroid cancer after 131I ablative therapy. J Nucl Med. 1999;40:1434–40.

Seo I, Del Priore E, Almonte A, Kappes R, Fedida A, Ong K. Extracardiac lesions: why more prominent on the rest SPECT? J Nucl Cardiol. 2005;12:S122 (abstr).

Shih WJ, Han JK, Coupal J, Wierzbinski B, Magoun S, Gross K. Axillary lymph node uptake of Tc-99m MIBI resulting from extravasation should not be misinterpreted as metastasis. Ann Nucl Med. 1999;13:269–71.

Shih WJ, Kiefer V, Gross K, Wierzbinski B, Collins J, Pulmano C, Ryo YU. Intrathoracic and intra-abdominal Tl-201 abnormalities seen on rotating raw cine data on dual radionuclide myocardial perfusion and gated SPECT. Clin Nucl Med. 2002;27:40–4.

Shih WJ, McFarland KA, Kiefer V, Wierzbinski B. Illustrations of abdominal abnormalities on 99mTc tetrofosmin gated cardiac SPECT. Nucl Med Commun. 2005;26:119–27.

Shuke N, Tonami N, Takahashi I, Kameyama T, Yokoyama K, Kinuya S, Nakajima K, Aburano T, Michigishi T, Hisada K. Prominent uptake of Tl-201 by duodenal leiomyosarcoma after exercise myocardial perfusion study. Clin Nucl Med. 1995;20(4):299–301.

Slavin Jr JD, Engin IO, Spencer RP. Retrocardiac uptake of Tc-99m sestamibi: manifestation of a hiatal hernia. Clin Nucl Med. 1998;23(4):239–40.

Smith JR, Oates E. Radionuclide imaging of the thyroid gland: patterns, pearls, and pitfalls. Clin Nucl Med. 2004a;29:181–93.

Smith JR, Oates E. Radionuclide imaging of the parathyroid glands: patterns, pearls, and pitfalls. RadioGraphics. 2004b;24:1101–15.

Soderlund V, Jonsson C, Bauer HCF, Brosjo O, Jacobsson H. Comparison of technetium-99m-MIBI and technetium-99m-tetrofosmin update by musculoskeletal sarcomas. J Nucl Med. 1997;38:682–6.

Sorrell V, Figueroa B, Hansen CL. The "hurricane sign": evidence of patient motion artifact on cardiac single-photon emission computed tomography. J Nucl Cardiol. 1996;3:86–8.

Strauss HW, Miller DD, Wittry MD, Cerqueira ME, Garcia EV, Iskandrian AS, Schelbert HR, Wackers FJ, Balon HR, Lang O, Machac J. Procedure guideline for myocardial perfusion imaging 3.3 (2008). J Nucl Med Technol. 2008;36:155–61. http://snmmi.files.cms-plus.com/docs/Myocardial%20Perfusion%20Imaging%203.3.pdf. Accessed 8 June 2015.

Sundram FX, Mack P. Evaluation of thyroid nodules for malignancy using 99Tcm-sestamibi. Nucl Med Commun. 1995;16:687–93.

Taillefer R, Robidoux A, Lambert R, Turpin S, Laperriere J. Technetium-99m-sestamibi prone scintimammography to detect primary breast cancer and axillary lymph node involvement. J Nucl Med. 1995;36:1758–65.

Taillefer R, Robidoux A, Turpin S, Lambert R, Cantin J, Leveille J. Metastatic axillary lymph node involvement technetium-99m-MIBI imaging in primary breast cancer. J Nucl Med. 1998;39:459–64.

Takekawa H, Shinano H, Tsukamoto E, Koseki Y, Ikeno T, Miller F, Kawakami Y. Technetium-99m-tetrofosmin imaging of lung cancer: relationship with histopathology. Ann Nucl Med. 1999;13:71–5.

Tallaj JA, Iskandrian AE. Extracardiac localization of technetium-99m sestamibi. J Nucl Cardiol. 2000;7:789–90.

Tallaj JA, Kova D, Iskandrian AE. The use of technetium-99m sestamibi in a patient with liver cirrhosis. J Nucl Cardiol. 2000;7:722–3.

Toran RE, Oates E, Dowling DJ, Udelson JE. Gallbladder nonvisualization during technetium-99m sestamibi myocardial perfusion imaging. J Nucl Med. 1997;38:74–5P. (abstr).

van Dongen AJ, van Rijk PP. Minimizing liver, bowel, and gastric activity in myocardial perfusion SPECT. J Nucl Med. 2000;41:1315–7.

Vijayakumar V, Gupta R, Rahman A. Pathologic extracardiac uptake of Tc-99m tetrofosmin identified in the chest during myocardial perfusion imaging. J Nucl Cardiol. 2005;12(4):473–5.

Wackers FJ, Berman DS, Maddahi J, Watson DD, Beller GA, Strauss HW, Boucher CA, Picard M, Holman BL, Fridrich R, et al. Technetium-99m hexakis 2-methoxybutyl isonitrile: human biodistribution, dosimetry, safety, and preliminary comparison to thallium-201 for myocardial perfusion imaging. J Nucl Med. 1989;30:301–11.

Watanabe N, Hirano T, Fukushima Y. Esophageal cancer detection with Tc-99m tetrofosmin SPECT. Clin Nucl Med. 1997;22:431–3.

Waxman AD. The role of (99m) Tc methoxyisobutylisonitrile in imaging breast cancer. Semin Nucl Med. 1997;27:40–54.

Weinmann P, Moretti JL. Metoclopramide has no effect on abdominal activity of sestamibi in myocardial SPET. Nucl Med Commun. 1999;20(7):623–5.

Williams K, Schneider CM. Increased stress right ventricular activity on dual isotope perfusion SPECT a sign of multivessel and/or left main coronary artery disease. J Am Coll Cardiol. 1999;34:420–7.

Williams KA, Hill KA, Sheridan CM. Noncardiac findings on dual-isotope myocardial perfusion SPECT. J Nucl Cardiol. 2003;10:395–402.

Wosnitzer B, Wray R, DePuey G. Photopenic mediastinum due to enlarged atria. J Nucl Cardiol. 2012;19(4):811–3. doi:10.1007/s12350-012-9557-2.

Index

© Springer International Publishing Switzerland 2017
M.E. Oates, V.L. Sorrell, *Myocardial Perfusion Imaging - Beyond the Left
Ventricle: Pathology, Artifacts and Pitfalls in the Chest and Abdomen,*
DOI 10.1007/978-3-319-25436-4